Improve, Perfect, & Perpetuate

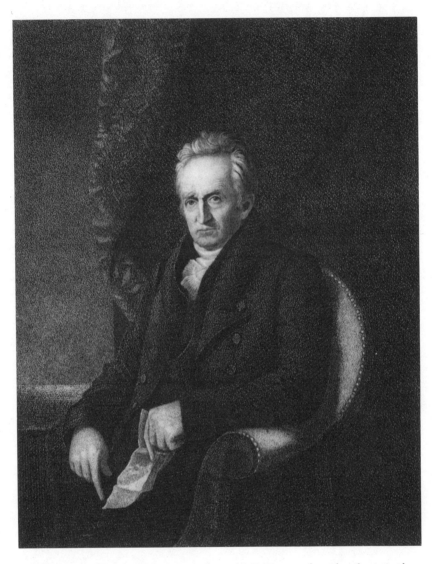

Engraving of Nathan Smith by S. S. Jocelyn and S. B. Munson, from the oil painting by Samuel F. B. Morse commissioned by the Yale University medical class of 1826.

Courtesy of Yale University, Harvey Cushing/John Hay Whitney Medical Library.

Improve, Perfect, & Perpetuate

Dr. Nathan Smith and Early American Medical Education

For Rosemary —
4 June 2011

OLIVER S. HAYWARD, M.D.

CONSTANCE E. PUTNAM

Foreword by C. Everett Koop

Introduction by Philip Cash

University Press of New England / Hanover and London

University Press of New England, Hanover, NH 03755
© 1998 by Constance E. Putnam
All rights reserved
Printed in the United States of America
5   4   3   2   1
CIP data appear at the end of the book

Publication of this biography of Nathan Smith has been
made possible by the generosity of the late
Elizabeth and Lane Dwinell.

PERMISSIONS

Permission to make use of material from the numerous articles on Nathan Smith
that Oliver Hayward published (most of which are cited or quoted in the footnotes, and all of which appear in the Bibliography of Works on Nathan Smith
[pages 346–47]) during the years he was working on the biography is gratefully
acknowledged. No permission was required by the *New England Journal of Medicine* (for mere reliance on material in or citation to articles published there), and
no response was received from the successors to the *Bulletin of the School of Medicine University of Maryland*. Permission was granted as follows:

"A Search for the Real Nathan Smith," in *Journal of the History of Medicine and
Allied Sciences* 15, no. 3 (July 1960): 270–81.
"A Student of Dr. Nathan Smith," in *Connecticut Medicine* 24, no. 9 (Sept.
1960): 553–59.
"What Nathan Smith Means to Me," in *Journal of the American Medical Association* 176, no. 1 (Apr. 8, 1961): 202, 204, 206; and "Jo Gallup, Epidemi-
ologist—1769–1849," in *Journal of the American Medical Association* 189,
no. 6 (Aug. 10, 1964): 81–82. Copyright 1961–64, American Medical Association.
"The Basis in Sydenham, Rush and Armstrong for Nathan Smith's Teaching," in
Annals of Internal Medicine 56, no. 2 (Feb. 1962): 343–48.
"Nathan Smith's Medical Practice or Dogmatism versus Patient Inquiry," in *Bulletin of the History of Medicine* 36, no. 3 (May–June, 1962): 260–67; and
"Three American Anatomy Letters," in *Bulletin of the History of Medicine* 38,
no. 4 (July–Aug. 1964): 377–78.
"Nathan Smith (1762–1829) on Amputations" (with Mather Cleveland), in *Jour-
nal of Bone and Joint Surgery* 43–A, no. 8 (Dec. 1964): 1246–54.

Continued on page 363

For Mary,

and

—in Memoriam—

William F. Putnam, M.D.

Contents

Illustrations

Foreword

C. EVERETT KOOP

W HEN I WENT to Dartmouth College in 1933 it was with the intention of taking a combined course of four years in the college and two years in the medical school, completing both in five years and thus saving one year of what was to be a great many in medical education. Dartmouth not only was an excellent medical school, still very much in the tradition of its great founder, Nathan Smith; it also offered the members of its small, select classes virtually certain entry to the third year at Harvard Medical School (or any other four-year school), thanks to the way Dartmouth had responded to Abraham Flexner's 1910 report on medical education in the United States and Canada. After having grown from its modest beginnings in 1797 into a four-year school (which became the standard across the country during the nineteenth century), in 1914 Dartmouth Medical School became a two-year school that gave concentrated basic science training to its students. Throughout its history as a two-year school, Dartmouth remained in the forefront of medical schools offering preclinical training exclusively.

I would have enjoyed being a student at Dartmouth Medical School— my Dartmouth ties are strong over three generations and have always been rewarding—but considering what happened with my life and career development, starting medical school elsewhere the year after I graduated from Dartmouth in 1937 was indeed the right choice. I have never regretted my wonderful training at Cornell University Medical School or the surgical training and career I had thereafter—a career that eventually took me back to Dartmouth in any case.

In 1973, Dartmouth Medical School was refounded as a four-year school, and Nathan Smith's dream of making a complete medical education available in northern New England came to life again. Two decades later, in 1992, I joined the Dartmouth faculty and became the senior scholar of the C. Everett Koop Institute there. When the time came to construct a seal for the Koop Institute, I chose as its centerpiece the image of the "New Medical House" that Nathan Smith built in 1811 and in which he held forth.

What a man he must have been! To found a medical school as Nathan Smith did two hundred years ago was awesome then; it is awesome now. But Smith went on to help found another school at Yale, a third at Bowdoin, and a fourth at the University of Vermont—certainly more than society should expect from any one physician. In addition, Nathan Smith was a demanding teacher, insisting his students have experience with preceptors (often even before they began their Dartmouth medical studies). Famously, he often traveled with an entourage of students in tow as he rode across the countryside on house calls, tending both the simply sick and those with complex surgical problems.

I have always been fascinated by the life of Nathan Smith; his emphasis on the patient's welfare is very much in tune with my own commitment to patient-centered care. I am delighted that Oliver S. Hayward and Constance E. Putnam have put this wonderful biography together. If I could I would like to be sure that it is read by every medical student in the country. Those Dartmouth medical students who read it will of course have a special infusion of pride, but there are many lessons here to be learned by every student of medicine. Especially in an era when there is so much doubt and uncertainty about the ability of doctors to stand out from a crowd, to accomplish their goals, and to achieve their professional purposes, the incredible contribution Nathan Smith made to American medical education in particular is a model that deserves to be better known.

Preface and Acknowledgments

CONSTANCE E. PUTNAM

My FATHER, William F. Putnam, a Dartmouth College graduate and later a general practitioner, began his medical studies in 1930 at Dartmouth Medical School (then a two-year school). As a youngster, I heard him talk about Nathan Smith and the legacy he had left for physicians, but I had only a vague understanding that Nathan Smith was the founder of Dartmouth Medical School. Still, I knew my father self-consciously and deliberately modeled himself after Smith, both in emphasizing the positive benefits of doing less rather than more and (above all) in adhering to the principle of *primum non nocere*. The doctor's first job, he always said, was to avoid making matters worse.

I also knew that my father's close friend, Oliver S. Hayward—a medical school classmate at Dartmouth, fellow intern at the Mary Hitchcock Memorial Hospital, and fellow New Hampshire G.P.—had developed a very particular interest in the life of Nathan Smith. He had written about Smith, and I recall learning that one of his papers on Smith had won the New Hampshire Medical Society's Pray-Burnham Prize.

Fast forward some thirty years. Having for a variety of reasons never brought to the point of publication the biography of Nathan Smith that he had been preparing off and on for decades, Oliver Hayward turned to me to help him finish the project. (How this all transpired—how we got in touch, what convinced Oliver that I was an appropriate co-author—is itself a complicated story, beyond what needs to be spelled out here.) Excited, challenged, honored, I agreed in principle to help Oliver, having duly warned him that other commitments would prevent me from turning my attention to Nathan Smith for some time. All too soon thereafter, before we had done more than exchange a very few letters on the subject of Smith and the book, this seemingly hale and hearty octogenarian died in January of 1990.

Sentimentally convinced that it helped Oliver in his last weeks to know that the Nathan Smith project would not die with him, I determined to fulfill my promise. I still did not have a clear idea what this might entail—not even when his widow, Mary Hayward, sent me boxes and boxes of files that included (among other things) several versions of more-or-less complete drafts of the life of Smith.

As an aside, it should be mentioned that some time around 1960 Oliver deposited copies of one version of his manuscript in several libraries— among them, appropriately enough, the libraries at Dartmouth and Yale. I know there is a copy also at the American Philosophical Society in Philadelphia and another at the Library of Congress; where else these early drafts can be found, if anywhere, Oliver's records do not tell me.

The above-mentioned prior commitments continued to keep me from doing anything beyond idly looking through some of the boxes occasionally, until the realization hit me that Dartmouth Medical School's bicentennial in 1997 was a good reason to take up at last a project with antecedents going back much further than I had initially realized. For once I began to familiarize myself with the materials that had been turned over to me, I discovered that during the 1930s Yale's Ashley W. Oughterson had planned to write a biography of Smith; some of his files had come to me as well. Further, Oliver's own work had for some years been done in collaboration with another great Yale physician-historian, John Farquhar Fulton; together, in fact, they had been recipients of a grant from NIH that facilitated major chunks of the work. Thanks in considerable part to that grant, Oliver had published more than a dozen papers on various aspects of Smith's career.

But a truly complete draft of the biography had never been finished. As I read the correspondence (most of it fragmentary) in what were now my files, I concluded this was largely a result of having too much of a good thing. Numerous physicians and medical historians at Dartmouth, Yale, and elsewhere—who shared Oliver's great enthusiasm for Smith the man, Smith the physician, and Smith the educator, and several of whom themselves had written one or more articles on aspects of the life of Smith or his descendants—had encouraged him with a variety of suggestions. Preeminent among these, perhaps, was historian Whitfield J. Bell, Jr., but there were others. Elizabeth H. Thomson, co-editor with Oliver of the *Journal of William Tully*, comes to mind, as does Herbert Thoms; I have a cartoon he drew to illustrate his felicitous observation that the same William Tully lies buried "just a bone's throw" from Nathan Smith. Librarians, journal editors, and research assistants also sustained Oliver. Staggering amounts of work were done by his faithful research assistant, Margaret Abbott, who—among other tasks—transcribed material for him by typing thousands of pages from books and articles (the research predates the easy days of word processing and photocopying).

Oliver himself did phenomenal amounts of research, following up every lead, learning more and more about eighteenth- and nineteenth-century medical history in general and Smith in particular. Everything seemed connected, and he made notes about it all—which created something of a challenge for me: Oliver's inimitable scrawl on scraps of paper (old prescription blanks, note paper from drug companies, pages from a loose-leaf ledger book) was not so easy to read as Ms. Abbott's perfect typing!

The question remains: Why, after all the work Oliver had done, was it left for another to complete the project? Simply put, I believe the answer lies in the fact that—in the end—he knew too much. Having to sort it all out, contemplating the need to omit some of what he had learned, giving appropriate balance to the materials collected, keeping in mind that readers would not perhaps even want to know all he had learned, and finally editing and revising (again) what he had written, became an overwhelming task. To his credit, he recognized he needed a new perspective to bring closure; whether he chose well I leave for readers to decide.

For me the work has been a curious mix of great delight and utter frustration. What I would have given to work side by side with Oliver, to have been able to ask directly whether changes I was proposing were acceptable to him! How I would have loved to have the long months of work that I put into this book enlivened by his wit as well as his wisdom. (Oliver was the only friend my father had who fully shared the zany sense of humor that proved a valuable release for both of them; the letter Nathan Smith wrote to his friend Mills Olcott on October 15, 1826 (see page 125) about the White Mountains having "gone to sea" could just as well have been from Bill Putnam to Ollie Hayward.)

On the other hand, there is no denying that being able to make changes in the manuscript unilaterally was a lot easier than it would have been to discuss with Oliver every one of the deletions and additions that I have made, or every bit of the re-organization—all of which resulted in substantial revision of his manuscript. I have tried, throughout, to be guided by what I believe was imperative for Oliver: Stay true to the story of Nathan Smith, and get it out.

And so, despite Oliver's having died before I really began work, this has been a collaboration. Although in the process of double-checking material Oliver had found I did considerable historical sleuthing of my own and uncovered a few items he apparently had not found (judging from his files), the bulk of the credit for relentless and dogged research goes to Oliver. Indeed, credit for the persistent dream of sharing the story of Nathan Smith in something like the detail it deserves also goes to Oliver. But perhaps understandably, much—perhaps even most—of the actual writing is mine. I have tried to keep Oliver's enthusiasm, respect, and admiration for Smith (which I came to share) even where I have not kept his "voice." I have also worked hard to make sure the solid basis for our shared respect and admiration for Smith is clear, by scrupulously documenting points that it appears Oliver believed were self-evident. Again, others must decide to what extent I have succeeded.

Some ten years before his death, after the Smith project had lain dormant for some time, Oliver turned his attention to it again. In a copy of one letter I found in his files (though whether it was ever sent, and if so to whom, is unclear), Oliver offered a great rush of reasons that a Nathan Smith biography was overdue:

Dr. Nathan Smith has never had the historical credit he deserves. Sir William Osler and I both believe he was the greatest physician of his time . . . . Yet there are few histories that mention him, few analysts who give him his due. He stood at the very center of tremendous change . . . and he deserves a biography [that shows him] understanding the epidemiology of typhoid fever as well as we do, using the natural force of healing and teaching it to his mixed bag of students, serving as the first of the great American [medical] consultants, launching four sons on medical careers, contributing significantly to the treatment of a dozen different diseases, and—perhaps his most significant achievement—by force of example showing how to be a good family doctor.

We can be confident, incidentally, given that last remark, that Oliver Hayward would be among those rejoicing in recent reports that ever-larger proportions of medical school graduating classes are entering primary-care specialties. And he would have been hopeful that at least some of those graduates and the students who follow them might find inspiration in the life and career of Nathan Smith, as generations of earlier students did—my father and Oliver Hayward among them. My fervent hope is that our book will increase the possibility of that happening.

A retrospective attempt to thank adequately the many people Oliver would have thanked had he lived to help write this portion of the book is doomed to failure. Still, mention must be made of some beyond those already named above. I know that the Grant RG-6625 from the United States Public Health Service, National Institutes of Health, came at a crucial time in Oliver's work; editors of the several journals who published his articles likewise played a critical role.

Among those who read drafts, encouraged, or otherwise supported Oliver's efforts are several writers with whom I have also been in touch. (One of them, the late William Field, never responded to my letter, perhaps owing to his illness. His attempt to tell the Nathan Smith story in his privately published book, *The Good Dr. Smith*, gives evidence of a too-close reliance on the copy of the manuscript Oliver had shared with him; only a few of the passages that clearly came from Oliver's work were acknowledged.) George H. Callcott had no way of knowing that his correspondence with Oliver and the marginalia he inserted in one draft of

Oliver's manuscript would be read by a grateful co-author years later; LeRoy S. Wirthlin kindly sent me a copy of his second article about Nathan Smith's encounter with Joseph Smith, the founder of all things Mormon. Without assistance from Ronald H. Fishbein and Christopher Longcope I would have been unable to produce the list of Smith family doctors in Appendix B; Caren Collier and Richard Behles at the University of Maryland Medical School and Margaret Burri at Med Chi in Baltimore also helped. Robert E. Nye, Jr., whose correspondence with Oliver and articles on Smith's study abroad and on Cyrus Perkins proved invaluable, added significantly to my understanding of several aspects of Smith's career at Dartmouth.

Additionally, I have other debts entirely of my own to pay. On the strength of what intuition Oliver Hayward concluded I might be able to help him, I have no idea; why he was willing to trust me with his magnum opus I will never know. But, hoping I have lived up to his expectations, I remain immensely grateful; it has been a wonderful ride. Mary Hayward, too, has earned my lasting gratitude for her faith in me and for her gift to me of Oliver's files, her only request being that I make a good-faith effort to finish the book and find a publisher for it. No doubt it was a relief to Mary to be able to empty out closets filled with boxes labeled "NS." Even so, her generosity and her repeated expressions of confidence in me have been more important than it is easy to convey. The rest of the Hayward family has also been supportive. Oliver's son John, a good friend as far back as our teen years—who, sadly, died before the book was finished—was especially so.

Dana Cook Grossman, editor of *Dartmouth Medicine*, made a persuasive case for my book to the Bicentennial Committee at Dartmouth Medical School (DMS); her efforts on behalf of my proposal gained me critical support from the chair of the committee, Heinz Valtin, and from committee member S. Marsh Tenney, former dean of DMS. Nor did Dana's aid end there. Always ready to confer, she has proved to be the very best kind of first-draft editor and negotiator-intervener-agent anyone could want. Conversation with Marsh Tenney confirmed my sense of his deep interest in history and commitment to the project; his comments on some early draft chapters did much to boost my confidence.

Katherine Swift Almy and Tom Almy encouraged me and gave specific help in interpreting, medically, the encounter between Nathan Smith and William Jarvis; Bill Bynum in London and my own physician, Henry Vaillant, answered other medical questions for me. The late Lane Dwinell, former Governor of New Hampshire—in honor of his wife Elizabeth Dwinell (now also deceased)—gave generous financial support toward publication of the book. He also treated me, in his ninety-first year, to a thoroughly delightful lunch during which we exchanged anecdotes about Nathan Smith as well as the New Hampshire political scene in the 1950s.

Reference librarians can make or break a research project of this magnitude; no doubt Oliver would have had his own long list of helpful librarians. Mine includes librarians whose names I never learned; I had the repeated pleasure of discovering that librarians near and far really are willing to help at the ring of a phone or the receipt of a letter. In addition to those at my home-town library, the Concord Free Public Library, I think of librarians at the public libraries in Boston and Worcester, Massachusetts; at the Episcopal Theological School and Harvard Divinity School as well as at Harvard University's Widener Library in Cambridge, Massachusetts; and of the librarians at Columbia University and the New York Academy of Medicine Library. All helped find materials, or confirmed that what I was after did not exist where I was looking.

Librarians whose names I *do* know performed a variety of services: Anne S. K. Turkos at the University of Maryland, Andy Harrison at Johns Hopkins, Stephen Nonack and Jim Woodman at the Boston Atheneum, John Stinson at the New York Public Library, and Emily A. Herrick at the Maine State Library. Tina Paquette at the New Hampshire Medical Society and Richard Schuldiner at Brooks Memorial Library in Brattleboro, Vermont, tracked down elusive old documents. Eric Albright at Northwestern University's Galter Health Sciences Library, Christopher Houlihan at the Edward G. Miner Library at the University of Rochester, and Kelly Brown, Susan Case, and Barbara Stevens at the University of Kansas Medical Center located student notebooks; Diana Yount at Andover Newton Theological School helped fill out the story of John Derby Smith. Carol Hughes at the Dana Medical Library at the University of Vermont was as disappointed as I when items I sought could not be located; earlier, David Blow at UVM's Bailey/Howe Library was able to find some of what I needed. Susan Ravdin checked and double-checked numerous items for me at the Bowdoin College Library with every evidence of good cheer.

This is not to say that I never visited libraries myself. Ask Virginia Smith and others on the staff at the Massachusetts Historical Society about the long list of requests I made there. Ask Stephen Greenberg and Elizabeth Tunis at the National Library of Medicine in Bethesda, Maryland, where I spent happy hours on several occasions—among other things, plying them and their colleagues with questions. At Yale, talk to Toby Appel at the Cushing/Whitney Medical Historical Library, who turned me loose in the files Oliver had collected and who provided valuable information that enabled me to identify which of Nathan Smith's publications had been translated into French and German; talk to Judith Ann Schiff and others—especially Bill Massa—in the Manuscripts and Archives division of Sterling Memorial Library; and talk to Vincent Giroud, Al Mueller, and Steve Jones at the Beinecke Rare Book and Manuscript Library. Lucretia McClure and numerous other librarians in the Rare Book Room at Harvard's Francis A. Countway Library of Medicine helped me solve one puzzle after another with energetic and creative approaches to problem-solving; Richard Wolfe gave early encouragement. Similarly, Anne Ostendarp and a dozen or so members of the staff in the Dartmouth College Archives at Baker Library came to know me and my project well. Among them, Barbara Krieger stands out for her extraordinary resourcefulness; her phenomenal grasp of Dartmouth's archival holdings is an institutional treasure. She and the others have earned my eternal gratitude.

The nonpareil reading room at the old British Library made me glad I had an excuse to look up, for example, the seventeenth-century poet John Collop. Several librarians at the Royal Society of Medicine in London assisted me (thanks are due my friend Leon Cobb, too, who graciously arranged for me to have a visitor's pass to that fine medical library); the biggest thrill there was reading Robert Houstoun's 1726 article, retrieved from the vaults just before closing time on my last day in London. The large staff of supremely helpful librarians at the Wellcome Institute for the History of Medicine, also in London, made an enormous difference to my progress. What a splendid place to work! After I returned home, Richard Aspin, Western manuscripts curator there, came to my rescue by looking up and copying materials I had run out of time to find. Matthew Derrick, at the library of the Royal College of Surgeons, solved mysteries by producing materials no one else had been able to find.

Nor was it only librarians who gave freely of their expertise and knowledge. Martin B. Green, biographer extraordinaire, read draft chapters and urged changes that resulted in pigs and prostitutes populating what had been a dull street scene. Joanne Phillips at Tufts University helped me track down quotations from Hippocrates, Pliny, and Cato; David Freeman found the passage from Maimonides I wanted. Barbara Blough found the list of Oliver's gifts to Dartmouth for me. Ralph Bloom, of Norwalk, Connecticut—with his steel-trap memory for dates—enabled me to find the news account of the Norwalk train disaster. Laurie Burt, court assistant at the Superior Court of Cheshire County, in Keene, New Hampshire, went through old records until she found confirmation of court cases from 1796 and 1797; Jeff Brown at the State Archives in Maine did similar work on *Lowell v. Faxon and Hawkes*. Christine Bastianelli did clerical tasks that kept me from drowning in paper at an early stage, and later—with Ben Swainbank—performed crucial macro magic to turn free-floating footnotes into endnotes.

Writer James B. Atkinson, president of the Historical Society in Cornish, New Hampshire, put himself at my disposal on more than one occasion; he and Gretchen Holm welcomed me into their house while I pored over old town and church documents. Jim also took me to meet Barbara Lewis, who lives in (and eagerly showed) the Salmon P. Chase house in Cornish; Dan Eastman, who lives in and takes loving care of Nathan Smith's own house in Cornish, served us tea at a beautifully laid table in one of the front rooms, enabling us briefly to imagine we were guests of Nathan and Sally Smith.

Other historical society librarians and volunteers helped in a number of different towns: Ellen Swanson and Greta Smith in Rehoboth and Taunton, Massachusetts, respectively; Virginia Putnam (no relation) in Walpole, New Hampshire; Brenda Davignon in the Rockingham, Vermont, Town Clerk's office; and John Leppman, president of the Rockingham Old Meeting House Society. Barbara M. Jones in Charlestown, New Hampshire, brought an unusual letter from Nathan Smith to my attention and tracked down several early nineteenth-century newspaper items for me. In Chester, Vermont, Andrew Ojanen answered more questions than I realized I had (never complaining when I wrote for "just one more thing"); he uncovered previously unknown material on Smith, doing it always with both alacrity and careful attention to detail. Brian Burford, Marilyn Christie, and Doug Gurley at the New Hampshire State Archives found what I needed there; Laura E. Beardsley at the Historical Society of Pennsylvania gave sympathetic assistance; Bill Copeley at the New Hampshire Historical Society confirmed holdings in that library; Marie E. Lamoureux at the American Antiquarian Society in Worcester, Massachusetts, uncovered elusive source materials. All of these librarians exhibited in exemplary fashion a collaborative and supportive approach to scholarly endeavors that was critical to my completing the book.

Rose Corbett-Gordon took on the task of finding appropriate illustrations for the book; her calm approach and expertise were most reassuring. My very supportive editor at the University Press of New England, Phyllis Deutsch, pressed me to tighten the tale and polish my prose. When I turned for assistance to Marian Weekly, she proved to be the kind of editor most writers only dream about; she sifted wheat from chaff with a sure hand and kept my spirits up when one more time through a chapter began to feel like too much work. In her I found a friend as well as an editor.

Others who deserve to be thanked, though it cannot be done adequately (never mind individually), are friends and family members who have listened with remarkable forbearance as I have raved on and on about Nathan Smith and nineteenth-century medicine and footnote verification. Their patience, sympathy, encouragement, and suggestions have been much appreciated.

Of course the one who has put up with the most is my husband, Hugo Bedau. I know it is traditional to end a thank-you list like this with something like "Above all, thanks go to my loyal spouse who thought I would never finish but supported me through thick and thin anyway." I could appropriately say that.

It would, however, be an outrageous understatement. Hugo read the entire manuscript three times; he read sections of it repeatedly. He helped edit, copyedit, and proofread, saving me in the process from most of my worst oversights and solecisms. More: He undertook secretarial tasks, making phone calls and drafting letters; he became a part-time word processor; he served as a research assistant. Finally, he never complained about the two other men in my life: Oliver Hayward and Nathan Smith have for months been virtual members of the household, and Hugo never objected. Instead, he was always ready to serve as a sounding board, whether the talk was of how to handle some aspect of the work Oliver had done or of my delight over some new-found tidbit about Nathan Smith. Hugo has been, in short, a critical part of making this book happen. For his unstinting and unselfish help I remain humbly grateful.

In the end, of course, most of the work and all the decisions about what needed to be done, when, have rested with me. Because Oliver died before he and I could work together, I alone remain responsible for a wide array of judgments that had to be made at every turn. Medical historians nonetheless owe Oliver Hayward a great debt. In addition to his published work, he gave a number of talks on Smith before professional organizations; he also discovered Smith artifacts that had been "lost." Having been given some of these (by a Smith descendant amusingly enough also named Hayward, though not related to Oliver), he made gifts to Yale (some silverware and a bleeding bowl), the Smithsonian (Nathan Ryno Smith's christening dress), and Dartmouth (tortoise combs, silver spoons, early tintypes and colored miniature portraits, and a manuscript letter to Smith from his son Solon). The Nathan Smith Exhibit that Oliver was largely responsible for having set up in the National Library of Medicine at NIH later went on display at Dartmouth. Without Oliver Hayward's sixty years of enthusiasm for Nathan Smith the man, to say nothing of his prodigious research efforts, this book would never have come to pass— and Nathan Smith would continue to remain a much more shadowy figure than ought to be the case with such a giant.

August 1997   *Concord, Massachusetts*

A Technical Note

I have maintained a flexible policy in handling grammatical and orthographic "errors" in quoted material. Many of the manuscripts on which I relied date from a period when spelling, capitalization, and punctuation were by no means so standardized as they are today; I saw little reason always to retain spelling that was likely to distract or—worse—confuse the modern reader. On the other hand, some of the flavor of the eighteenth- and nineteenth-century material would be lost if all the nonstandard spelling, grammar, and technical details in the quoted documents were corrected. Thus I decided to follow a very loose rule of thumb, which was to correct without comment the most distracting or confusing "errors" and to leave some of the more charming oddities for flavor. I used "[sic]" sparingly, only where it seemed necessary to keep the reader from stumbling or thinking what appeared was a typographical error. Of course my judgment on any or all of these points could be challenged, and I have admittedly tampered with what purists might consider the authenticity of the quoted material; authenticity can be checked via the footnotes, however, and my goal was to make the material accessible and the reading a pleasure.

Introduction

American Medicine and Doctors, 1790–1830

PHILIP CASH

THE POST-REVOLUTIONARY WAR medical stage on which Nathan Smith played out his career was richly adorned and crowded. But it portrayed a world of medicine very different from what we know today. The American Revolution itself influenced medical practice in the new nation in three important ways.

First of all, nearly 40 percent of the doctors practicing during that time saw some sort of military medical service in the Continental army, Continental navy, state militias, state navies, on privateers, or with the British forces. For many of them this service was a highly rewarding experience, providing opportunities for surgical operations, encountering and treating a wide variety of diseases, gaining exposure to hospital medicine, and meeting better-trained and more-experienced medical men; this was especially true for those serving with the British forces. All of this made them better and more-aware doctors than they otherwise might have been. Furthermore, the devastation and upheaval caused by our second-longest, second-bloodiest, and most-exhausting war resulted in the loss of a large number of established physicians, providing unusual opportunities for medical newcomers. In 1775, Boston, a city of sixteen thousand permanent inhabitants, was served by twenty-one doctors, and there was little chance of a new doctor setting up a successful practice there. Between then and 1780, three of these physicians died, all from war-related causes, and four went into exile. Another returned home from the army broken in health. During this time their place was taken by six young newcomers, four of whom had served in the Continental army. Lastly, most American doctors, as was the case with a majority of other citizens, were exhilarated by the overthrow of British rule and sobered by the challenge of creating a viable new nation.

These factors did much to shape American medical practice through the early years of the nineteenth century. The medical men of this era were apprehensive but self-confident, concerned about the present but optimistic about the future, competitive but possessed of a heightened professional awareness.

In 1790 there were roughly four thousand physicians ministering to the medical needs of a population of almost four million Americans, a doctor-patient ratio of one to one thousand, as opposed to around one to six hundred in 1775. By the early nineteenth century the ratio had fallen, in New England, to one in five hundred, and by 1820 it was one to four hundred. Throughout the nineteenth century this type of doctor-patient ratio created chronic problems for the regular medical profession and was a mixed blessing for patients, but proved to be an opportunity for the sons of poor farmers and laborers to engage in some forms of "irregular" medical practice. It also set a pattern of medical practice in which well-connected and well-educated physicians were able to establish stable and successful practices, while the poorly educated and economically disadvantaged were forced to move to the frontier or some other undeveloped region, move about within a region, combine practice with another occupation, or abandon the practice of medicine altogether. Still, Barnes Riznik's "Professional Lives of Early Nineteenth-Century New England Doctors" (1964) showed that at least two thirds of them were unable to set up practice in one place and stay there. Many of them had practices of three to four hundred families and individuals. Only a few doctors were wealthy, however. In 1830 it was estimated that most regular practitioners in New England earned about $500 a year counting both money and payments in kind—about the same as a skilled laborer, though the social status of a physician was higher. During this period it was common for accounts to be settled on an annual basis. Leaving debts to be paid out of one's estate was also standard procedure. One half of Riznik's doctors owed between $2,500 and $10,000 at death. But despite this relative lack of wealth, physicians at the time played a disproportionate role in the founding of humanitarian and cultural institutions and in the promotion and development of the sciences.

Heightened professional awareness among American medical men following the Revolution was most clearly visible in the founding of medical schools, societies, and journals, and in the passing of licensing laws. The purposes of these instruments of professionalism were the same as they are today: to raise professional standards and improve the quality of medicine, advance and disseminate medical knowledge, increase collegiality, advise and lobby the public and the government, limit competition, and in general protect the profession's interests.

The movement to found professional institutions actually began in 1752 with the establishment (through the efforts of Benjamin Franklin) of the admirable Pennsylvania hospital. By the outbreak of the Revolution, in addition to that hospital there were two medical schools—established in Philadelphia in 1765 and New York in 1767, one major medical society (New Jersey, 1766), and two licensing laws (New York city, 1760—never enforced; and New Jersey, 1772). Because of the Revolution, the two medical schools and the medical society were forced to begin all over again, this time within a national rather than an imperial context (though the school in Philadelphia managed to keep going throughout the transitional period).

Immediately after the War of Independence, the two most-active areas of professionalization were the founding of state medical societies and the passing of state licensing laws. These activities reflected the tension for a doctor of being both benefactor and businessman. Within a decade after 1781, five new medical societies were founded, and the society in New Jersey was reactivated. These societies often played a role in the healing process between Whig doctors (who were generally younger, more aggressive, and strongly nationalistic) and the remaining Tory medical men (who tended to be older, better educated, and more cosmopolitan in outlook).

The first of these societies to be founded was the Massachusetts Medical Society, which was incorporated in 1791 and is the oldest medical society in the United States whose meetings continue to this day. By 1815 nearly all states had state medical societies, which were eager to promote professional solidarity and interests. Their efforts met with mixed results. Of the 896 doctors in Riznik's New England study who practiced between 1790 and 1840, more than four hundred were not members of any medical society. A similar pattern prevailed elsewhere. All too often bitter and vitriolic quarrels among doctors were carried on in public. As time went by the public became less sympathetic to the values and interests of the regular medical profession.

One economic interest that was left to local medical societies was the creation and enforcement of fee bills or rate of charges. This was so because these arrangements proved effective only on the local level. After 1808, state medical societies began promulgating codes of medical ethics and behavior based on the British model published by Thomas Percival in 1803. These codes dealt more with professional etiquette than with ethics, however; one of the chief objectives was to distinguish members of the "regular" medical professional from a growing list of competitors.

Between 1781 and 1830, thirteen of twenty-four states adopted medical licensing laws. Some states, following the lead of New Jersey, placed the enforcement of these laws in the hands of independent state boards. Others followed the example of Massachusetts and assigned the task to the state medical society. After 1820 the practice in Massachusetts of automatically licensing graduates of medical schools became more generally accepted. By the end of the 1830s, only three states lacked a medical licensing law.

At the opening of the Civil War, however, no state had a working law, for several important reasons. Such laws went against the spirit of Jacksonian America, which prized experience and intuition over expertise and erudition, equality over quality, and opportunity over stability. The burgeoning medical sects exerted formidable political pressure to repeat these laws or render them ineffectual. Most important of all was the widespread recognition that, aside from outright quackery (often hard in any case to determine), the knowledge and therapies of orthodox medical practitioners could not be shown to be clearly superior to those of their medical competitors.

The basic form of medical education in America from earliest times to the Civil War was the apprenticeship system. The advantages of this system were that it was readily available and relatively inexpensive, gave considerable practical experience, and helped develop a sense of professional identity. The disadvantages were that there was no uniformity or quality control, the amount of medical knowledge that could be passed on was limited (especially if the preceptor was himself only apprentice trained), and a strong temptation existed for the preceptor to exploit his charges. In defense of preceptors, however, it should be pointed out that they often also had to assist poorly educated pupils in making up deficiencies in languages, mathematics, and the sciences. And Riznik found that fewer than 10 percent of the New England doctors he studied held an A.B. degree. Apprentice fees were an important part of the income of many doctors, however, just as apprentice labor was highly prized.

This type of medical education was particularly well established in New England, a fact of which the region's medical schools were well aware. Indeed, the first medical schools were founded to supplant the apprenticeship system; only later were they intended to complement it. (As late as the 1840s a graduate of a medical school would have spent more than 80 percent of his time studying with a preceptor.) After 1820 the number of doctors trained exclusively by the apprenticeship method declined, and the importance of medical schools rose accordingly. Precisely when those doctors who were trained solely by apprenticeship became fewer than those who took a medical degree is not known. Riznik found that of 215 doctors practicing between 1790 and 1840 in Worcester Country, Massachusetts, 152 were exclusively apprentice trained.

By 1810 there were six medical schools in the United States. They were, in order of their founding: the University of Pennsylvania (1765), Columbia (1767), Harvard (1782), Dartmouth (1797), the College of

Medicine of the University of Maryland (1807), and the College of Physicians and Surgeons (also 1807)—which merged with Columbia six years later. (The medical college of the University of Transylvania, in Kentucky, had been founded in 1799 but was not fully in operation until 1816–1817.) In 1810 these schools together had 650 students and graduated about 100, but 406 of these students were enrolled at Pennsylvania, then the country's leading medical school. All of the schools except Dartmouth were in urban centers, and all but the College of Physicians and Surgeons (founded under the auspices of a county medical society) were affiliated with academic institutions. None was in the South or the West.

By the 1820s there were almost twenty medical schools scattered around the country with about two thousand medical students. Most of them were still affiliated with colleges. In 1820 New England had five; those medical schools granted 44 degrees (Dartmouth 14, Harvard 12, Brown 9, Yale 7, and Castleton 2). By the end of the decade the number of medical schools in New England had risen to seven, and they awarded 207 degrees (Bowdoin 46, Yale 36, Castleton 34, Berkshire 34, Harvard 23, Dartmouth 18, and Vermont 16). From 1830 until 1906 the number and variety of medical schools in the United States grew at an astonishing rate, greatly increasing accessibility but lowering the overall quality of medical education, and hampering medical reform.

Until after the Civil War, virtually all teachers in American medical schools were practicing physicians. Except in anatomy (and sometimes obstetrics) classes, lecturing was almost the sole teaching method. Clinical, tutorial, and laboratory instruction were highly limited. Even in anatomy, the irregular supply of cadavers—most obtained illegally from among the poor, blacks, and immigrants—hindered laboratory work; the amount of dissecting it was possible for students to do was directly dependent on the number of cadavers available.

Throughout the colonial period and the nineteenth century, western Europe provided a positive example for American medical education and practice. From 1730 a small but important group of elite American medical students went abroad for advanced study and training (fewer European doctors came to New England, and fewer students from that region went to Europe to study medicine than from the middle and southern colonies). The numbers declined between 1775 and 1795 and then rose again until the beginning of the twentieth century. Until the early years of the nineteenth century a majority of the students went to London, Edinburgh, and Leyden; after 1820 the focus shifted to Paris, and after the Civil War to the German-speaking countries.

Following the Revolution, an improved postal service, better transportation, greater literacy, and a growing population resulted in a proliferation of newspapers and a wide variety of periodicals, including medical journals. These provided a significant but often underestimated vehicle for the professionalization of American medicine. By serving as forums for discussion and advocacy concerning current medical issues, reporting on medical news from abroad and at home, providing information about medical societies (as well as schools and hospitals), disseminating medical knowledge (especially current research) and case reports, and publishing book reviews, the journals helped make a place for American medicine on the contemporary stage. Many of these journals were short lived, however, and most had only a small circulation.

Medical journals were published in the United States only a little later than in Europe—the first was the *Medical Repository* in New York in 1797—but by 1850 approximately twice as many such journals were appearing in America as in Great Britain. Before 1820 almost all of these journals emanated from the Northeast; Philadelphia was the center of American medical journalism, just as it was home to the leading medical school.

The use of hospitals in America developed very slowly despite their widely recognized value in teaching medicine and the prestige that being on a hospital staff brought to doctors. There were good reasons for this. The new Republic was overwhelmingly rural and largely undeveloped, and hospitals were an urban institution. This country lacked the great concentrations of public and private wealth that characterized the older European societies. The function of hospitals at this time was as much custodial as curative; anybody who could afford private doctor visits was treated at home. As a result, hospitals were chiefly for the poor—and America also did not yet have the great reservoirs of poor that Europe did. There were no religious orders to found and staff hospitals (that would come later). Lastly, the political and economic ideologies and social dynamics of the post-Revolutionary era weakened the sense of paternalism and community.

As late as 1810 the United States had only two general hospitals: the one already mentioned in Pennsylvania that had been opened in 1752, and one in New York built in 1774 but not opened until 1791. (The Charité in New Orleans had burned in 1809 and did not re-open until 1815.) Both of these hospitals were used for teaching purposes. Massachusetts General Hospital (MGH), which opened in 1821, provided Harvard with a badly needed major teaching facility. This hospital quickly adopted innovations that were not found in most American hospitals until much later. They included special provisions for the training of both undergraduate and graduate medical students, emergency service at all hours provided by physicians who were always at the hospital, an out-patient department with hours designated for different types of specialty services, admission of paying patients (also a policy of the Pennsylvania hospital from its founding), and maintenance of detailed case records. An indication of the relative lack of clinical need for general hospitals at this time is found in the fact that while MGH had beds for ninety-seven patients, it received only twelve during the first year and grew but slowly over the next decade.

After 1800 specialized hospitals also began to appear. In 1802 the United States government ordered marine hospitals to be built in Norfolk, Virginia, and in Charlestown, Massachusetts. The latter, which had a capacity of about thirty patients, offered opportunities for clinical observation to Harvard medical students. In 1824 Massachusetts Eye and Ear Infirmary opened. In 1832 New Haven Hospital—which was to serve as a teaching hospital for Yale medical students—was founded, and in 1833 Boston Lying-In Hospital—which averaged only twenty-seven deliveries annually during its first twenty-two years—was opened. As late as 1873 there were only 178 institutions providing in-patent care for the sick in the United States, and fifty-eight of these were asylums.

During the period 1790–1830, infectious disease continued to be the nation's number one health problem. Tuberculosis was by far the most important of these diseases, especially in New England. It was so prevalent that it was an important factor in shaping the culture of that period. Malaria had virtually disappeared from the Northeast, but continued to be a serious health problem elsewhere. In the 1790s the coastal cities of the United States were ravaged by violent outbreaks of yellow fever, leading to the establishment of boards of health in Philadelphia (1794), New York (1796), and Boston (1799). The outbreak in Philadelphia, then the nation's capital, was perhaps the most catastrophic epidemic in American history. After 1825, yellow fever disappeared from the North, but it continued to plague the South for the rest of the century.

Although the impact of smallpox gradually decreased during the eighteenth century thanks to greater use of inoculation (making use of pus from smallpox victims to build up immunity), this was an expensive and dangerous procedure. In the early years of the nineteenth century a significant improvement was made in combatting this loathsome disease by the adoption of the safer and less costly vaccination (using noncontagious cowpox rather than smallpox to develop immunity). Unfortunately, smallpox continued to be prevalent in the urban areas to which poorer immigrants flocked. Also, many Americans were not vaccinated until an epidemic threatened. Further compounding the problem was the country's deep commitment to a democratic-libertarian ethic, resulting in strong opposition to compulsory vaccination.

Respiratory illnesses such as influenza, pleurisy, and pneumonia were widespread. Diarrhea and dysentery were gradually lessening in significance. Typhus/typhoid (the two had not yet been clearly distinguished) was largely an affliction of the poor. Childhood diseases like cholera infantum, scarlet fever, and diphtheria took a grim toll. Erysipelas and hepatitis were also common, and dietary deficiencies, worms, and chronic diseases further compromised the well-being of the citizenry.

An especially serious health problem of this era was the enormous amount of alcohol imbibed, never equaled since. Between 1790 and 1830 the annual per capita consumption of alcohol was nearly four gallons, more than the English, Irish, or Prussians, and equal to the Scots and the French. By 1850, the temperance movement had succeeded in reducing the annual per capita consumption by almost half.

In attempting to explain illness, medical thinkers and practitioners of the eighteenth and much of the nineteenth centuries drew on a wide range of theories and speculative systems. They recognized five basic but overlapping external causes of diseases, each necessitating its own preventive measures. One cause of illness was thought to be a justly wrathful deity; such a cause could best be prevented by prayer and penance. A second notion was that the body was assaulted by poisons (called miasma effluvia) released into the air by filth and decaying matter (especially of the vegetable variety); appropriate remedies were flight, fumigation, and personal and public hygiene. A third concept was that of contagion, the spread of illness by either invisible *animalculi* or chemical poisons that came from contact with animals, inanimate objects, or other patients; here the remedies were quarantine or (again) flight. A fourth theory held that the human body was adversely affected by specific climatic conditions, especially excessive heat, cold, wetness, or dryness; avoiding these extremes would prevent their associated disorders. A final related theory proposed that the fundamental cause of widespread epidemic disease was some drastic change in the quality of the atmosphere produced by celestial occurrences, like comets and meteors; by certain alignments of heavenly bodies; or by natural disasters such as earthquake, volcanic eruption, flood, and drought. Nothing could be done about these causes; the only remedy for their supposed effects was diet, rest, exercise, and improved hygiene. As the nineteenth century progressed, the miasmatic and contagious theories came to predominate.

Doctors explained their patients' symptoms in terms of chemical and structural theories that had their roots in ancient Greek thought. One theory was that the body contained four "humors": blood, phlegm, black bile, and yellow bile. Symptoms associated with a corruption or imbalance of any of these humors could result in excessive heat, cold, wetness, or dryness, depending on which humor was affected. Advances in chemistry and physiology during the seventeenth and eighteenth centuries led to increased emphasis on the role of the blood in illness, and to a new chemical theory of disease that centered on the relative acidity of the stomach.

Another theory postulated that the body—especially the blood vessels and the nerves—was composed of fibers, and that sickness was the result of excessive tension or weakness of these fibers. Still other theories questioned whether illness involved the whole body or only a particular system or organ, and whether diseases were specific entities or simply different manifestations of a generalized pathological condition. Heredity, environment, and lifestyle received heavy emphasis in all questions of sickness and health.

The therapy employed in treating illness at this time reflected contemporary medical theory. If humoral imbalance or corruption were produced by something in the blood, then the offending "poison" should be expelled by bleeding it out, or by drugs that purged, puked, or sweated it out. If the body was excessively hot or cold, wet or dry, then foods and medicines that were thought to counteract these conditions should be administered. If the body fibers were too tense or too weak, then they should be relaxed or stimulated by appropriate depressants or strengthening tonics. Bleeding could also be employed to relax the circulatory system. It was all very rational and logical. Since the true source of most illness was not known, doctors treated their patients' symptoms. Of course, drugs that eased pain were always in demand; opium was a staple.

Pain, blood loss, and infection (whose bacterial causes were unknown) placed great restrictions on the surgery that could be performed in the period 1790–1830. Skin and wounds could be treated, cataracts and superficial tumors removed, teeth pulled and bones set, and hernias crudely repaired. Surgeons could also amputate, trephine (bore holes in the skull to relieve pressure), and cut for the bladder stone. However, to operate in the interior of the chest and abdomen would have meant almost certain death for the patient. Still, despite surgery's limitations and horrors, surgeons were able to save lives and improve life for the injured.

The quality and effectiveness of surgery at this time was heavily influenced by the experience and skill of the operator. Only a few doctors were bold enough to perform major operations. The surgical tools and supplies available, and the conditions under which an operation took place (including the number, skill, and experience of the surgeon's assistants) were important. Other variables included the cleanliness of the surgeon, the approach he took to wound treatment, and the physical and psychological state of the patient. American surgeons of this era enjoyed a better reputation at home and abroad than did physicians.

As had been the case throughout history, most care and treatment of the sick and injured was done by the women of the household. Doctors were resorted to only in serious cases. Except for the very poor, most households owned a domestic health guide or manual. Two of the most widely used were John Wesley's *Primitive Physick* (which went through thirty editions in England and the United States between 1747 and 1848), and William Buchan's *Domestic Medicine* (of which there were no fewer than 142 British and American editions between 1769 and 1871). In addition, medical preparations and advice were found in newspapers, magazines, and (to a lesser extent) almanacs. A typical household would also have on hand a small number of medicines, mostly herbals and tonics, many of them prepared at home. After the Revolution, numerous inexpensive patent medicines, almost all made in America and peddled with lively imagination and entrepreneurial ingenuity, were readily available and widely used. Also, between the family and the physician stood a group of poorly educated but not necessarily unskilled purveyors of inexpensive and limited medical services. These included herbalists, midwives, bleeders and cuppers, and bonesetters.

During the middle half of the nineteenth century orthodox medicine was confronted with a serious challenge from the medical sectarians of the period: Thomsonians, Eclectics, Homeopaths, and Hydropaths. (The only one of these sects that was of any importance before 1830 was the Thomsonians; they were a force in American medicine by 1815 and a menacing harbinger of difficult times for orthodox medicine.) These sects capitalized on the growing doubts about traditional medicine and the new spirit of reform, democracy, and free enterprise that exploded in the Age of Jackson. They took advantage of the decline of licensing laws and the ease with which medical schools could be established. They also appealed especially to women.

In the fifty years after Nathan Smith's death in 1829, the aspirations and goals of the post-Revolution medical generation were weakened and sometimes even temporarily abandoned. Nonetheless, it was the medical leaders of that generation—Nathan Smith among them—who had repaired the losses and exploited the opportunities of the War of Independence to lay the foundations of the American medical profession. Their accomplishments and dreams have inspired their successors down to this day.

August 1997   *Ashland, Massachusetts*

PART I

THE ROAD TO DARTMOUTH

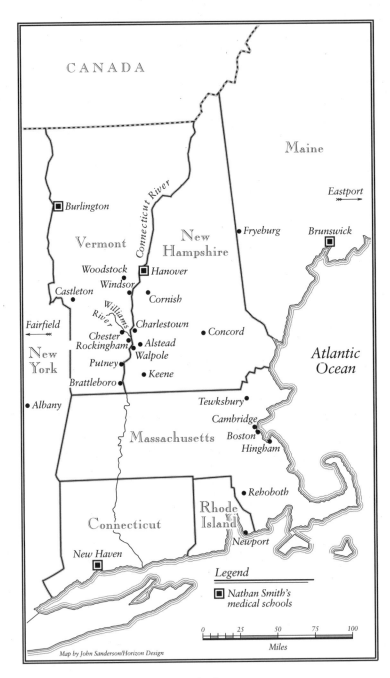

CANADA

Maine

Eastport →

Burlington

Vermont

Connecticut River

New Hampshire

Fryeburg

Brunswick

Woodstock
Windsor
Hanover

Castleton

Cornish

Williams River

Charlestown

Concord

Fairfield ←

Chester
Rockingham

Alstead
Walpole

New York

Putney

Keene

Brattleboro

Albany

Tewksbury

Massachusetts

Cambridge
Boston
Hingham

Atlantic Ocean

Rhode Island

Rehoboth

Connecticut

Newport

New Haven

0   25   50   75   100

Miles

Map by John Sanderson/Horizon Design

Nathan Smith's New England. Courtesy of Horizon Design.

CHAPTER ONE

The Early Years

Much has been said about the inspiration of genius. [But t]he greatest efforts
that have ever been made . . . were the result of hard study and patient labor.
— SAMUEL D. GROSS [1]

S OME FAMILIES SEEM destined to produce physicians; some young
people, even without being members of those special families, seem
nonetheless destined to become doctors. Life stories in such cases
have vigorous beginnings, an apparent inevitability about the general direction they will follow.

Then there are those who become doctors against all odds, as Nathan
Smith did. How did he come to be the kind of man he became? What in
his heritage explains his extraordinary energy and vision? What curious
combination of genetics and geography turned this New England farm
boy into a physician and medical educator for the ages? Clear answers
elude us, but the effort to find them yields a picture suggestive of certain
conclusions.

Family Background

On an early autumn day in 1762, John and Elizabeth Smith welcomed
their fourth child, a son, into the world. They named him Nathan. For
John, this was his eighth child, the sixth son. All four of his children by his
first wife—also named Elizabeth—had died before reaching the age of
ten: John at two, Nicholas at nine, Nathaniel before his first birthday, and
Elizabeth in her tenth year. After their deaths, John used two of the boys'
names again: another John, another Nicholas. But, perhaps not wanting
to tempt fate, he named his second daughter Hannah and altered the ill-

fated "Nathaniel" to "Nathan"; both Hannah and Nathan would live well into the next century.

Rehoboth, Massachusetts, where Nathan Smith was born in September 1762,[2] was one of the Bay Colony's largest townships. Sprawling inland from the northeastern shore at the narrow tip of Narragansett Bay—which exposes the towns along its reaches to Rhode Island Sound and the wide open sea—Rehoboth was well situated, though it was not marked by many events of great historical importance. Thirty-five miles south of Boston and twenty miles from the thriving center of colonial life at Newport,[3] the town was a point of disembarkation for families arriving from England. Many were Smiths; by 1750, southern New England boasted at least nine thousand of them.[4] Dr. Nathan Smith's forebears were among the immigrants who used Rehoboth as a staging area, staying for a time before seeking more fertile lands in the interior.

Nathan Smith's great-great-grandfather Henry Smith landed in Hingham, Massachusetts, in 1638. Rehoboth had already been settled two years earlier, so he might well have gone there directly. The town was incorporated in 1645, and by 1662 the Smiths were sufficiently well established for Ensign Henry Smith, Jr., to represent Rehoboth in the General Court, the legislative body of the province. He also surveyed the town, work that found an echo when his grandson—Nathan's father—became a road developer and town "fence-viewer" in Vermont roughly a hundred years later. Ensign Smith's son (another Henry) was a deacon, further evidence of Smith involvement in town affairs.

John Smith, in the fourth generation, may have been prompted to leave the town of his forebears by the same desire for greater elbow room that, over generations, opened the West. Or perhaps he had an urge to be more of a pioneer—like his surveyor grandfather—than was possible in Rehoboth by the 1760s. When Ensign Smith was surveying Rehoboth, after all, it was still very much on the frontier; neighboring Rhode Island was not granted a royal charter until 1663.[5] Whatever the reason, in Nathan's tenth year the family moved to Chester, Vermont. Town records there indicate that John Smith bought "just one hundred acres" from John Chandler on July 23, 1772.[6]

At the time, Chester existed principally as township boundary lines on the royal maps of the proprietors of the Colonies, empty even of the Native Americans who had greeted the earliest settlers. Most of the Indians had retreated when the fortunes of the French and Indian War (1756–63) went against them. Moving permanently to northern hunting grounds, they later visited the Connecticut Valley only briefly as war parties for the British during the War of Independence; local tribes up and down the eastern seaboard were effectively wiped out by smallpox.[7] The country was thus poised and waiting for young settlers, though land claims came through two different agents of the British crown—one in Portsmouth, New Hampshire, the other in New York City.

Certainly the region was attractive. In addition to being comfortably reminiscent of the English countryside by virtue of its green rolling hills, the rich bottom land was readily accessible by canoe or barge. What is known today as the Williams River runs through Chester into the Connecticut River; families who turned their watercraft northwest out of the Connecticut found it a welcoming place to settle. The contrast to Rehoboth, an established town with a settled population in 1765 of 3,690,[8] would have been dramatic.

John Smith threw himself into town affairs. Shortly after arriving in Chester with his family, he was elected fence-viewer. He was also chosen member of a committee that called a Town Meeting to discuss whether "the inhabitants of said Town will agree to Purchase a Tract of Land for the use and service of a Minister . . . And to built [sic] a School House"; he was subsequently voted onto a committee to pursue these points. On August 9, 1773, he was made moderator. At other times he was "Overseer of the Poor" and "Commissioner of Highways." In late November of 1774, it was voted that "Meeting for public worship" would be at "the Dwelling House of Mr John Smith" until such time as the school "could be made comfortable for that purpose."[9]

Not quite three years after moving to Chester, however, John Smith died on January 13, 1775, at age fifty-seven.[10] Given his involvement in town activities, one has to conclude that the death of this citizen was a great loss to the community. It must also have been a blow to his family, though we have no record of how they reacted. Nathan, twelve at the time, seems not to have spoken much about his father in later years. One of the men who knew Nathan best as an adult (and knew his mother, too —"I was well acquainted with [her] for some years. She was a very sensible and respectable Woman") said of Smith's father, "I . . . do not recollect having heard anything in particular said with regard to him."[11]

Growing Up

Despite being the youngest child, Nathan would certainly have been called upon to help on the family farm, the more so given his father's death; yet once again we have no record. Among the tales told about Smith over the years—generally without attribution—this one stands out: Nathan is supposed to have been "reared an unsophisticated country boy, with a limited education . . . whose irrepressible genius first found employment in stealthily breaking the legs of his father's lambs and sheep, and then humanely offering to patiently mend them."[12]

Be that as it may, in the meantime, it was presumably from his mother that Nathan got his rudimentary education; it will be remembered that when the family moved to Chester, there was no school. Elizabeth Smith must have done well by Nathan, because at the age of thirteen he is said to have had enough book learning to teach in a nearby school.[13] (He presumably had also grown tall and sturdy; in early colonial schools, full of rough and ready farm boys, book knowledge was often less important for a teacher than a strong right arm.[14]) No accounts of Nathan Smith ever having attended a school himself or of his success as a teacher have survived. Given Smith's persistent efforts to advance his own education in the years ahead and his steadfast determination to share his knowledge with others, however, it seems safe to assume his early experiences as both student and teacher were rather more satisfactory than not.

Shortly after Nathan turned seventeen, his mother remarried (on October 12, 1779), taking as her husband Samuel Parker of Walpole, New Hampshire, himself apparently just widowed after a marriage of mere months.[15] On the same day, she deeded the Chester property over to her son John,[16] the eldest, and moved to Walpole with her new husband.

Our chief source of information on Nathan's youth, either before or after his mother remarried and moved, is a book by his granddaughter-in-law, Emily A. Smith, written in 1914. The little volume includes extracts from numerous letters, but it is based largely on undocumented family lore and anecdotes heard by Smith's first medical mentor and other friends —sometimes directly from Smith—but not recounted publicly until much later.[17] The anecdotes provide a very fragmentary picture of Smith's early life on the Chester farm. They include reports of him listening to his mother tell stories of her experiences as a midwife (though town records in Chester and Walpole provide no information confirming that she practiced midwifery), hearing political stories from his neighbors (the uncertainty of political authority in the region gave plenty to politic about), serving in the Vermont militia when he was 15, and even being shot at by Indians.[18]

Since Nathan Smith had a well-developed sense of humor and was quite capable of embroidering a story, as is evident both from the letters he wrote as an adult and from stories recounted about him, it is questionable how much of this can be believed—in particular, the claim that he was an Indian fighter. The tales he himself told about hardships and privations he endured as a very young man, whether while hunting or as a Vermont militiaman, are best taken as illustrative material for points he wished to make rather than as strictly factual accounts. The extant records of his 150 days of service in the Vermont militia in 1782, for instance, give no indication that he was anything other than a common soldier (along with his brother Nicholas and two others from Chester) or that his duties were other than routine.[19] Strikingly, Smith made no mention of either of his parents in any surviving sources, and he apparently left no written record of this period of his life.

Encounter with Josiah Goodhue

The only firsthand account we have of Smith's life in those early years is a letter written by Josiah Goodhue forty-five years after the fact, telling of his initial encounter with Smith in 1784.[20] The letter is extremely valuable to us, because the meeting between the two men turned out to be a turning point in Nathan Smith's life. Central to the importance of the story is that Goodhue (twenty-five years old at the time, and thus three years Nathan's senior) was a doctor.

Josiah Goodhue (1759–1829) had received his early tuition from the Reverend Samuel Whiting in Rockingham, Vermont. In 1775 young Josiah had been at Harvard College, briefly, but the disturbances occasioned by the War of Independence had sent him home and a "white swelling of the knee" (probably a consequence of rheumatic fever or tuberculosis) resulted in his being sent to the care of Dr. Kittredge in Tewksbury, Massachusetts.[21] For two years, Goodhue studied medicine with the famous bonesetter and surgeon. A popular teacher, Kittredge is said to have had but a small library,[22] hardly unusual for the day. He was thus forced to rely on his wits and experience rather than the written opinions of professional medical men.

Goodhue, too, when he first set up practice, apparently had only about six books,[23] but he knew their value. There is reason to suspect that when he did his first amputation he had never seen the operation performed; he may have been "guided only by his books."[24]

A major operation such as an amputation was a solemn occasion in a frontier town. The patient would usually have already endured many months of suffering, innumerable family conferences, and several professional consultations before consenting to such a desperate procedure. Anxiety over the pain the patient knew he would have to undergo—there was of course no anesthesia available beyond that provided by large doses of whiskey or, for the fortunate few, a little opium—necessarily loomed large. So did the predictably high mortality rate. Only when it seemed that death was certain if the amputation was *not* performed would anyone submit to it. Public prayers for divine intervention might be offered.

The whole town would typically turn out. Some, to be sure, were drawn by genuine sympathy; others would appear out of morbid curiosity. Farmers who had to do their own operating on livestock would come, not only to evaluate the doctor for their family, but also to learn what they could to increase their veterinary skill. From the surgeon's point of view, it was useful to have a few strong-armed men in the crowd, for unless he had apprentices, the doctor rarely brought assistants with him. Thus he was sure to need volunteers at the very least to hold the patient, who—even with the help of drugs or alcohol—could not be counted on to lie perfectly still. Depending on the complexity of the operation, the surgeon might even need to turn to the crowd for assistance in exposing the tissues around an incision, or in tying off arteries. Surgery was often an amateurish affair.

Today, a surgeon can afford to take an hour or more for an amputation, supported by a highly trained surgical team and equally sophisticated anesthesiologists. When Josiah Goodhue arrived in Chester, Vermont, to amputate a leg, however, he would have known that an operation of more than a few minutes would be unthinkable. A truly skilled surgeon would take only forty or fifty long, shriek-filled seconds.

Whether or not Nathan Smith had been schooled in midwifery by his mother (as Goodhue later said he believed), which might have sparked the youth's interest in medicine, it was he who stepped forward to help Goodhue with the operation. We do not know how much he actually did. All the descriptions we have are second- or third-hand at best; some are almost certainly the products of overactive imaginations. For example, Henry I. Bowditch in 1851 gave an account he said he got from Joseph Perry, who in turn claimed to have it directly from Goodhue. In 1879, Oliver P. Hubbard retold the story, citing Bowditch citing Perry citing Goodhue (New England doctors all, and all fans of Smith). Hubbard's version was that "Goodhue was struck with the apparently intense interest that he [Smith] took in the proceedings, and with his unflinching steadiness of nerve. Smith even tied the arteries . . . and did so without a tremor."[25] In a famous 1928 address, the great medical man Harvey Cushing similarly focused on the youth's steadiness, saying that Nathan Smith "stepped forward and accepted the trying task without flinching."[26] Cushing may have been relying either on Hubbard or on the account Smith's granddaughter-in-law gave (itself probably inspired by Hubbard): "Nathan Smith stepped boldly forward and with unflinching nerve gave his aid, even so far as to tie the arteries without a tremor."[27] Other writers since have clearly relied on one or another of these versions of the story. Thomas F. Harrington, in a multivolume history of Harvard Medical School, devoted more than the usual amount of space to the tale, spinning it out in imaginative detail:

When all was finished and the curious villagers had departed, Smith remained. To him, at least, the day was more than a casual holiday, the event more than a subject of village gossip. To him the surgeon was a ministering angel of comfort, the workings of the human body more marvelous than he had dreamed.[28]

In any case, meeting Josiah Goodhue under these circumstances seems to have been a transformative experience. Nathan Smith was overcome with the conviction that he wanted to be a surgeon. Virtually unlettered, certainly almost penniless, grown into full manhood though still without a family, this Vermont farmer-schoolteacher was about to set off on the long road to becoming one of the young nation's great physicians.

Preliminary Studies

Like most other medical men of the day, Josiah Goodhue—barely eighteen when he set up practice as a physician—soon had apprentices of his own. Indeed, he became so popular that "students flocked" to him;[29] he obviously took seriously the part of the Hippocratic oath that says, "I will hand on precepts, lectures and all other learning to my sons, to those of my master and to those pupils duly apprenticed and sworn."[30] He worked steadily to improve his skill both as a surgeon and as a preceptor. The importance to him of the latter role is evidenced by his words when he was inaugurated in 1823 as president of the newly chartered Berkshire Medical Institution in Pittsfield, Massachusetts: "It has for many years been my delight to see young men, well started with medical knowledge coming forward in the world."[31]

By the day in 1784 when he traveled to Chester to amputate a leg, Goodhue seems to have had an instinctive sense of what it would take to assure that a given young man was being "well started with medical knowledge." Moreover, he had behind him seven years of strenuous country practice and probably some experience as a preceptor. After the amputation was over, it appears that young Smith told the surgeon of

his desire to engage in the study of medicine, and requested permission to enter his office as a student. —The Doctor judiciously inquired of him, for they were almost strangers to each other, what had been his previous course of life, and what were his acquirements. The reply was, until last night, I have labored with my hands during my life. Dr. Goodhue told him kindly, that he was not in the habit of receiving young men as students, who had not received some preparatory education. Giving him as the reason for this, that the profession of medicine was in a low state in that part of the country, and that to elevate it in reality and in public estimation, young men properly qualified only, should be encouraged to engage in it. In conclusion, he stated to Mr. Smith, that if he would place himself under the tuition of some person capable of instructing him, and acquire so much literary information, as would enable him to enter the freshman class of Harvard College, he would then receive him as a student.[32]

One can imagine that this advice might have discouraged a less resolute youth. With no formal education, Nathan Smith was being told he must qualify for entrance to Harvard before his chosen mentor would even consider taking him on! But Smith apparently was undaunted. Furthermore, more by good luck than as a result of careful consideration, he had chosen his mentor well. He had no way of knowing when he asked Goodhue to take him on as apprentice that Goodhue's judgment that the "profession of medicine was in a low state in that part of the country" was made in sadness mitigated by the conviction that he could do something about it. The two men had much in common; they would become close friends. Goodhue was later said to have "always regarded" Smith

with that esteem and affection which can be excited in the mind of an instructor only by diligence and good conduct on the part of the pupil. These feelings were fully reciprocated by Dr. Smith. [Smith] always spoke of this, his early friend [Goodhue], in the warmest terms of esteem and gratitude, as well for his early advice, as for his subsequent instruction and for his countenance and support after he engaged in the practice of his profession.[33]

First, however, Josiah Goodhue suggested that Smith go to Rockingham, Vermont, to the Reverend Mr. Samuel Whiting—the man who had prepared Goodhue himself for Harvard. Whiting was probably the first truly educated man Nathan Smith had ever even met, let alone become acquainted with.[34]

Having decided relatively late (by the customs of the day) to become a doctor, Smith was a ready pupil, and Whiting seems to have taught him well. In later life, though the colloquial speech that betrayed Smith's background continued to be evident, he always spoke grammatically; his words were well and carefully chosen, his arguments cogent. He also demonstrated an ability to modulate his manner and tone so that he could variously comfort and advise patients, inspire students, or persuade boards of trustees and legislative bodies, as the situation demanded. How much of this he acquired from his teacher we do not know, but given Whiting's reputation as a preacher and experience as a tutor, it is reasonable to imagine that the minister coached his pupils in classical rhetoric along with Latin (for the teaching of which he is said to have had a great facility). Further, given the air of religious liberalism that surrounded Whiting, Smith was probably exposed to the ways of "free thinkers" as well as to standard Congregationalist doctrine.

The few months Smith spent with Whiting are the only formal instruction he had before going into medicine, but it sufficed. Not only was

Goodhue then willing to take him on, but when Smith decided to attend Harvard Medical School in another six years, he passed the entrance requirements. Whether his manifest abilities were due primarily to native talent or to the Rev. Mr. Whiting's tuition matters little now; the results in any case were excellent. Later in life Smith's lectures gave evidence of his having been trained to think clearly, to set his ideas down in logical order, and to express himself well. (A comment once made—by someone with greater social advantages and a more systematic formal education—that Smith was "illiterate" was certainly not based on fact.[35]) Smith's surviving letters make pleasant reading, though they tend to be rough-hewn and show no particular flair for style. He did have a keen sense of irony, however, and his dry wit frequently burst forth like a pent-up geyser.

Apprenticeship

When Whiting pronounced him ready, Smith presented himself once more to Josiah Goodhue, at his home in Putney, Vermont; this time, he was accepted. He remained formally Goodhue's apprentice for three years. During that time Goodhue sent him to Brattleboro, Vermont, twenty-three miles to the south for six months of specialized obstetrical training from Dr. Lemuel Dickerman of that town. (Smith probably walked from Putney to Brattleboro, just as he would have walked the eight miles from Chester to Rockingham and presumably then walked the twenty additional miles to Putney.)

That Goodhue should have decided this particular area of medical practice required special training—roughly equivalent to today's rotation on the obstetrical service—is somewhat surprising. Not only had he, as a popular physician, probably done a fair number of deliveries himself; it was also common practice to rely on midwives. Nonetheless, when Goodhue took on his own brother, Joseph, as an apprentice a few years later, it was again only after first sending him to Whiting and then to Dickerman. Clearly Goodhue had considerable confidence in this three-way division of the task of instructing would-be physicians: With help from Whiting and Dickerman, he thus succeeded in creating a kind of rustic faculty for his pupils. Judging by the results in Smith's case, at least, the system worked well. And to the extent that this was a sign Goodhue knew his own limitations and appreciated superior skill in others, he set an example that Smith would follow in the years to come, however unconsciously.

Dickerman (1751–1832) must have been, in his own way, quite as stimulating as Whiting; certainly he had an unusual background for a medical man, even for those days.[36] Having left the security of a settled town in

Massachusetts (Stoughton), where he had completed an apprenticeship as a shoemaker, Dickerman had come to Brattleboro about 1765. He first hired out as a farm hand and then as an apprentice to Dr. Henry Wells. Dickerman shortly did so well that Dr. Wells eventually lost most of his practice to him. The old doctor moved to Massachusetts, leaving his apprentice a thriving practice and a position as town leader. He was famous enough to have had his portrait (now lost) hanging in the Town Hall and respected enough to head the list of those who (in 1806) endorsed the use of cowpox inoculations against smallpox.[37]

The only record we have of the three years Smith spent with Goodhue is receipts Goodhue signed in 1804 and 1813—long after Smith had completed his apprenticeship—indicating that Smith had paid first $35.00, and then ("in full of all amounts and demands to this day") $50.00.[38] These payments presumably were for tuition, fee plus interest—more than a quarter of a century late!

The extremely late payment accords with much that was to come, and with Goodhue's assessment at the time of Smith's death that "Smith's faults . . . were as few as generally fall to the lot of humanity. He had, however, a very prominent one . . . . He was a bad paymaster." How much Smith's poor record on paying bills had to do with his own early experience with poverty—Goodhue said he "was often poorly clad for a Vermont winter"—and how much with poor habits, bad luck, or a genuine character fault, is unclear.[39]

Though we do not know the particulars of Nathan Smith's apprenticeship, much has been written on the general subject.[40] The details of the work or training and the overall quality of the experience of "reading with the doctor" and then "riding with the doctor" varied considerably, largely depending on the extent of the preceptor's own education and personal qualities. Some apprentices were given opportunity to do little more than keep the office clean, prepare and perhaps dispense medicines, and drive the horse and buggy so the doctor could sleep en route to a patient's house. A few talented and industrious young men overcame poor experience in this regard: Charles Caldwell, in his day a very distinguished physician, studied with a preceptor (around 1790) who, though intelligent and attentive, had "no library, no apparatus, no provision for improvement in practical anatomy, nor any other efficient means of instruction in medicine."[41] In general, a preceptor was "entitled to the student's services in preparing and dispensing medicines, extracting teeth, bleeding, and other minor surgical operations, and, when more advanced in studies, in attending on the sick."[42]

Occasionally apprentices either kept a diary or later put their recollections down on paper. Daniel Drake (1785–1852), later an eminent physician and medical school teacher, was apprenticed at the age of fifteen to Dr. William Goforth in Cincinnati. In his memoirs he wrote about his early days of apprenticeship:

My first assigned duties were to read Quincy's Dispensatory and grind quicksilver into UNGUENTEM MERCURIALE; the latter of which, from previous practice on a Kentucky hand mill, I found much easier of the two. But few of you have seen the genuine, old Doctor's shop of the last century; or regaled your olfactory nerves in the mingled odors which, like incense to the God of Physic, rose from brown paper bundles, bottles stopped with worm-eaten corks, and open jars of ointment, not a whit behind those of the Apothecary in the days of Solomon; yet such a place is very well for a student. However idle, he will always be absorbing a little medicine; especially if he sleeps beneath the greasy counter . . . . It was my allotted task to commit to memory Cheselden on the bones, and Innes on the muscles, without specimens of the former or plates of the latter; and afterwards to meander the currents of humoral pathology, of Boerhaave and Vanswieten; without having studied the chemistry of Chaptal, the physiology of Haller, or the Materia Medica of Cullen.[43]

Drake obviously had access to more books at Dr. Goforth's than most apprentices did. (Goforth, educated in New York, seems to have been fairly affluent.[44])

Mindful of the frustrating handicap under which he had studied, with access only to Kittredge's small library, Goodhue eventually developed a good one of his own. It is unlikely, however, that he had a very substantial collection of books by the time of Smith's apprenticeship,[45] though both he and Smith probably read every medical book they could get their hands on. A good picture of the kinds of books an apprentice in the 1780s might have had access to comes from the list kept by Thomas Eaton, apprentice to Dr. Elijah Butler of Francestown, New Hampshire, in 1792–93, in his diary.[46] (Two of the volumes Smith later bequeathed to the medical library at Yale[47] were on Eaton's list: Gerard Van Swieten's *Diseases Incident to Armies* and John Freind's *Emmenologia* [disorders of menstruation].) Quite probably Smith read at least some of the better-known and more important books Eaton mentioned, like William Cheselden's anatomy text and William Cullen's *Materia Medica* (roughly, the study of herbal remedies and what today would come under the rubric of pharmacology), *First Lines*, and *Synopsis of Nosology* (a "nosology" was how doctors classified diseases).

Whatever Smith read, he must have gained by it at least as large a stock of misinformation as of useful guidance. Reading was then as it is today only one part of a medical education. The far more important contribution of the preceptor was the experience his practice provided for the preceptee. Here, certainly, Smith was fortunate. Goodhue was later described by a younger contemporary, Yale medical professor Jonathan Knight, as "the most celebrated surgeon in that region [northern New England]."[48] Some physicians of the day, with a lesser reputation than Goodhue, might have been able to show their students only an endless stream of patients with grippe or gripes and the inevitable *exitus*.

Goodhue almost certainly had much more. We know his practice was large and included a varied number of serious problems and considerable surgery.[49] But Goodhue himself attested, fifty years later, to another critical factor in the success of Smith's education, something for which the mentor took no personal credit:

While Smith lived with me the country was new, the roads were bad, . . . [M]y pupils . . . sometimes objected on account of the road, or inclemency of the weather, but it was not so with him; it was enough to say he might go, and he was gone. Neither the darkness of the night, the mud to his horses knees, or the violence of the storm were any impediments to him . . . . If it should be asked what laid the foundation of Doctor Smith's eminence, the answer is industry. If it should be asked what brought him to the pinnacle of the profession the answer is the most unremitting industry.

Goodhue also recounted in that same letter another episode that transpired during the apprenticeship, which he believed helped show the measure of the man (and which may, if Goodhue was right, also have been the origin of Smith's intense interest in anatomy). After a particularly taxing ride, Smith faced the need to destroy his overworked horse. "[H]e felt rather bad for a few minutes," Goodhue wrote,

but soon concluded to turn his loss to good account, and converted the dead horse into a subject for dissection; to which he immediately proceeded with perhaps as high a degree of interest as ever he felt in dissecting a human subject.

When Nathan Smith had completed his apprenticeship with Josiah Goodhue, he was as well prepared as any apprentice of the day could have hoped to be. Soon his excellent grasp of the fundamentals of "physic" (or "physick"—in either case meaning the art or science of healing diseases, the art of medicine and therapeutics) and of epidemiological principles would show Whiting and Goodhue had done their jobs ably.

CHAPTER TWO

Newly Minted Doctor

[A]ll the knowledge of [nature] is to be had only from experience . . . . [A]ll the
philosophy of a physician consists in searching into the history of diseases,
and applying such remedies as experience shows to be curative thereof; observing . . . the method of cure, which right reason, . . . not . . . vain speculation, points out.   —THOMAS SYDENHAM [1]

Opening a Practice

IN THE 1780s, three years was a fairly standard medical apprenticeship,
although some young men spent more and many prospective doctors
spent less. Nathan Smith may have begun to be restless and eager to go
out on his own or to think he had learned all he could from Josiah Goodhue. There was in fact no easy way to determine whether an apprentice
was ready to begin practice; there were no state boards or licensing procedures in 1787. Instead, preceptor and preceptee together had to decide
when the moment had arrived. If the preceptor had poor prospects for attracting another "pupil," he might cling to one already on hand. Eminent
doctors like Goodhue, however, could count on being able to draw more
apprentices and might well have several students at once, who would constitute "a small class . . . drilled as regularly in their studies as they would
be in college," according to medical historian and physician N. S. Davis,
who wrote nearly a century later.[2]

We know that Josiah Goodhue, widely respected as both physician and
surgeon, was adamant about the importance of education and the need to
improve medical care. He would probably have been happy to see a trainee
of his as self-assured and competent as Smith go out on his own, helping
to improve the sorry state of the profession. Thus it may have been Goodhue himself who suggested that Smith should start putting into practice
what he had learned from Goodhue.

Smith had, of course, already had opportunities to play the role of physician. Goodhue remarked years later that, while Smith lived with him, he often relied on his students to see patients on their own. "Physicians [were] scarce," he observed; "it often became necessary to send my pupils to visit the sick, sometimes a considerable distance."[3]

When Smith did decide to leave Goodhue, he did not go far. He moved across the Connecticut River and a few miles north to Cornish, New Hampshire; there, by his own account, he started practicing medicine in 1787. Soon he was seeing patients in an area he later told students was probably about "fifty miles [in] diameter."[4]

Cornish would prove to be a happy choice. Not only is it unusually beautiful, "a lovely place, diversified by hill and dale, woods and dells and brawling streams . . . [with] the charming cone of [Mt.] Ascutney" rising to the west across a broad bend in the Connecticut River.[5] (The exceptional beauty of the geography was attested to in dramatic fashion by the formation a century and a half later of the "Cornish Colony," which drew a wide range of artists, first as acolytes to the sculptor Augustus St. Gaudens and then simply because they could not stay away.[6]) The area was also hardly overburdened with medical practitioners. To be sure, there was a Dr. James Moore in Hanover, but that was some twenty or twenty-five miles (and a good half-day's ride) to the north. Besides, by 1795 Moore seems to have left Hanover to practice elsewhere (his Hanover journal ends on October 2, 1794).[7]

Cornish itself also had a physician. Dr. Solomon Chase had moved to Cornish prior to the Revolution, during which he served first as a company commander in a militia regiment raised by his brother, Colonel Jonathan Chase, then as a physician and surgeon with General John Stark's brigade, and finally with the Continental Army itself as Surgeon General in the Northern Department.[8] When Solomon Chase returned to Cornish, he may have continued to practice medicine until near the end of his life in late 1828. By 1790, however, he was devoting time to managing the store owned by his brother Jonathan, and it seems plausible that he would have welcomed the assistance of the new young doctor who showed up in town. Evidence of interaction between the two is sketchy at best, however. Occasional references in Smith's 1792 accounts to financial dealings with Solomon Chase, for example, and a receipt Chase gave Smith for a payment of $1.00—the latter dated years after Smith had moved away from Cornish—merely prove that they knew each other.[9] And although the records of the Old Chase Tavern make clear that both men frequently ate and drank there, no indication is given that they did so together.[10]

Smith had barely arrived in Cornish when he found himself caring for the Spaldings and the Chases, two of the most prominent families in town. This helps explain the rapidity with which he came into favor particularly with the extended Chase family, town leaders by every measure. Chases were among the earliest settlers in the area, and several members of the family (including Jonathan's father, seventy-year-old Judge Samuel Chase) served with distinction in the War of Independence.

Town records consistently show Chases holding one local office after another. Colonel (later General) Jonathan Chase, for example, repeatedly served as town treasurer, moderator, and selectman.[11] Several Chases typically held office simultaneously; at any one time, two or more of the selectmen were likely to bear the Chase name.[12] Chases were also frequently chosen as moderator, warden, or clerk—or all three—of the local church (variously called the Episcopal Society of the Church of England, Trinity Church, and the Protestant Episcopal Society).[13] Nathan Smith's association with this distinguished family progressed satisfactorily; he soon married into it.

The young doctor's first task on arriving in Cornish was to make the availability of his services known. With a senior physician already on hand for emergencies, Smith had to do something to establish his reputation. Two hundred years ago most people hesitated (with good reason) to trust a new doctor; the odds were good that their own home remedies would be as effective as any the doctor might propose.

The fact that Nathan Smith understood and liked country people would not have been enough to ensure employment. In addition, he needed to show the townspeople what sort of a person he was. In this he received a fortunate boost, if a story preserved in the annals of Cornish is not apocryphal. Even if the account is not literally true, the fact that it was told and retold hints what Smith was like and how people thought about him in those early years:

While the newly fledged doctor was patiently waiting for business, a company of young men concluded to have a little fun at his expense. Their plan of procedure was suggested by the sight of a goose with a broken leg. Taking the tavern keeper into their confidence, they caught the limping bird, and as soon as all arrangements were complete, a messenger was dispatched in haste to tell Dr. Smith that a patient who had unfortunately broken his leg desired his services at the tavern immediately. The doctor was promptly on hand, but began to suspect a trick as he came in sight of the house. Preceded by "mine host," and followed by a crowd, all ready to burst with delight at the anticipated surprise and chagrin of the doctor, he entered the great hall where, sure enough, lay the poor goose, extended in all honor upon a bed.

The doctor, without the least hesitation or show of surprise, advanced to the bed, and having, with scrupulous care, examined the broken limb, prepared his splints, reduced the fracture, and bound it up in the most scientific manner. He then, with extreme gravity, directed the tavern keeper to pay strict attention to the patient, on no account to suffer him to be moved from the bed for at least a week, but to feed him plentifully with Indian meal and water.

There was not much laughter when the doctor went away, though thus far all had gone well enough; but the next day the joke really became serious, when a good round *bill for professional services* came to the landlord, which he found himself obliged to pay.

The affair soon got abroad, and the shrewd and level-headed young doctor suddenly found himself famous. People said, "There's a man who knows how to take care of himself." Everybody respected him, and the foundation of a lucrative practice was laid for the young physician.[14]

The best records of Smith's first years in practice are to be found in his account book that begins in 1792 and runs through 1794. Frequent entries of "to visit and advice [sic]" remind us there was often nothing a physician could actually do. On the other hand, we also learn that the young doctor was more actively tending to a variety of minor ailments: "dressing & opening a sore," "dressing his knee," "to visit & dressing a sore," "to visit & extracting a tooth," "fractured finger," and "visit, dressing a wound & cerate" (a common medicinal preparation for external application). More substantial problems are noted as well: "fistula in ano" (anal ulcer) and "extracting a foetus" (in other words, delivering a baby) on one day, and "reducing [setting] a fractured thigh" on another.[15] Time was spent in travel, too. Even a quick perusal of Smith's day books, ledgers, and accounts between 1790 and 1794 shows that he had patients scattered over a wide area: in the New Hampshire towns of Croydon, Newport, Claremont, Plainfield, Lebanon, and Hanover, and across the river in Windsor and Hartland, Vermont. Clearly it was no exaggeration to speak of a fifty-mile diameter for the practice.

No contemporary account remains to tell what prompted Smith to suspend his practice abruptly less than three years after he began, but the reason is evident: He had decided to attend lectures at Harvard Medical School, more than a hundred miles to the south. The decision must have been difficult from a financial point of view. Though he seems to have laid a solid "foundation of a lucrative practice," he is said to have sold his horse to finance the trip.[16] And if Goodhue's latter-day recollection is to be trusted, when Smith left Cambridge after receiving his degree, he had only 25¢ in his pocket.[17]

Josiah Goodhue may deserve some credit for Smith's decision to take the big step of going to Cambridge. For although Smith had always had a restless thirst for knowledge and must have been growing acutely aware of how much he did not know, Goodhue—himself thwarted by illness from completing his Harvard education—would almost certainly have urged his ambitious and talented protégé to think about attending the still-new medical school there, at that time the only one in New England.

Goodhue knew from his own days at Harvard and from his three years with Smith that the younger man's preliminary education with Whiting was as good as that of many Harvard students; he would have been confident Smith could learn much that was useful at the medical school.

Off to Harvard

In the autumn of 1789, Nathan Smith arrived in Cambridge to begin his formal education at Harvard Medical School, where the central figure in the enterprise was John Warren (1753–1815), a man of considerable reputation. Warren had apprenticed under his talented brother, Joseph, who died at the Battle of Bunker Hill. He took further study under Edward Augustus Holyoke (1728–1829), the impressively long-lived and distinguished doctor of Salem, Massachusetts (recipient in 1782 of the first honorary M.D. degree awarded by Harvard); and he had spent long years of hard work in Cambridge at the Base Hospital of the Revolutionary Army.

In May 1782 the Harvard Corporation formed a committee that described the requisite professorships for a medical school; action was taken promptly. That Warren should be appointed the first professor, of anatomy and surgery, was virtually a foregone conclusion; he had already had great success in giving anatomy lectures in the military hospital. Though others were actively involved in the early planning stages as well,[18] Warren's importance warrants his being credited with founding Harvard Medical School.

John Warren proved to be a man to capture student loyalty. His effect on Smith's near contemporary, Jacob Bigelow (1786–1879), was striking:

I believe that my original distaste for the profession of medicine was removed by the eloquence of Dr. John Warren, the eldest of a line of distinguished physicians, who at that time, lectured on anatomy to the senior class of undergraduates. I thought I discovered that a physician might be fluent and accomplished, and serve his generation in other ways than as a mere vehicle of pills and plasters. I began to think that if a man could obtain foothold in a city, and diversify his calling with the additional function of a lecturer or professor, he might find his position agreeable and advantageous.[19]

The next choices for faculty members at Harvard's new medical school were also excellent, even though one of them would prove problematic. The appointment of Benjamin Waterhouse (1754–1846) as professor of the "Theory and Practice of Physic" made great sense, on the face of it; by the standards of the day, he had "superior scientific qualifications."[20] On the other hand, he was by some standards no patriot, which one might have thought would be a consideration so soon after the War of Independence. Yet there was a connection between his lack of "patriotism" (or at least his unwillingness to fight against the Crown) and his fine medical education. As a Quaker, he had sat out the entire war, spending seven years beneficially in the three most important centers of medical education of the day: London, Edinburgh, and Leyden. He was a cousin of the English Quaker physician John Fothergill (1712–1780); being sponsored by him and John Coakley Lettsom (1744–1815), another Friend numbered among England's most outstanding and important medical practitioners, helped give Waterhouse entrée wherever he needed or wanted it. No one could have received a better medical preparation anywhere else in the world of that day.

Benjamin Waterhouse, however, was opinionated and cantankerous; he showed little of the gentleness of spirit generally associated with the Quakers.[21] Not a little of the man is revealed in a letter he wrote Lettsom in November of 1794:

Should I ever execute what I am constantly revolving in my Mind, "A View of Society and Manners, with the Natural History of New England," I should send it to England, and publish it there without a name. The fact is, I have no taste for the practice of physic as it is conducted in this country. It is not worth a man's attention. I feel such a mighty difference between transcribing from the great volume of Nature, and practicing among the very vulgar, that is conforming to the whims and nonsense of old women and silly people, that I am sometimes almost determined to renounce it for ever. I know how a London physician gets his bread, but with us it is widely different: a man like me of a weakly frame, addicted to study, is liable to be called out five or six miles on horseback in a severe winter night, and to remain out all night, and to receive (in the course of a year) a guinea for it! We are obliged to be physician, surgeon, apothecary, and toothdrawer, all under one; and if we are not attentive to small things, and if we do not give consequence to trifles, we are dropped for some one who does.[22]

Given this, it is perhaps not surprising to learn that Dr. Waterhouse, among his other distinctions, holds the rare one of "being discharged from a professorship solely because his fellow professors disliked him."[23] Another historian has concluded that, "knowing the basic facts, the physicians of Boston were fully justified in regarding Waterhouse with suspicion and hostility."[24] Though Waterhouse was difficult to get along with (Smith was not alone in finding him insufferable), he was friends with both Thomas Jefferson and John Adams, and he had genuine medical skill. He was a major force in American medicine for half a century.

The third member of the Harvard medical faculty was Aaron Dexter (1750–1829). Having received his Harvard A.B. in 1776, he spent a year apprenticing with Samuel Danforth before marrying and opening a practice in Boston. Reputedly a fine physician with many interests, he was an incorporator of the Massachusetts Medical Society and a member of sev-

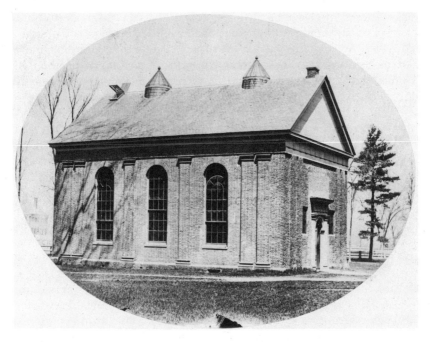

Holden Chapel, first site of Harvard Medical School, where Nathan Smith would have attended lectures. Photo courtesy of Harvard University Archives.

eral learned societies. At Harvard he was professor of chemistry and "Materia Medica" from 1783 to 1816, where he was known as an outstanding scientific chemist (not at all to be taken for granted among physicians of the day).

Some idea of the sort of man he was can be gleaned from a story about him given currency by Oliver Wendell Holmes, a Harvard medical graduate. The chemist's demonstrations were said, Holmes recounted, to be of "startling precipitations, of pleasing changes of color, of brilliant coruscations, of alarming explosions and above all of odors innumerable and indescribable." But when one experiment—which Dexter had promised the class would result in a powder bursting into a "sudden and brilliant flame"—produced nothing, he was unperturbed. " 'Gentlemen,' " Holmes reported that Dexter said "with a serene smile, 'the experiment has failed; but the principle, Gentlemen — the principle remains firm as the everlasting hills.' "[25]

This trio of faculty members gave the lectures that comprised medical education at Harvard in the 1780s and into the 1790s. Smith also attended the course on "Natural Philosophy" given by Professor Samuel Webber in the college.[26] With Dexter's chemistry course, this would have been all the "science" Smith studied. His name appears in the official record of graduates;[27] beyond that, the publication of his "inaugural dissertation" (more akin to a student essay today than to a modern doctoral dissertation) in the first two numbers of the *Massachusetts Magazine* for 1791 is the only direct evidence of Smith's time at Harvard. He grandly dedicated the dissertation to the "Rev. J. Willard, S.T.D. Prof.," president of the university,[28] and gave it a title of sweeping promise—on "causes and effects of spasm in fevers"—that might well lead one to expect something more substantial than the paper of roughly 2,500 words he actually wrote. In the essay, he concerned himself primarily with the kinds of speculations on etiology and classification of diseases promulgated by the Edinburgh professor of materia medica, William Cullen (1710–1790), whose books (as we have seen) were read by apprentices of the day, and who was the acknowledged expert of the day on fevers. Some of what Smith wrote was arrant nonsense, some absolute error; for the most part, he was probably repeating what he had learned from Waterhouse (who had studied under Cullen). Smith's paper—given its brevity, superficial treatment of the subject, and lack of independent research—would not be acceptable even for a bachelor's degree at a respectable college today. These realities notwithstanding, an eager note (signed "A.Z.") to the editor of the *Magazine* headed the published paper: "I have long wished that your medical department might consist of American papers. To accomplish this desire, I forward Dr. Smith's Dissertation, delivered at a late publick examination, Harvard University, for the degree of Bachelor of Physick [sic]."[29]

The only other reaction to Smith's dissertation of which we know was a "critique" by an anonymous author (who signed himself "Philozetemia") that ran five months later in the *Magazine*. The debate continued over the next two years, first with an answer by Nathan Smith (he signed himself this time in Latin, "Nahum Smith," perhaps in mocking response to his critic's having chosen a Greek pseudonym), then with a second criticism by Philozetemia and another reply by Smith.[30] The eighteenth-century language and style of the controversy are probably of greater interest today than its inadequate scientific content. And, in light of the absence of any particular originality on Smith's part, we have to conclude that Philozetemia's criticism lacked perspicacity when we read what he wrote at the end of his second attack: "Doctor Smith's medical ingenuity will never be contested. The sentiments of his dissertation are original, ingenious, chimerical; and present greater occasion to admire his ingenuity than applaud his judgment."[31]

The one hint that the "dissertation" accurately reflected the work of Smith the practitioner is to be found in the places where he implicitly showed a reliance on what he had himself seen: "I think it may be observed as a rule in practice," for instance, and "this is not the case, so often, as some would have us believe." In the third section, he also used his own considerable personal experience with influenza as evidence for what he had to say (though even then he hinted only very tentatively at disagreement with Cullen).[32]

On the whole, the thesis is lucidly written and no less impressive than the typical "inaugural dissertation" of the day, even if much of it was misconceived. "Pronounced" at Cambridge on July 5, 1790, this thesis—in conjunction with the credit Smith was given for his time with Goodhue and his years of private practice (he had returned to Cornish to care for patients between terms)—sufficed to earn him a Bachelor of Medicine degree. He was only the fifth man to receive the degree from Harvard.

Exactly what or how much Smith actually learned at Harvard Medical School is unclear, however. John Warren was in a peculiar position. During the Revolution, he had taught surgical procedures by using cadavers and by taking his students into the Boston Almshouse to watch him operate. Already in 1782, he had lectured at public dissections. But popular opinion began to turn against such demonstrations. The overseers of the Almshouse were among those who had trouble getting along with Waterhouse; they were therefore not disposed to cooperate with anyone at the medical school. Those factors in turn helped create controversy over the use of the Almshouse patients for teaching purposes in general, let alone the use of their bodies once they had died. For years, therefore, surgery was taught largely via lecture. So great was public disapproval of "cutting up" the dead that dissections required great secrecy. During Smith's time at Harvard, there were neither laws to protect the dead from the anatomist nor laws to shield the anatomist from public disapprobation.[33]

It is doubtful, therefore, whether Smith could say of his stay in Cambridge what John Johnston (an almost exact contemporary) wrote to his father in 1790 after five months as a student at the Medical Department of the College of Philadelphia: "I have an opportunity of seeing every kind of operation that can be performed on the human body, also the treatment of every kind of disease that is incident to the human system."[34] Johnston may of course have overstated Philadelphia's medical munificence, but certainly Harvard could not—or did not—use much clinical material. Moreover, looking back eighteen years later, Smith was quite prepared to criticize the Harvard professors' medical lectures. If what a student of Smith's wrote in his journal in 1808 is accurate, Smith apparently said the Harvard faculty had been delivering the same lectures for twenty years. The student journalist did not reveal what evidence Smith had for this claim, or even whether Smith bothered to elaborate.[35]

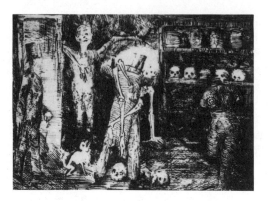

"A Midnight Foray into Holden Chapel":
A nineteenth-century artist's view.
Photo courtesy of Harvard University Archives.

Smith himself left no written record of his experience at Harvard. Fortunately, Moses Appleton, a 1791 Phi Beta Kappa graduate of Dartmouth, kept an account of *his* studies at Harvard four years later (during 1793 and 1794), which fills in the gap for us. Lecture outlines and questions from the final examination in 1795 appear in Appleton's diary. From his notes, researchers tell us,

> it appears that Dr. Warren's lectures on anatomy, midwifery, and surgery dominated the teaching of the Harvard Medical School of the 1790s. . . . That Dr. Warren's teaching of anatomy was not entirely didactic is indicated by Appleton's description of an autopsy performed during the course of his lectures.[36]

Appleton's transcript of the final examination supports the judgment that Warren's work was the centerpiece of the curriculum. The questions on anatomy and surgery take up more space than Waterhouse's questions on the theory and practice of physic and Dexter's on chemistry and materia medica combined.[37]

One reason Smith may have been disappointed with his time in Cambridge can be found in a number of his letters—mostly from several years later—that hint at financial difficulties and attest to Waterhouse's irritability. The most comprehensive statement of the sore point between the two men, though put somewhat obliquely, is in a letter Smith wrote to Waterhouse at the end of 1794 (more than four years after he had finished at Cambridge): "I readily grant that either you or or [sic] I have been greatly abused," wrote Smith; "I have been very much mortified . . . ." He went on to make several further points: Waterhouse had proposed letting Warren and Dexter determine the amount of Waterhouse's fee for private instruction; Smith had never intended to leave it up to Waterhouse; furthermore, although Waterhouse claimed Dexter said the fee should be £20, Dexter and Warren both said they had never discussed the matter with him. Finally, Smith insisted his poverty was so manifest that Waterhouse should have offered him money rather than used "improper means" to get it from him.[38]

Although it appears Smith considered his grudge against Waterhouse a serious one, it is difficult to be sympathetic. If he had been misled by Waterhouse with respect to who would set the fee, he was perhaps entitled to some annoyance. Beyond that, however, the fee itself does not seem unreasonable, and Waterhouse was surely quite within his rights to ask for payment. (Not everyone could be expected to wait as patiently as Josiah Goodhue did.) Moreover, when Smith noted in a letter to John Warren that he had paid Waterhouse the basic lecture fee and sixteen shillings toward private instruction,[39] he seemed implicitly to acknowledge that he had been the beneficiary of more than routine instruction.

Smith had also boarded with Waterhouse while he was in Cambridge. Why he should have balked at paying extra, and why the dispute over the bill should have vexed him so much and rankled so long, is unclear. But both Smith and Waterhouse were stubborn men, and despite Smith's later reputation for being able to get along even with the most difficult people, it is quite possible that he simply did not like Waterhouse. Was it because he felt Waterhouse looked down on him? Writing to John Warren in February 1791, and again in March, Smith used strong language, speaking of his "contempt" for Waterhouse and asking whether Warren thought he should proceed with court action against Waterhouse. Clearly, Smith believed he had been maltreated:

Does Dr. Waterhouse think the young men from this part of the Country are fools that they will suffer themselves to be imposed on in such a futile manner—I think . . . I shall take some active measures to expose him & bring upon him that contempt which he so justly deserves.[40]

The matter dragged on. Waterhouse also turned to Warren, complaining five years later as follows:

[I ask you] . . . Whether the charge I made Dr. Smith for the time he resided in my family as my pupil (from Nov. to Commencement, 4 or 5 weeks absence excepted) of *twenty pounds*, was in your opinion unreasonable, or any way extravagant and whether my voluntary unsolicited abatement of eight pounds of the twenty, making the charge to Smith but *forty dollars*,[41] was not low beyond any rate for pupillage among your physicians?[42]

On April 23, 1796, Waterhouse wrote once more to Warren: "I called this day on you respecting that ungrateful business of Smith's . . . . Can you . . . write your declaration and bring it to [Justice Greenleaf] . . . . Your atten-

Transcript of a medical examination
before the Professors at Cambridge University.
1795

Anatomy. Doct. John Warren

What is understood by anatomy?
The general divisions of anatomy what?
What the composition of the bones?
Describe the bones of the head.
. . . . . of the trunk
. . . . . of the extremities
Upon what mechanical principle are the bones acted
upon?
What are the different kinds of articulations?
What are the Fluids in the body? ———
The composition of the blood what?
What phenomena does the blood when newly drawn
exhibit? ———
What the difference between the crassamentum
serum and Lymph? ———
What are the component parts of the most simple
fibre?
What is a fibre? What a Muscle? Mention

Surgery. ———
What are the usual Phenomena in recent Wounds?
What is the difference between a Phlegmone and an
Erythema? ———
What are the external applications for promoting
resolution in a Phlegmone? ———
What to induce Suppuration? ———
How is a Gangrene to be prevented?
How many kinds of fractures are there? ———
What is the difference of treatment in a simple or
compound fracture? ———
Describe the operation of Trepanning.
. . . . . . Lithotomy.
. . . . . . Couching.
. . . . . . Amputation of the Thigh
. . . . . . Reduction of the luxated humerus
What are the different kinds of Bandages? ———
. . . . . . Sutures ———

*Notes by Moses Appleton on
his examination at Harvard
Medical School, 1795.*
Used with permission of the
Francis A. Countway Library
of Medicine.

tion to it will further oblige your friend, B. Waterhouse."[43] Then in February of 1797, he had this to say to Warren:

Behold me once more plaguing you on the ungrateful and odious subject of Dr. Nathan Smith! I never meant to make a serious defense until the matter came before the superior court [of New Hampshire] and now I intend to go up . . . . As Smith and others are taking steps to establish medical lectures at Dartmouth College, should he be successful in making people believe *that the resident Prof. at Cambridge under the cloak of kindness, defrauds needy students who put themselves under his protection* very few will be disposed to make the trial. . . . I mean to call on you in a few days, but I thought I would write this much that you might think a little on the subject, previous to my seeing you. In the interim I remain your friend and humble servant.[44]

Apparently Dr. Warren was neither persuaded by the reasoning nor impressed by the protestations of humble friendship. His respect for and loyalty to Nathan Smith turned out to be stronger than any sympathy he might have felt for his colleague, and his eventual deposition was decidedly in Smith's favor.[45] The suit itself fizzled out on its second appeal, neither side appearing for its continuance.[46] That notwithstanding, the social strain between the men never healed. In a letter to John Warren early in May of 1797, Smith pointedly did not mention Dr. Waterhouse even as he asked to be remembered to both Mrs. Warren and Dr. Dexter.[47]

Marriage and Family Life

When Smith returned to Cornish, New Hampshire, in the summer of 1790 with his new medical degree, he had himself become a most attractive potential preceptor. He knew he would have at least one student immediately: Lyman Spalding, scion of Cornish's other leading family. Though still a very young man (he was barely sixteen when Smith returned from Cambridge), Spalding was ambitious, idealistic, and already planning to study medicine at Harvard. Jo Gallup also came, from Vermont. He had been practicing medicine for eight years, but he was eager to be exposed at least indirectly to a Harvard education.

The likelihood that the Harvard degree coupled with the reputation he had already established would bring Smith apprentices in Cornish does not appear to be all that drew Smith home. His mother lived not far away, in Walpole, New Hampshire, and he stopped to see her on his way back from Cambridge. But Cornish was where he had put down roots, and within six months of his return—on January 16, 1791—he married Elizabeth Chase. She was the second daughter of Jonathan Chase and his first wife, Thankful Sherman Chase. Thus this man whose parents and siblings

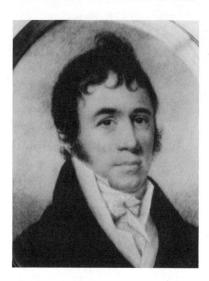

Lyman Spalding, 1775–1821.
Used with permission of the Francis A.
Countway Library of Medicine.

are largely lost in the mists of migration and mishap acquired an established family with a vast number of sisters and cousins and aunts (to say nothing of brothers and uncles) close at hand, very visible, and perennially active on the local scene. Elizabeth was not yet twenty-six; no one could have guessed that she would live to enjoy little more than two years of married life. On April 24, 1793, she died.[48]

Elizabeth and Nathan had had no children, leaving him quite bereft,[49] except for the extended Chase family. Given their numbers and prominence in town, the intimacy that had developed between Nathan and his in-laws, and the generally accepted view that it was not right for a man to remain unmarried for long—both his father and his father-in-law had married again shortly after being widowed—it is unsurprising that he soon turned his attention to another Chase. This time it was his late wife's considerably younger half-sister, Sarah, who caught his eye.

Actually, it may have been Nathan who caught Sarah's eye more than the other way around. She had been, we are told, "a mere child [probably sixteen] at the time of her sister's marriage, on which occasion she is said, in her admiration for Dr. Smith, to have pushed her way in beside him and stood for a while between the bride and groom."[50] She was, perhaps, a young woman who knew her mind. In any case, Sarah came doubly of prominent stock. Her father was the same General Jonathan Chase who had remarried two years after Thankful Sherman Chase died, and her mother was Sarah Hall, the daughter of the Rev. David and Elizabeth Prescott Hall (another name that figures frequently in Cornish history).

Regardless of who caught whose eye first, a letter that Nathan wrote to "Sally" (as she was generally called) less than a year after Elizabeth's death shows he was ready to open a new chapter in his life:

Cornish, N.H., January 22, 1794

Sally:

You will excuse the precipitancy with which I proceed in my endeavors to accomplish my connection with you. I expected last evening to have set off for Hanover this morning, and I could not endure the least uncertainty till I returned, therefore I have discovered my wishes respecting you to your Sire and Marm last evening, and they have generously given me leave to marry with you.

I hope I shall never meet with your disapprobation. Transported with Joy and Expectation I am

Your sincere Lover
Nathan Smith[51]

They were married the following September 16. In sharp contrast to her half-sister, Sally Smith was long lived (she did not die until 1848, thus outliving her husband by more than the thirteen years or so that separated them in age). She also gave birth to their ten children.

In light of this enduring and fruitful marriage, it is frustrating to have so little information about Sally. Few documents even mention her name; few letters to or from her exist. We are told the "marriage proved a happy one in every way, Sarah being a true helpmeet in the home of her husband"—which sounds like generic words of praise for the largely invisible eighteenth- and nineteenth-century wife. Though the author of that line gave no evidence to support her claim, beyond Sally's having borne and reared the numerous children, we know at least one student saw Smith asking Sally's advice and generally relying on her.[52] How pale, even transparent, the picture that emerges of a great man's wife often is! The lack of a clear and focused image of Sally Smith is especially disappointing when one considers how this mother of ten must have been largely responsible for her husband being able to devote himself so thoroughly to his career.

From scattered fragments of information we must try to infer the kind of woman Sally Smith was. She gave birth to their first child, a boy, almost exactly nine months after the marriage. He was given the ponderous name of David Solon Chase Hall Smith. She was pregnant with the second child when Nathan went abroad (see chapter 3). A telling anecdote, one of the few to give us insight into Sally's character, concerns this second (and much-favored) son—but whether it shows a sense of humor or veiled resentment at having been left on her own temporarily is not clear. When Nathan came home, Sally is said to have tested him by "borrow-

ing" for the occasion several neighborhood babies to create a line-up of
infants. She then directed her husband to pick out his own new son, born
while he was abroad. One cannot but wonder what Sally would have said
or done had Nathan failed to identify his child—but he did not fail. He
succeeded, he claimed, by picking "the prettiest" one.[53]

This second son was with prescient appropriateness named Nathan,
but called always by his middle name, "Ryno," to distinguish him from
his father. "Ryno" was taken from the poetry of Ossian, as were the middle names "Malvina" (used for the third child, Sally, born in another two
years) and "Morven" (for the third son, James). The source of the children's names is not of great significance, except for the extent to which it
hints that at least Sally was attuned to the popular poetry of the day.[54]

Like so many other women, Sarah Chase was kept busy by pregnancy,
giving birth, and raising children; the ten were born over a span of two
dozen years. We have no record to tell us how she felt about this or how
she reacted to the death of her third child (the first daughter, her namesake). We know only that at the time she had eight other children ranging
in age from twenty down to three, and that four years later she gave birth
to her tenth child (and sixth daughter)—also named Sarah in memory of
her dead sister (as well as for her mother).

We are likewise left to infer what we can of Sally's child-rearing abilities and attitude toward her husband's career from the fact that all four
sons became doctors. While the accounts of Nathan Smith's life credit
him for creating a medical dynasty, Sally must at the very least not have
spoken out against medicine as a career. Nathan's frequent and sometimes extended absences from home might have given her cause to rail
against the demands the job put on her husband. But it seems she did not,
for there is no reason to think the mother's support for the sons' careers
was less influential than the father's example. In particular, Nathan Ryno
—the one whose medical career most closely rivaled the senior Smith's in
importance—was a great admirer of his father;[55] Sally likely was responsible in part for Ryno's following in his father's footsteps.

On the other hand, lack of evidence must lead us to suspect that Sally
Smith played little or no direct part in her husband's career. A comment in
the student journal referred to earlier is informative if not dispositive: Arriving at Smith's house in Hanover to meet his "instructor that was to
be," the student observed that he and those with him were "not likely to
be burdened with compliments, for, all this while, [Smith] had not introduced us to the ladies of his family, and three were sitting, silently, engaged in some kind of needle-work."[56]

Perhaps the greatest insights into Sally's character and the role she
played as a doctor's wife come from the fact that she did not automati-

cally pack up and move when Nathan changed the location of his practice and his residence. In the first instance, having already experienced what it was like to be at home in Cornish with children during her husband's absence abroad, and having presumably coped satisfactorily (no doubt thanks in part to the presence of her extended family), it is hardly surprising that she hesitated to move to Hanover when Nathan began the shaky enterprise that was to become Dartmouth Medical School. Though a college town, Hanover could offer little to a young mother that Cornish could not, and the uncertainty of Nathan's undertaking must surely have raised doubts about how prudent it would be to move.

Nathan Smith was like many modern doctors in having an unpredictable schedule. He had no hospital rounds to make, but he was frequently off on long horseback trips to care for patients in distant villages and on remote farms. Sally may have believed that where she lived made little difference in how much she would see of her husband. She appears not to have assisted with the doctoring (except by occasionally boarding students or patients or both), nor was she usually able—because she was not at his side—to advise, encourage, or discourage him when he was faced with career choices. Her world remained the hearth and home; his was teaching and practicing medicine.

CHAPTER THREE

New Ventures

Qui sapientes volunt esse
Laborare est necesse.

[For those who would be wise,
Work begets the prize.]
—GEORGE W. PUTNAM [1]

Practicing Medicine, Dreaming of a Medical School

FROM THE SECOND and longer period of Smith's practice in Cornish, beginning with his return from Harvard in 1790, there is little information pertinent to his medical practice apart from his own records. The first official confirmation that he was practicing in Cornish is a notice of action taken by the selectmen in August of 1790: "Voted that Nathan Smith M.D. shall have liberty to erect a pest house and inoculate for the small pox in Cornish."[2] This is a striking indication that Nathan Smith was being drawn into town affairs, just as family practitioners are today when dealing with birth and death certificates, well-child clinics, and school inoculations. The action by the selectmen implied confidence in their local doctor; many towns would not allow inoculations for fear that careless medical intervention would spread true smallpox.[3]

We know Smith tried unsuccessfully in February 1791 to get instruments for couching cataracts and for midwifery,[4] indicating he must already have had call for both eye surgery and obstetrical services. Smith's daybooks, ledgers, and account books give an indication of the medical problems he encountered, as well as what he charged and (sometimes) where the patients came from. As his practice grew, the pages filled up, and he carried accounts for a patient or a family forward (often into another book altogether); they become ever more difficult to read and interpret.

Still, there is much to be learned from Smith's records for those willing to study them. The following excerpts from 1792 show, among other things, how little a late eighteenth-century doctor would earn for "reducing" a fracture or "extracting a foetus" (fees are in pounds, shillings, and pence):

> Noah Cady of Wethersfield
>   to visit & reducing a fractured thigh, and camphor   0 - 7 - 0
> Dan Clark of Wethersfield,
>   extracting a foetus   0 - 12 - 0
> John Dutton of Claremont
>   to visit & reducing a difficult arm   0 - 4 - 0[5]

We also know from the accounts of the Chase Tavern in Cornish that Lyman Spalding, one of Smith's first apprentices, was his occasional social companion. Tacked on to Smith's bill (for "1 Gill rum, 2 meles victuals") at the Chase Tavern one day in November 1792, for instance, is a notation of payment due, "2 Glasses Ginn for Spalding."[6] Still only seventeen, Lyman may well have accompanied Smith with some regularity on medical calls. Indeed, he would soon take over as Smith's *locum tenens,* as we shall see.

In many ways, Cornish and its environs might have seemed a most satisfactory place for Nathan Smith to settle and spend a long career. The excitement of general practice lies in getting to know people and helping to relieve their problems; certainly the accounts show Smith was finding the opportunity to do that. Later in 1791 Smith wrote to Warren inquiring again for help in of obtaining ophthalmological and obstetrical instruments,[7] even though charges for "extracting foetuses" largely disappeared from his account books some time after 1790. Perhaps he made use of a midwife. (Interestingly enough, this would not prevent his being appointed "Professor of Obstetrics" in later years, nor would it keep him from lecturing on obstetrics and midwifery or giving his students "Directions to the Accoucheur."[8]) Boston was the closest source for pharmaceuticals, so Smith may have made up his own or received assistance from someone locally. But by 1806 he was including in his lectures his own recipes (as well as those of others) for numerous medications. One Smith recipe, for example, yielding a dozen pills "for violent cough," called for 20 grams of Ipecac, 6 grams of Calomel, and 6 grams of opium. He also recommended 10 drops twice a day of Balsam Copaiva.[9]

Smith's account books give considerable evidence that he was busy and working hard. Entries such as the one for January 30, 1798, a charge to Jonathan Whitney of Tunbridge ("to board Medicine & attendance for his daughter for 10 Days")[10] indicate that Nathan and Sally may have boarded patients who needed close watching. While that would save house calls, it was also bound to be a burden, especially for Sally. In any case,

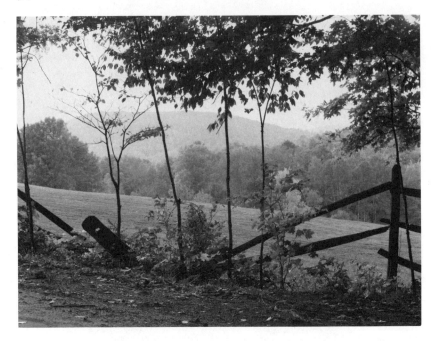

Nathan Smith country, Cornish, New Hampshire.
Photo courtesy of Jeffrey Nintzel, Grantham, New Hampshire, © 1997.

what evidence we have gives us every reason to think that Nathan Smith was indeed becoming "successful and popular," as we have been told.

In addition to the challenges that life in Cornish presented, the north country was beautiful. Riding horseback fifty miles to see a patient was not all hardship. In the winter, with snow bending the branches of the trees so that the trail was fairly blocked until the rider had dumped the snow, branch by branch—much of it down his boots or down his neck— even then there were scenes of pure delight, and the horse's feet would fairly dance through the snow if the drifts were not too deep. Busy country doctors working in northern New England long after Smith's day continued to go about their work with zeal and a gladness of heart, inspired by being out in the natural world.[11]

In the spring, rides were magnificent. Anyone who has ridden over the old roads of the region on horseback knows that the trees then take on a number of pastel shades and cover the hills with a gentle beauty that quickens the blood. Summertime brought rich beds of wildflowers, many of them represented in the pharmacopoeia of the day, to brighten the way.[12] And autumn gave the landscape a whole new explosion of colors and a brisk clearness in the air unmatched elsewhere. Furthermore, Smith also often had company on his rides. He took his students along with him (one such student wrote home: "Now I [must close as] I am obliged [to] ride with Dr. Smith"[13]), to enhance their medical experience but also, one suspects, to share with them the beauties of the countryside.

Why would Smith have considered going elsewhere, or starting a new venture? No doubt the very students who accompanied him were part of the reason. For although we have no idea how many of them came or from how far away, we know they did come. Earnest fellows from the backwoods, they wanted facts and treatments that would work—and Smith supplied both. By the time he had been in practice six or eight years, he certainly knew most of the problems these students were likely to meet in their own practices. He knew how to treat patients; he found he knew how to teach. He had a healthy skepticism that appealed to young men. Above all, he seemed to know instinctively when to follow traditional practices and when to ignore them.

Still, his apprentices quite likely worried him in many ways. What Josiah Goodhue had said more than a decade earlier about the profession of medicine in New England being in "a low state"[14] was still true, at least as a later retrospective account has it:

At this period the medical profession, in that vicinity, was at a low ebb. . . . The large majority of the physicians were uneducated and unskilful. . . . This state of his favorite profession was painful to the benevolent and enterprising mind of Dr. Smith. Instead of merely taking advantage of it, to elevate himself by the ignorance of others, he early engaged, with his usual vigor, to correct it. The most obvious and effectual means to remedy this evil, was to furnish those who were about to enter upon the profession, with an opportunity of obtaining a correct professional education.[15]

In November 1790 Smith wrote to John Warren that "Two young gentlemen are studying with me who purpose to attend your medical Lectures at Cambridge this Autumn." We don't know who they were or whether they did go to Harvard, but nine months later Smith wrote again to Warren concerning "several [other?] young men, waiting for me to procure a Library, when they purpose to commence the study of Physic with me, & to finish their Education at Cambridge."[16] He may by then have had as many as a dozen "pupils"; the vision of a true medical school was taking shape.

The idea that Smith might affiliate himself with an educational institution and then not need to send his students on to Harvard "to finish their Education" seems to have occurred to him at least as soon as the mid-1790s. Several possible reasons existed for wanting to teach under the auspices of an established institution. For one thing, Smith knew students needed to be able to carry out dissections and to practice surgical technique, and he may have hoped being associated with a college would protect him and his students as anatomists. Bodies were notoriously hard to find, and "grave watchers" were often hired to guard the cemeteries.[17] (In March of 1796, the town of Cornish voted that the selectmen be requested to punish any persons who dug up the dead from churchyards[18] —a hint that some midnight requisition may have been taking place in town, possibly for the benefit of Smith's pupils.)

Another consideration was the expense of medical books.[19] Smith may have hoped that his becoming connected with an existing institution would make a genuine library accessible to him and his students. Finally, having taken the trouble to earn his own M.B. from Harvard, he would have been sensitive to the desire of students to have a college degree as evidence of their hard work.

But why should they have to go as far as Cambridge, Massachusetts? Knowing the financial hardships that would mean for many prospective doctors, Smith apparently concluded there was no reason not to provide "pupils" with an educational opportunity closer to home. The only candidate was the sole institution of higher learning in all of northern New England: Dartmouth College, in Hanover, New Hampshire.

By 1797, Smith was spending considerable time in Hanover. His periodic presence there is attested to by the running account the enterprising Jedediah Baldwin carried for him in his jewelry shop, where tinkering and —more surprising—postal services were also offered.[20] Perhaps Smith was testing the waters by familiarizing himself with the College. Superficially, it must have seemed like an attractive place to be for those engaged in teaching. The newly built Dartmouth Hall was impressive, and the generous room it would provide for classes was easier to contemplate than the $4,000 debt it had saddled on the College.

The advantages of moving apprentices from Cornish to Hanover and forming a medical school around them were more apparent than real, however, though Smith could not know it. Dartmouth students in those early years brought little cash money into town; no Dartmouth student at the end of the eighteenth century would have been eager to spend extra money on medical lectures. Furthermore, Dartmouth offered no science courses that could serve as premedical work or supplement what Nathan Smith would teach.[21]

Dartmouth as an institution was desperately poor, in no position to pay a salary to a medical professor—much less to hire him an assistant. Quite the contrary: The College was holding back the salary of the three professors it already had, and it was struggling to meet the expenses incurred by the building of beautiful Dartmouth Hall.[22] As much as her president may have wished to make the institution into a university, Dartmouth was not even a well-organized college.

Nevertheless, Dartmouth was showing some increased prosperity. Where there had been only a handful of students in 1780, there were around a hundred in 1795.[23] To Nathan Smith and his little band of loyal apprentices in Cornish it must have looked like a great seat of learning, a thriving educational institution. Moreover, the need to train young men who could not afford to go to Boston or Philadelphia was of paramount concern to Smith, not only because his impecunious background helped him understand the financial considerations; he also knew the virtues of the countryman's mind. Smith was apparently confident he could train talented country boys to become good physicians. He knew how to speak their language, and he probably delighted in their independence and ingenuity. He certainly hoped many would stay on to care for backcountry folk.

Even so, it must have been with some trepidation that the young doctor, with no undergraduate degree and bearing only the M.B. to show for his seven months' stay at Harvard Medical School, approached the "Board of Trust" of Dartmouth College with his bold proposition. Nathan Smith's idea was no less than that the Board should appoint him Dartmouth's fourth professor and let him create a school of medicine under the College's auspices.

Shortly prior to the August 1796 meeting of the Board of Trust, Smith presented them with two documents. The first was his "Proposal for [a] Medical Institution." Relying on his own experiences at Harvard, he explained to the Dartmouth trustees the arrangements at Harvard, using them as a guide for the new medical school he intended to found at Dartmouth:

The Medical Institution of Harvard College is governed by the Authority of the College

The Medical Professors receive a certain stipend from the College and are obliged to deliver one complete Course of Lectures every year & two if required by the Authority.

Those who attend the medical Lectures are required to pay a certain fee to the Professors, viz. to the Prof.[r] of Anatomy £7. to the Prof.[r] of Physic & Prof.[r] of Chymistry £4:8:- each, for every course of Lectures

The Sen.[r] Class in College are admitted for half the above fees. None but the Sen.[r] Class of Scholars in College [no other undergraduates] are admitted to attend Medical Lectures.

All persons except those above excepted who have a good Moral Character are admitted to attend the medical Lectures, on paying the fees. But in order to obtain a Degree in Medicine it is required that they study 2 years with some able Physician and attend 2 courses of Medical Lectures. Those who have not had a public Education are required to understand the Latin Language sufficient to enter College & to understand the rudiments of Mathematics & Natural Philosophy & to attend one course of Philosophical Lectures in the College for which they pay to the College £2: they also pay the College £7 for their Degree.

All who offer themselves for Degrees are examined before the President the Professors & Tutors of the College Those who have had a Public Education are examined by the Medical Professors on the several Branches of Medicine & if found worthy they have a Degree But those who have not had a Public Education are examined by the authority of College on Latin, Erethmatic, Mathematics & Natural Philosophy if approved the medical Professors proceed to examine them on the Several Branches of Medicine.

The Authority of College attend the medical Lectures without expence All students while attending the Lectures are admitted to attend the Professors practice free of expence.

Those who have attended two courses of Lectures may attend as many more as they please without any additional cost.[24]

The accompanying document was more personal, a letter in which Smith laid out what he was prepared to do as his contribution to the proposed enterprise:

To the Honble Board of Trustees of Dartmouth College
Gentlemen—
Relying on your Patronage, and being confident, that you will favour any measures, which are likely to promote useful Science, I have ventured to make certain proposals, which, I now present for your consideration.

As we have no medical school in this State where Students in Physic can be regularly instructed in the several Branches of that Science, I propose, if the Honble. Board will establish a medical school in this College and will honour me with an appointment in it, that I will go to Edinbourgh in Scotland, and will attend to the Several Branches of Medicine as taught and practiced there & will then return to this College where I will commence public teaching as soon as may be after my return

I am with due Respect your Very Humble Servant

Nathan Smith
Hanover Augt. 25th, 1796

P.S. I do not consider the Board of Trustees, if they should incourage me in the pursuit of Medical Knowledge as under any obligations to pay any part of my expenses which will accrue in going to Europe, and shall acquiess in their determination respecting a medical Institution at my return.[25]

Nathan Smith

Understandably, the Board hesitated. Despite Smith's promise that he would pay his own expenses for further study, the Board passed a resolution to defer consideration to the next annual session (in August 1797), saying that they could not at the present time

promise any pecuniary compensation, yet from a view of the extensive usefulness of such an institution under proper regulations, the board of trustees do approve of the general object of M.r Smith. And from the opinion which they have of his character & medical knowledge they could wish that the encouragement for the establishment of such a Professor may in some future time be inviting. And they feel themselves disposed to afford him all such encouragement and assistance in the laudable pursuit as they shall think and determine their circumstances may admit and his qualifications merit.

By order of said Trustees
B. Woodward Secr'y[26]

To a man of Smith's determination, it was enough. Furthermore, Smith then received, quite unsolicited, a letter of introduction from President John Wheelock to give to the Reverend Mr. Samuel Peters, a useful friend of Dartmouth in England. Wheelock's letter read in part as follows: "Permit me, Sir, to introduce . . . Dr. Nathan Smith [who] by a resolve of our Corporation, stands now as the only candidate for the Chair of Medical Professor at this University."[27]

There was of course no such "Chair" at Dartmouth as yet, and with no graduate schools at all—never mind a school of medicine—Dartmouth was no "University." It may be that President Wheelock was so eager to preside over a university that he stretched the facts in his endorsement to suit his own purposes. He similarly overstated the matter of the trustees' commitment to the project; nowhere had they referred to Nathan Smith as the "only candidate for the Chair of Medical Professor."

Study Abroad

Having studied under men who had themselves trained in Europe, and knowing that the institutions teaching medicine in Edinburgh and London were considered the best in the world, Smith must have expected to profit from some time abroad himself. Edinburgh, especially, ranked at the very top in medical education in that period. Even after the most famous of its medical teachers—William Cullen—retired, "Edinburgh was preeminent."[28] A novelist's judgment written twenty-seven years earlier was still applicable: "The University of Edinburgh is supplied with excellent professors in all the sciences; and the medical school, in particular, is famous all over Europe. The students of this art have the best opportunity of learning it to perfection, in all its branches . . . ."[29]

Nathan's family (Sally was pregnant for the second time) and his busy practice could have made him hesitate, and of course money was always a problem. But with the hope that he might begin a formal school at Dartmouth, two more reasons for making the trip emerged: A European sojourn would give him added prestige at Dartmouth, and he had grounds for believing he would pick up much that was useful for his teaching (as well as his practice) in those great centers of learning.

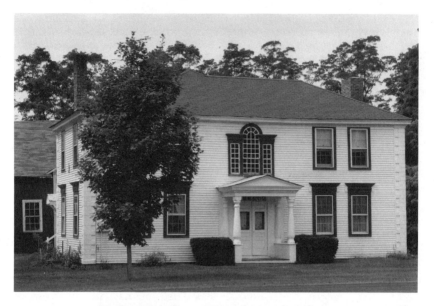

Nathan Smith's home in Cornish, New Hampshire.
Photo courtesy of Dartmouth College photographer, Joseph Mehling.

We have no way of knowing whether Sally was opposed to her husband's plan to be away for several months, for there is no record of her views. Nathan could in any case be very convincing when he had a purpose in mind, and Sally's parents probably encouraged him. The Chases were an unusually well-educated clan for the day and wise enough to understand the value for their son-in-law of further formal education. They could also be counted on to care for Sally's material wants (as they probably had been doing to some extent since her marriage—the Smiths had been living in a Chase-owned house, for instance); the extended family could be counted on to rally around.

Sally also had the company and protection of Lyman Spalding (by this time he was twenty-one), whom Smith explicitly asked to handle the practice and watch over the family in his absence. By mid-November 1796, Smith had completed his preparations for Europe, and he wrote to Spalding: "I believe it is the wish of many people in this neighbourhood that you should stay in town till I return which I wish you to do if you think it will be consistent with your interest. . . . I wish you to attend to my family if you should stay in Cornish & if they should be sick."[30]

In the same letter, Smith alerted Spalding to some unsettled accounts (this would prove to be a typical pattern) he hoped Lyman would take

care of for him: "I have directed [my attorneys] to call on you and hope
you will attend to it as you are better acquainted with my business than
any other man." Among the "unsettled accounts" was money he had borrowed in Cornish, almost certainly with help from his father-in-law and
quite probably from Sanford Kingsbury, a lawyer in Claremont.[31]

On December 11, 1796, Smith was in Boston waiting to sail; he put
further pressure on Spalding in another letter. "I have still a greater reason now to wish you to [stay in Cornish] than when I wrote before for I
conversed with your Father & found that he was very much opposed to
your going away this Winter . . . ."[32] In a second letter written the same
day, he re-iterated the themes: "I wish you to do what you can towards
settling my accounts while I am gone. Am glad to hear that you are at my
house and hope you have enough business to make you contented."[33]

If Smith was nervous in anticipation of making the great voyage, he
showed it only in his repeated instructions and stubborn assertions of optimism. The same three letters just quoted contain remarks such as these:
"Our business at the College increases very fast and I hope will succeed
better than we feared"; "The information I have recd. here respecting the
success of my project is flattering"; and "I have obtained a number of
very good letters from Gentlemen in this town to Gentlemen in England,
Drs. [John] Smith and [Thomas][34] Bartlett have given me Letters of Credit
and thro' their means I can import such preparations of the Humane
Body as I shall want. I think my prospects of success are very good I
shall persevere with confidence and submit the ISSUE to God and my own
good judgment."

Perhaps he was trying to re-assure himself and boost his own spirits.
Certainly his farewell letters to his wife were "full of tender solicitude for
her and his little son." Using the delay in sailing to write yet again ("I
have lately sent you two letters"), Nathan wrote to Sally on December 17,
1796, the day before the *Hope* finally set off: "All my anxiety is for my
family. I fear no danger but on their account. . . . Do, my dear, remember
me. You are ever on my mind. . . . Do be careful of our dear little son."[35]

The mood was the same in a letter he wrote from Edinburgh two
months later, in February 1797:

I am quite homesick . . . my thoughts continually turn on you and our dear little
son . . . . [W]atch over him with maternal care, kiss him for me a thousand times
each day and tell him that his papa is coming soon.[36]

Almost no evidence remains of Nathan Smith's stay in the British Isles.
In the letter to Sally just quoted Nathan barely mentioned the topic that
was the reason for his trip, saying only "I am now in Edinburgh, shall stay
here but a few days [an attack of homesickness had apparently struck

him; he stayed considerably longer], shall then go to London . . . . I have had no material misfortune since I came here; have become acquainted with the Medical Professors here, and am attending their lectures. I have a prospect of accomplishing my purpose to my mind."

In general, the few letters Smith wrote during his nine months' travels that have survived tell little about his studies or his relationship with his teachers or fellow students. Given that the academic sessions in Edinburgh began in November and lasted about six months, he presumably missed at least half the standard course.[37] Furthermore, he left no discoverable traces of his visit: He does not appear to have formally matriculated at the university, nor—as far as extant records show—did he sign up for any of the lecture courses.[38] It may have mattered little; he was unimpressed by what he did hear. Shortly before returning to America he wrote a letter to his respected Harvard professor, John Warren, filled mostly with a discussion of the political situation in London. Of his medical experiences he said only this: "I have attended the Medical Lectures and surgical operations in Glasgow, Edinburgh and London and am much disappointed to find that the faculty in this country who have been so much looked up to by our country had so little real merit."[39]

Though he may have learned less than he had hoped to, the trip was not entirely without value. If, as has been said,[40] he sat in on the anatomy and surgery lectures of Alexander Monro *secundus* (1733–1817)—of the brilliant Scottish anatomical dynasty established when John Monro arranged for his son, Alexander *primus*, to begin teaching in 1720 (the incompetent Alexander *tertius* would follow his father and grandfather)— he was probably keeping company with nearly four hundred other eager students. Physicians, surgeons, and all manner of would-be doctors came from far and wide for the privilege of listening to the energetic Monro.[41] Joseph Black (1728–99), whose chemistry lectures Smith also may have heard,[42] was even more likely to have taught Smith some things he did not know (chemistry was never his strength, as we shall see). At the very least, Nathan Smith's horizons were being broadened as he was exposed to new ways of looking at old problems. If he came away "much disappointed," it may have been because his expectations were too high.

Some inkling of what the experience in Edinburgh may have been like for Smith can be gleaned from a collection of letters written by William Quynn, a Maryland student almost exactly Smith's age. Fourteen years before Smith's arrival in Edinburgh, Quynn had gone there for a full three-year course leading to an M.D. His letters give insights into life at the university in Edinburgh for a young American in the late eighteenth century:

This University flourishes more now than has been known since its first Institution — the number of students that appeared at the three first Introductory Lectures were to the number of 500 — and they are now so numerous that Dr. Monro [*secundus*] is obliged to enlarge his theatre and Cullen lectures in the Episcopal Chaple . . . .

There seems to be a great spirit of Emulation prevailing here among the students who shall excell in Medical researches, they seem to be Indefatigable in their pursuit after knowledge and [I] am in hopes they will have their labours rewarded with Laurels they deserve —

There is a great spirit of controversy among our Professors. New theories appear daily, but I believe they commence Authors more for a display of ingenuity— than from any real benifits that society can possibly derive from it.[43]

Some of the student enthusiasm that Quynn raved about might have faded by the time Smith arrived, of course. Cullen had died; Monro had aged appreciably. Controversy among the professors probably still existed, however. Within the university, the faculty—a self-perpetuating caste (one need think only of the Monro family)—"tended to view medical knowledge as a strictly finite resource," and to display "a strongly territorial attitude to medical knowledge."[44] At the same time, however, extramural teaching was also going on. Smith's sojourn in Edinburgh fell during the period when John Allen (1771–1843) was engaged in giving the "first freestanding course of lectures in physiology,"[45] and he may have attended some of those. But one historian's judgment that Smith's "visit to Europe was attended with the most beneficial results"[46] does not accord with what Smith himself wrote home.

A passport issued to Smith in London on April 25, 1797 (he had already been in the British Isles for months) gives one of the few physical descriptions of Nathan Smith (and the only official one) to be found anywhere:

I RUFUS KING, Minister Plenipotentiary of the United States of America, at the Court of Great-Britain.

DESIRE all whom it may concern, to permit Nathan Smith a citizen of the United States of America, to pass without giving or suffering any molestation or hindrance to be given to him; but, on the contrary, affording him all requisite assistance and protection, as I would do in similar circumstances to all those who might be recommended to me.

The said Nathan Smith is Thirty four years of age, Five feet ten inches (English) in height, blue eyes, small mouth, Aquiline nose, high forehead, round chin, fairish complexion, brown hair and eyebrows, and long face.

In witness whereof, I have delivered to him this Passport, to be in force for Three Months Dated in London, this 25th day of April,

One thousand seven hundred and ninety seven

Rufus King, GRATIS.[47]

A student description of Smith given roughly a decade later in Hanover, though not inconsistent, was far less complete: "He is a man of medium height, rather thin, and spare."[48]

Nathan Smith's passport, issued when he arrived in London,
1797. Courtesy of Dartmouth College Library.

Smith may also have attended the lectures of James Gregory (1753–1821). Gregory had succeeded Cullen as professor of the "Practice of Physic," and one ground for thinking Smith might have heard his lectures is the intimate knowledge of Cullen's theories that he later exhibited in his own lectures, when he used Cullen largely as a foil, criticizing and countering what he said.[49]

Exposure to Cullen could also have come from another professor whose lectures Smith may have attended. The young Alexander Philips Wilson

Philip—eight years Smith's junior—devoted considerable time to the study of fevers (an interest inspired by Cullen, who had supervised his education from the age of twelve on); in the summer of 1796 he gave his first course of lectures in Edinburgh, illustrating them with physiological experiments. Given that Smith later edited the second American edition of Wilson Philip's magnum opus on febrile diseases (first published in 1799), it seems reasonable to guess the two men might have met in Edinburgh; it would help explain Smith's familiarity with that work, as well as why he chose to edit it and felt free to make additions of his own. Smith and Wilson Philip would in any case have been kindred souls. Both were imaginative, busy practitioners; both were dedicated to careful observation of the patient and to exploration of new methods in medical pedagogy. Smith's interest in the new science of pathology mirrored the younger man's interest in physiology.[50]

Smith's most valuable experience abroad, at least in his own mind, seems to have been his friendship with John Coakley Lettsom. It was he—along with John Fothergill (dead by the time Smith was in London)—who had helped Benjamin Waterhouse gain entrée to London medical circles; Waterhouse had no doubt frequently mentioned Lettsom in his lectures. Lettsom was also known for helping American medical students (a colonial from the West Indies, he thought of himself as American), which would have made it easy and prudent to look him up. Smith no doubt used his letter of introduction from Wheelock to the Rev. Mr. Peters, and it may have been Peters who showed him around London (where he apparently spent three months engaging in hospital work and consorting with "eminent physicians"[51]); it may have been Peters who actually introduced him to Lettsom, though Smith also had letters to Lettsom from both Warren and Waterhouse.[52]

In any case, it was almost certainly Lettsom who took Smith to meetings of the Medical Society of London, where physicians met surgeons and apothecaries in a collegial search for knowledge; we know it was Lettsom who nominated Smith for membership. The Council's approval of Smith as "a proper person to become a corresponding member of the society" was "signed by Doctors J C Lettsom   James Sims   Sayer Walker. Thomas Wheeler Register" on May 22, 1797, and referred to the Society;[53] before leaving London, Smith was duly voted a corresponding member of the Society and given a "diploma" to make it official.[54]

Lettsom did more than carry out a ceremonial function, however; it has been said that he played a crucial role in the development of American medicine by being "spiritual father" to both Smith and Waterhouse.[55] Furthermore, when Smith undertook to buy books and instruments for his new school, "he found Lettsom's help and advice . . . useful. Lettsom told him what books to purchase. He also helped him generously from his own Library, and assisted him to pay for much of the apparatus. . . ."[56]

Smith's affiliation with the Medical Society of London gave him a lasting souvenir of the trip abroad in a sequence of initials to mark the affiliation, which he sometimes thereafter appended to his name. The initials were used inconsistently, however, and when they did appear following his name—usually written as "C.S.M.S.Lond."—they were not always in the same sequence. One wonders how much stress Smith laid on precisely what they stood for or how much he cared. Yet more than one student who dedicated his thesis to Smith added the initials, and students sometimes included them after Smith's name and the "M.D." in the heading of their lecture notes. When Smith's byline on a published article included the initials, that may have been the editor's doing rather than the author's.[57]

Smith arrived back in Boston on September 11, 1797, and promptly wrote Lyman Spalding that he was out of funds—no surprise there—and would need money before he could stir from Boston, presumably to pay "the expenses of my voyage and freight for my goods"[58] as well as Dr. Bartlett's note.

Tradition has it that Smith had acquired a skeleton and books valued at thirty pounds sterling, which he "sent home to the college library," and chemical, anatomical, and surgical apparatus that he "deemed indispensable for commencing the proposed medical institution" (the items Lettsom helped him choose). As usual, however, Smith hoped someone else would pay for these treasures, since, as he saw it, he "could ill afford to bear the expense himself."[59] Money was an issue when he left home; money was the first issue when he returned.

CHAPTER FOUR

The Founding of
Dartmouth Medical School

Quam multa fieri non posse, priusquam sint facta judicantur?
[How many things seem impossible until they are judged to have been done?]
— PLINY THE ELDER [1]

S MITH IMMEDIATELY FACED the problem of how to get the medical school started. Traditionally, a course of lectures commenced in the autumn, then as now, and although Smith did not return from Great Britain until late September, he was eager to begin. The Board of Trust at Dartmouth met only once a year, however, in August. With Smith not even in the country in August of 1797, they had some justification for taking no further action on his proposal. (A year earlier, it will be recalled, they had agreed in principle, without going so far as to make it official.)

Anything that might add to the College's expenses had to be undertaken with caution. When Nathan Smith proposed a medical school, John Wheelock had been Dartmouth's president for eighteen years, and during most of that time he was in difficulty. Not least of his problems was that the school was poverty stricken. Wheelock had gone to England in 1783, hoping to raise more money from loyal benefactors there, and he had had some success. But the ship on which he returned, the brig *Peace and Plenty*, was wrecked off Cape Cod, near Provincetown, and John Wheelock escaped with nothing but the clothes he was wearing; his hard-won donations were lost.[2]

President Wheelock did bring the useful information that government-run lotteries in England were raising the equivalent of one and a half million dollars a year in revenue. Why not try something of the sort to bolster Dartmouth's fortunes? Although Wheelock's first attempt to do so was as dismal a failure as his English trip had been, a second lottery did better.

Coupled with a state grant, private subscriptions, and close attention to finances, the result was just enough money to replace the old school buildings (little more than rough-hewn cabins) with an ambitious copy of the handsome and imposing Nassau Hall at Princeton. The new Dartmouth Hall (the present structure of that name is a close imitation) was three stories high, one hundred and fifty feet long, and fifty feet wide. Now Dartmouth at least *looked* like a real college. In 1797, Dr. Timothy Dwight saw the six-year-old building and pronounced it to have "a decent appearance," praise indeed (if somewhat grudging) from the president of Yale.[3] But the College at that point still owed $4,000 for the structure, and among the financial maneuvers needed to pay off that sum— accomplished two years later—was the already-mentioned postponement of roughly $3,000 in professorial salaries.

First Classes

When Smith came home, he no doubt found his apprentices as eager to benefit from his travels as he was to share what he had seen and done and learned. That autumn of 1797, he began making the twenty-five-mile trek between Cornish and Hanover with considerable frequency. The trip could be arduous, especially in bad weather; roads were little more than lanes, bridges were unreliable, and streams sometimes had to be forded. But it must have seemed important to him to go. Whether he was actively negotiating with Wheelock or members of the Board of Trust, or merely trying to organize on his own a time and place to get started with his new enterprise, is not altogether clear. But in Hanover, Rufus Graves[4] came to the rescue. It was he, we know from a charge early the next year, who boarded Smith.[5] Thus Smith was set to begin lecturing in Hanover, two months after having returned from London and more than nine months prior to the offer of an appointment from the College's Board of Trust.

And so there it was: In the autumn of 1797, Nathan Smith was giving medical lectures in Hanover, New Hampshire. With his eyes clearly on the future, he was teaching medical students in the shadow of Dartmouth, if not strictly *at* Dartmouth. The trustees had not officially sanctioned a medical school any more than they had appointed him to teach in it, but Smith simply would not be deterred. "You know I am not easily beat down in my projects," he once wrote to Lyman Spalding, "and tho' sometimes slow in execution, yet keep the object in view."[6] Thus Dartmouth Medical School came into being. Subsequent events would show that those November 1797 lectures were, indeed, the beginning of something finer and longer lasting than even Nathan Smith could have anticipated.

What a pity that Smith did not write down some of what he was think-ing on that November day when he gave his first medical lectures in Hanover! (If he did, the evidence has not survived.) Did he attribute as great a significance to the fact that he was at last lecturing in Hanover, as future generations have? Was he so naive (or so confident) that he as-sumed all would fall into place when the Board of Trust next met? Or was he deliberately pressuring the Board by presenting it with a fait accompli? Was he nervous? Was he excited? Or was he just continuing what he had been doing for several years, now in a different venue, with the same commitment to raising the "low state" of the medical profession?

Whatever Smith's thoughts, having already taught a number of ap-prentices during his years in Cornish, he was unlikely to find intimidating the idea of teaching in this slightly more formal setting. Certainly he would have been comfortable with the clinical side of medicine. The non-clinical subjects would have been harder for him even given his recent time in the hallowed lecture halls of Glasgow, Edinburgh, and London. Abstract and theoretical courses were considered important there; they were designed to give students background information and a sense of the history of the profession.

The gap between theory and treatment was wide and confusing, how-ever; Smith wanted his students to focus on the very concrete and practi-cal matters of patient care. The problem was mainly one of emphasis. He had plenty of answers, at least with respect to country practice. Still, he was perhaps more influenced than he realized by what he had been ex-posed to in Edinburgh. Harvard, with its three faculty members, had been in a position to offer only a minimum of specialization; at Edinburgh the faculty probably numbered closer to ten, and one result was the possibil-ity for each professor to concentrate on a narrower field. Separate lectures on chemistry, for instance, seem to have made an impression on Smith, showing him the value of acquainting his students with the nature of, say, virgin sulfur—in addition to learning its use in the treatment of, for ex-ample, scabies (a contagious form of dermatitis).

This may well be why Smith almost immediately asked his young pro-tégé, Lyman Spalding, to lend a hand. Spalding had recently earned his own M.B. at Harvard, and he apparently had a greater interest in (and perhaps a greater flair for) the still primitive science of chemistry than Smith did. In any case, we know that Spalding gave Smith assistance that first year as a lecturer and demonstrator in chemistry. His nearly contem-porary report fills in a critical piece of the picture of what went on in the first term of Dartmouth Medical School. In early 1799, he wrote from Walpole, New Hampshire—where he had by then established himself in practice—bringing a Boston friend up to date on his recent activities: "I have resided at Dartmouth College for a few weeks . . . . While at Hanover, I prepared all the Chemical Suspensions . . . for Dr Smiths Lectures in the fall of 97 . . . . The fall course I had the soul [sic] management of as well as profit—I expect to continue in this branch."[7]

How many students attended Smith's first lectures we do not know. We can be reasonably sure they were a mixed lot: some with college degrees, some without; some experienced in medical practice, others in the midst of an apprenticeship; still others drawn by the mystery of the subject matter but with no particular desire to become physicians. Lyman Spalding, with his newly minted medical degree, probably sat in; since all the students would be listening to Smith whenever he was lecturing, the chemistry lecturer might as well do so, too.

We know there were at least two students in the first group at Dartmouth who did have some medical experience. Joseph ("Jo") Gallup, at twenty-eight, had already been practicing medicine in Vermont (where he would return to spend most of his quite distinguished career); he had also spent time in Cornish under Smith's watchful eye.[8] Levi Sabin was even older; at thirty-three, he was barely two years younger than Smith himself. What his motivations and qualifications were prior to attending Smith's lectures, we do not know. As it turned out, he would live only another ten years, having practiced in Windsor and Windham counties in Vermont.[9]

These two were the first students to be awarded the Bachelor of Medicine degree by Dartmouth's Board of Trust at its August 1798 meeting. The College's willingness to grant these degrees is significant: They were voted at the same meeting during which the Board finally appointed Smith to a professorship and approved the creation of a medical institution,[10] as we shall shortly see. Awarding the two earned degrees to Gallup and Sabin is thus another critical part of the school's history; this act of the Board of Trust constituted an ex post facto ratification of what Nathan Smith had done, a kind of acknowledgment that his first lectures in Hanover, in 1797, really were under the auspices of Dartmouth College.

How much did Smith actually teach his first students, and especially these first two Dartmouth medical graduates? His time abroad gave him a wider perspective than either of them could have had, but Gallup certainly had almost as much practical experience as Smith. Still, numerous stories attest to Smith's unusually good diagnostic skills,[11] and listening to him describe how he elicited the presenting complaint from a patient certainly would have been helpful even to practicing physicians.

The real significance of those first classes, however, lies less in what transpired in the makeshift classroom in a private home than that they took place at all. Smith, by lecturing in Hanover, was demonstrating his

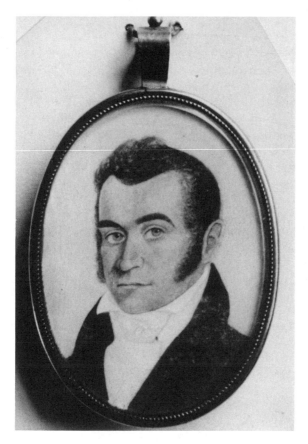

Jo Gallup, 1769–1849.
Courtesy of the Woodstock Historical Society.

conviction that country doctors could and should set about learning their skills in a systematic way. Of course, attending lectures or even earning a degree no more guaranteed a skillful practitioner in 1797 and 1798 than it does two centuries later. But the very fact that education of a formal sort was being made available in a remote country town by a practicing country physician for country practitioners signaled a dramatic shift in educational geography: Philadelphia, New York, and Boston no longer had a monopoly on medical education. From then on, northern New England's sons (and—*much* later—daughters) would be able to study medicine taught by a northern New Englander, in northern New England, above all for northern New Englanders.

Appointment as Professor

The Medical School was soon enough fully legitimized. No doubt there was a connection between the Board's being prepared to award medical degrees to Gallup and Sabin and its willingness to take action on Nathan Smith's proposal. Certainly he had done everything he could to show good faith. Having promised that he would go to Edinburgh to expand his education "if the Hon'ble Board will establish a medical school in this college and will honour me with an appointment in it," he had gone them one better by setting off for Scotland with Wheelock's letter of dubious authority and an indication from the Board only that such an establishment would be considered. Having promised to "commence public teaching as soon as may be after my return," he began lecturing within weeks of his arrival back in the United States. Having promised not to consider the Board "under any obligation to pay any part" of his expenses, he had paid out of his own pocket (never mind that it would take him twenty years to pay off the debts incurred by the trip[12]). He had, furthermore, responded to a request from the College in the spring of 1798 "to deliver a science course," as we learn from the letter already quoted that Spalding wrote to his Boston friend. In this, too, Lyman Spalding "took an active part, composing & delivering one third part of the Chemical Lectures."[13] The Board was apparently quite happy to take advantage of Smith's presence in town—and, thanks to him, Spalding's as well—to gain extra instruction for the College undergraduates even before they had appointed Smith a professor or officially settled the issue of whether there was to be a medical school.

Smith had also promised—no doubt because he assumed the answer would be favorable—to acquiesce in the Board's "determination respecting a Medical Institution." The annual meeting in August 1798 was a critical time for both parties. Smith's optimism was, however, vindicated. The Board duly appointed Nathaniel Niles and the Reverend Mr. Eden Burroughs "a Committee to arrange and report a system to carry into effect a medical establishment at this University,"[14] and history was in the making.

Now it was the Board of Trust's turn to go Nathan Smith one better. Anticipating that a satisfactory "system" would be found, the Board of Trust at the same session awarded an A.M. degree to Nathan Smith. Three years later, Dartmouth voted to award an honorary M.D. to her professor of the "Theory and Practice of Medicine"—who by that time was also professor of surgery, chemistry, materia medica, clinical medicine, and medical jurisprudence, and what was tantamount to dean and treasurer of the medical school.

All that lay in the future. The trustees at their August 1798 meeting

Entries in one of Nathan Smith's Day Books, 1798. Courtesy of Dartmouth College Library.

voted "that this board now proceed to the choice of a professor of Medicine at this University [sic]. The ballots being taken Nathan Smith A.M. was unanimously chosen." Smith thus became a recognized member of the Dartmouth faculty. For the country doctor, just shy of his thirty-sixth birthday, it was a great moment: He was a professor at last, de jure as well as de facto.

The Board voted further "that the professor of Medicine be authorized to employ such persons to assist him in the duties of his office as he may judge necessary" (thus again ratifying ex post facto an action of Nathan Smith's—hiring Lyman Spalding during the previous academic year), "provided this board incur no expense in consequence thereof." This latter proviso throws light on Smith's reaction three and a half years later, when Spalding told Smith that he—Spalding—had in effect been fired by the president. Smith replied firmly (and sensibly enough):

I do not think the President or the Board of Trust have or ought to have any control over your lecturing. It was I who employed you, and they had no business with you respecting it, nor do I think till they give us some money for our services that they ought to set bounds to our performances, provided we do not injure the Institution . . . . I will say this to you in Confidence: that you are at liberty to come and deliver the Chemical Lectures at what time and as long or short a Course as you please . . . and I will give you all the support I can.[15]

Such future irritations notwithstanding, a workable system was found for "carry[ing] into effect a medical establishment at Dartmouth," complete with a reasonably thorough set of rules and regulations. Nathan Smith was to give "public lectures" on anatomy and surgery, chemistry and materia medica, and the theory and practice of physic. The Board's stipulations were set out in some detail:

1.—Lectures shall begin on the first day of October annually and continue ten weeks, during which time the professor shall deliver lectures on the three branches each day Saturdays and Sundays excepted as shall be agreed by him and the president and other executive officers.

2.—In the lectures on the Theory and Practice of Physic shall be explained the nature of diseases and method of cure.

3.—The lectures on Chemistry and Materia Medica shall be accompanied with actual experiments tending to explain & demonstrate the principles of chemistry and an exhibition of the principal Medicines used in curing diseases and also an explanation of their Medicinal qualities & effects on the human body.

4.—In the lectures on Anatomy and Surgery shall be demonstrated the parts of the human body by dissecting a recent subject if such subject can be legally obtained, otherwise by exhibiting anatomical preparations and which shall be attended by the performance of the principal capital operations in Surgery.

5.—The Medical professor or professors shall be entitled to the use of the library and apparatus equally as the other professors and to all honorary privileges attached to a Collegiate profession.

6.—Medical students under the private instruction of a Medical professor and all students while attending lectures shall be entitled to the use of books from the College library under such regulations as the President shall direct they having given suffi-

cient bonds to the Treasurer for the payment of all fees fines &
forfeitures.

7.—Medical Students shall be subject to the same rules of Morality
and decorum as Bachelors in Arts residing at College.

8.—No graduate at any College shall be admitted to an examination for the degree of Bachelor in Medicine unless he shall have
studied Medicine with some respectable practising physician or
Surgeon two full years and attended two complete courses of
public Medical lectures at some University.

9.—No person not having received the degree of Bachelor of Arts at
some University shall be admitted to an examination for the degree of Bachelor of Medicine unless he shall have studied Medicine three full years with some respectable practising physician
or surgeon, attended two complete courses of public Medical
lectures at some University and shall appear upon a preparatory
examination before the President & Professors to be able to parse
the English and Latin languages to construe Virgil and Tully's orations, to possess a good knowledge of common arithmetic, Geo-
metry, Geography, and Natural and Moral Philosophy.

10.—All examinations for a degree in Medicine shall be holden publicly before the executive authority of College by the Medical professor or professors, at which time each candidate shall read and
defend a dissertation on some medical subject which shall have
been previously submitted to the inspection & approbation of
the Medical professor or professors & President.

11.—Every person receiving a degree in Medicine shall cause his dissertation to be printed and sixteen copies thereof to be delivered
to the President for the use of the College and Trustees.

12.—The fee for attending a complete course of Medical lectures to
any person not a member of some class in College shall be fifty
dollars, that is, for Anatomy and Surgery twenty-three dollars,
for Chemistry and Materia Medica seventeen dollars, and for
the theory and practice of physic ten dollars.

13.—The fee to be paid by the members of the two Senior classes in
College who shall attend those lectures shall be twenty dollars
for a complete course, that is, for Anatomy & Surgery eight dollars, for Chemistry and Materia Medica seven dollars and for
the Theory and practice of physic five dollars.

14.—Any person having attended two complete courses of public
Medical lectures in any University shall be admitted *gratis* to any
lectures.[16]

The above-mentioned fees, following the Harvard model Smith had
presented to the Board at the time he made his initial proposal, were to be
paid directly to the professor. Most tuition, however, like many other
debts of the day, was paid by promissory notes. While notes were fairly
negotiable, they were also typically hard to collect—as Smith knew well
from his own experience. He had paid his tuition at Harvard in notes, and
although Waterhouse got his money within a year because of the legal un-

pleasantness that arose between him and Smith, Warren had had to wait a long time.[17] The College also stood to benefit financially from a medical school; the minutes of that same August 1798 Board meeting went on to specify "that one half part of the fees for conferring the degree of Bachelor of Medicine pro meritis be perquisite to the President and the other half to be a perquisite to the professor of medicine."

Exactly how these regulations were hammered out, we can only guess. The substantive content specified for the several courses, though hardly amounting to a syllabus, was nevertheless too detailed and technical to have been written without Smith himself having helped to formulate it. The regulations concerning how many courses students would be required to attend and how many years they had to study extramurally with a "respectable" physician in order to qualify for a degree bear a marked resemblance to the Harvard requirements Smith had described in his August 1796 report to the Board.

The importance of the Board's document thus lies not in its originality but in the extent to which it attempted to formalize medical education in the backwoods of New Hampshire. And this is probably precisely what Nathan Smith wanted. *His* students would not be mere medical apprentices of unknown and inadequate background; they would be College Men, members of an educated elite with a professional understanding of what it meant to be a physician.

And so it was done! In 1798, the second year of the medical school, the course was to begin in early October, according to Nathan Noyes, a prospective student. Noyes, who had already attended lectures in the fall of 1797,[18] was restless and eager for classes to begin after having spent "23 days [quarantined] under the operation of small pox" (which in his case had turned out to be a "mild disorder"). In his mid-August letter to his parents, he continued: "On my return . . . [to Hanover I had to wait] till the establishment of our medical professor or professors here shall be completed. It is now in contemplation to have the lectures commence on the fifth of October and continue ten weeks. If this should be determined I shall probably continue here till their conclusion."[19]

Clearly Noyes did stay the course; the next year he was one of the second group of students to earn a medical degree from Dartmouth. In August 1799, the Bachelor of Medicine degree was voted to Nathan Noyes, Daniel Adams, and Abraham Hedge.[20] All three had probably been apprentices of Smith's; certainly Noyes had been. It was he who ended the letter home quoted above with the remark about being obliged to ride with Smith—a clear indication that he was accompanying Smith on calls as would have been expected of an apprentice.

At the same meeting where those degrees were awarded, the Board of

Trust also voted "that the room No. 6 in the lower storey in the College" (i.e., Dartmouth Hall) be "devoted to the use of Professor N. Smith for the purpose of lecturing." With this vote, the medical department became even more explicitly a part of the College. A further vote of confidence in Smith's enterprise was that the Board went on to say "that the Agent be requested to cause [the room] to be repaired and accommodated with seats and such other conveniences as may be necessary."[21] The trustees must have been more than satisfied with the way things had gone in the first two years.

Nathan Smith should also have been pleased. By August of 1799, he had been teaching in his own medical school for two years, and he had five students with medical degrees to prove it. For the erstwhile farm boy from Chester, Vermont, a new career was unfolding in New Hampshire. From now on, it was not just "Dr. Smith" in some little New England village. It was Professor Nathan Smith, M.B., A.M., Corresponding Member of the Medical Society of London, of Dartmouth Medical School.

PART II

PROFESSOR OF MEDICINE

CHAPTER FIVE

The Heart of the Matter

Theory and Practice

I combat opinions on the certain ground of practice, and not on the uncertain ground of theory; for which reason, the highest authority upon earth could not persuade me to admit a doctrine which disagrees with my own experience.
— ALEXANDER GORDON [1]

Teaching Medicine

IN MEDICAL SCHOOLS of the eighteenth and nineteenth centuries the central course was "Theory and Practice of Physic." As the title clearly implies, the theory behind medicine was considered at least as important as its practice. Theoretical constructs concerning health and illness were a powerful organizing feature of the way medical students were taught.

Nathan Smith was as aware of the prevailing medical theories of his day as the next medical man, and we will explore at a later point (in chapter 9) how his critical view of those grand theories influenced—or failed to influence—the way he practiced medicine. Of course, since the medicine Smith practiced played a major role in the medicine he taught, separating discussion of one from the other is a bit arbitrary. Given that a dominant feature of Smith's approach to medicine (as we have already seen) was a steady undercurrent of basic common sense rather than any abstruse theory, however, this approach makes sense. Elisha Bartlett—whom the brilliant medical teacher William Osler called a "philosopher," and whom one historian considers among the most distinguished graduates of Rhode Island's first medical school[2]—expressed views in his mid-1840s "Essay on the Philosophy of Medical Science" that Smith would have understood and supported:

Medical doctrines, as they are called, are, in most instances, hypothetical explanations, or interpretations, merely, of the ascertained phenomena, and their relationships, of medical science. These explanations consist of certain other assumed
and unascertained phenomena and relationships. They do not constitute a legitimate element of medical science. All medical science is absolutely independent of
these explanations.[3]

The contrast between the Smith-Bartlett view of medical science and that
typical of Benjamin Rush (1745–1813) and most others who returned to
practice following their study abroad is considerable. All too often, these
proud worthies thought of themselves as a genus apart (we saw this in
Benjamin Waterhouse)—skilled thinkers who should be sought out and
obeyed unquestioningly for their great knowledge.

Nathan Smith's attitude was different; he knew that he had to teach his
students a searching, critical appraisal of the actual practice of medicine if
he was to keep them from accepting mere dogma. Thus there are grounds
for thinking what he taught was always going to be quite independent of
the theories propagated by the dogmatists of the day—and reason enough
to focus in this chapter on aspects of Smith's teaching that emphasize his
pedagogy rather than its philosophical underpinnings.

Smith's lecture style has been preserved for us by students who wrote
down his lectures in their notebooks; letters his students wrote home, and
reminiscences of former students and colleagues, show that the responses
of those who heard him varied. One of his students in 1808, William
Tully (who had come to Dartmouth from Yale), recorded in his diary his
reactions to the first day of class. While waiting for Professor Smith to arrive, he surveyed the room and assessed his fellow students:

Such a motley collection I am sure I never set my eyes on before. Some seemed to
be so awkwardly put together that, at first view, one would almost suppose that
chance was the agent in their formation. The Clothes of some . . . were, in general,
so ludicrously put on that I hardly dared trust myself with a second view.

Given that mood and tone, Tully's initial disappointment over Smith himself is not surprising:

Doctor Smith, after a while, slipped into the room and seated himself almost without our knowledge. I had really been expecting some . . . majesty and grace, and I
felt a kind of disgust from my disappointment. His introductory address was altogether extemporaneous and couched in the most colloquial phrases. It was pithy,
however, and in spite of its want of elegance, I could not but like it tolerably well.
By this time I had got past being disappointed at anything that I should meet in
Hanover, and I made up my mind to be attentive to the matter only and not the
manner of what my instructor and fellow students should say.

So Smith could grow on one! The disgruntled young man at least had

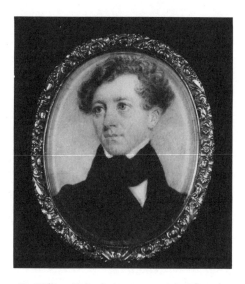

Dr. William Tully, Jr. (*1785–1859*) *by Thomas
H. Parker.* Photo courtesy of Yale University Art
Gallery, Lelia A. and John Hill Morgan Collection.

the honesty to acknowledge that style and substance might warrant different responses:

As I had just got into this frame of mind, the embarrassment of the Doctor's first
address was over, and the man of true erudition, and the master of his profession,
was manifest. He seemed determined that every one should have the full benefit of
his instructions, however triflingly he [the student] had prepared himself to attend
such a course.[4]

What in the "introductory address" Tully found so appalling, we do not
know. Certainly the one such lecture of which we have what purports to
be the full text—Smith's "Introductory Lecture on the Progress of Medical Science" (probably the first lecture he gave at Yale years later)—
though hardly a brilliant piece of work, is a long way from being an embarrassment. A clear (if too brief) history of medicine designed to whet
student appetites for what is to come, it ends, neatly, with the observation
that "[w]e seem now to have arrived at the proper point for starting."[5]

Further testimony to Smith's interest in the history of medicine is found
in a ledger he kept in 1800; it contains "Heads of Lectures" for his course
at Dartmouth. The first lecture was on anatomy and opened with the
Greek derivation of the word, a later writer tell us; "as was Dr. Smith's
custom in all that he did or said, he commenced at the very foundation of
things and traced the history in outline along from the ancients to the day
in which he was lecturing."[6])

More common than misgivings like those William Tully expressed are former students' remarks full of praise. A. T. Lowe, looking back years later, recalled Smith's lectures as having been "delivered in language clear and strong."[7] And Ezekiel Dodge Cushing, who attended the medical school at the University of Pennsylvania after having studied under Nathan Smith at Dartmouth, wrote to his father comparing Smith favorably with Philadelphia's famous medical professors: "Dr. Smith gives infinitely better lectures on surgery than Dr. [Philip Syng] Physick and certainly more useful ones on the theory and practice of physic than Dr. [Benjamin] Rush."[8]

Smith spoke primarily from experience, citing his own cases freely—which did not mean his lectures were always sober affairs. Isaac Patterson, another student recalling those lectures years later, recounted the following:

He related one anecdote which I remember, that a boy went out into the yard with a bridle in hand and salt to catch a horse. The horse kicked the boy in the head, his friends informed the Dr. that the horse had knocked out a piece of the boy's skull which they had picked up and brought in. The Dr. called for some warm water, washed off the blood when lo & behold a great lump of Rock Salt. He said to his class, "I would have you know that the human skull is not so thick as a big lump of salt."

He would sometimes joke the class upon the practice of physic, saying that it was questionable whether they could do any good or not, that it was a plesant thing to be called Dr.—sent for & consulted [but] that in his own case, if anything was the matter of his family he did not give medicine, but sent for old Mrs. Dewey—Dea[con] Dewey's wife.[9]

One of the eulogies given on the occasion of Smith's death stressed both his reliance on experience and the good humor in his lectures:

His object was to instil into the minds of his pupils the leading principles of their profession . . . . These principles he would illustrate, by appropriate cases, furnished by a long course of practice; related always in an impressive, and often in a playful manner, so as at once to gain the attention, and impress the truth illustrated, upon the mind.[10]

The most remarkable feature of what Nathan Smith taught is that from his own careful examinations of patients—his down-to-earth assessment of what he discovered patients were actually experiencing—an understanding of disease processes emerged that placed him surprisingly close to modern medical thinking. Today, obscure difficulties of immunity in infectious diseases and cancer, in diseases of the endocrine glands, and even in organic heart disease, have forced a general acknowledgment that it is possible to focus too minutely on cells and subcellular particles, which in turn has led to the bio-psycho-social approach to disease in human beings prevalent today. The overlap with the concerns that drove Nathan Smith is notable, and his attempt to treat the whole patient is suggestive of today's emphasis on "total care." He often spoke of the importance of good nursing.[11]

At the opening of the nineteenth century, Smith and his fellow physicians stood on the threshold of a world where revolutionary ideas were being vigorously advanced. For generations, disease had been seen as largely a matter of the derangement of the parts of the body. One view was that the body was possessed by demons; another was that it was disturbed by the imbalance of "humors." Wild and fearsome curative procedures were sometimes advocated to shake the body free of disease—nor were the violent evacuations and vomiting ("purging and puking") often induced in Nathan Smith's day very far removed from the devil dance and the chant of medicine men. All were designed to help the body adjust. Slowly, however, a few practitioners were beginning to explore different approaches. Smith was among those who understood that just because bleeding and other "depleting remedies" might be inappropriate, it did not follow that strong stimulants would be useful.

Being on the frontier of society as Smith was had its disadvantages. But given his imaginative and independent mind, and his uncannily accurate diagnostic skills, the isolation may have saved him from blunders that others made, influenced as they were by some of the more spectacular theories and trends of the day. Smith taught that the wise physician takes advantage of every healing mechanism, while watching carefully for undesirable side effects. This is the essence of the new outlook Smith presented in his lectures. In his practice he confirmed by experience what he saw he needed to teach his eager students (see chapter 7 for a fuller discussion of Smith's relationship with some of his students and their subsequent careers).

Before we turn to the actual content of Smith's courses, several aspects of the way medical schools were organized in his day deserve comment. The formal lectures in medical schools of the time were typically presented within a brief ten-week span (sometimes given a second time in the academic year); students were expected, and usually required, to attend two such courses. For most young men, despite that heavy concentration of the academic work, medical study was a year-round activity. Many of the students stayed at the end of the term and saw patients with their professors, or they went home and apprenticed themselves to local physicians. Those in the most dire financial straits could not afford this, however; they studied ten weeks and then returned to farming or some other occupation between terms. We know that by 1809, at least, this had become an all-too-common practice. Ebenezer Adams, a member of the college faculty, wrote to a former medical student and friend, saying "[o]ur students are, as usual at this season of the year, considerably scattered over the country, discharging the humble but useful office of Pedagogues. This, I believe, is a growing evil . . . ."[12]

At first blush, the requirement that students attend the same set of lectures more than once seems unreasonable. If the lectures had all been like the ones at Harvard that Smith later said (as one student claimed) had "varied not at all for twenty years,"[13] the repeated attendance could have been deadly boring. But students were generally not required to attend both sets of lectures at the same institution; in any case, Smith kept his own lectures up to date and revised them in light of his recent experiences. According to a student at Dartmouth in 1812, for instance, Smith opened the eighth lecture of the autumn course with the topic "*Contraction of the Esophagus*"; the subject seems to have been chosen simply because Smith had just dealt with a case that provided him a timely example. "A man came to me today with this complaint . . . ," he began, and then expanded on what he had done for the patient by reference to previous experience: "I have known 3 or 4 cases of this kind." Another student noted similar presentations of actual cases: "A young man who had many symptoms of Phthisis Pulmonalis . . . ," and "A young woman in the last stages of Phthisis Pulmonalis . . . ."[14] Notes recorded by a student at Yale the next year provide several further examples of the use of current cases: "Saturday about 5 o'clock [Hezekiah Smith] fell from a horse and was taken up to appearance dead . . ."; "On Saturday Morning Moses Richards was attacked with the Cholera . . . ."; "On Sunday Morn Mr. Stevens was taken with frequent discharge downwards (without pain) . . ."; "On Wednesday Evening I was called to visit [Mrs. Nettleton] with all haste, the Messenger reporting that they thought her a Dying. I accordingly rode there as quick as possible, and found her very low from flooding."[15]

Such reports were bound to give the students a sense of immediacy in what they were learning. Lectures filled with vivid accounts from Smith's own practice made medicine come alive. This was not dry and outdated theory; these were real cases of patients who were living, breathing—and sometimes dying. As the student Isaac Patterson once said, Nathan Smith might be

deficient in classical education, but [he was] a genius highly gifted—he usually commenced [his lectures] with some anecdote that happened in his practice and proceeded in a conversational style—his talk was full of practical instruction. You could not hear him without being convinced how thoroughly he understood his subject—he seemed to hold all the knowledge contained in the Books & in other sources in solution—he would tell you how far the authors went & how far short they came of imparting full information—His keen observation went far beyond the medical authors of his day.[16]

Listening to Smith's lectures more than once would not likely have been dull. Quite apart from his lively (if plain-spoken) style and the ever-changing content of his lectures, one must remember that students in those days had no textbooks. When famous authors of standard printed works were quoted or cited, few students would have had access to the source. Knowing this, lecturers paced their oral presentations in a manner that made it possible for their auditors to take nearly verbatim notes, a practice already widely used by professors in every academic field by the time Nathan Smith engaged in it.[17]

Despite the fact that student notebooks exist for many professors' courses in a number of medical schools, however, we have little direct knowledge of what use students made of their own notes. Some apparently copied theirs over at a later date.[18] Sometimes they copied notes from others (just as students today are apt to do, if they miss a lecture) or added commentary based on their own experience.[19] Amazingly, there is internal evidence in some student notebooks to suggest that Smith himself, even midway and late in his career, read his students' notes and corrected them, adding points he thought needed stressing.[20] How he found time to do this staggers the imagination.

The Lectures

We will begin by taking a quick look at what Smith had been appointed to teach and what else was on his agenda (at least in later years) before turning to student lecture notes to see what he actually said. Dartmouth's Board of Trust, it will be recalled, specified that Smith was to give "public lectures" on anatomy and surgery, chemistry and materia medica, and the theory and practice of physic. Leaving the teaching of anatomy and surgery for later, what was to be included in the other courses?

The agreement drawn up by the Trustees, it will be recalled, had stipulated that the lectures on the theory and practice of physic should explain "the nature of diseases and method of cure," and that the lectures on chemistry and materia medica should be accompanied with "actual experiments tending to explain and demonstrate the principles of Chemistry and an exhibition of the principal medicines used in curing diseases and also an explanation of their Medicinal qualities & effects on the human body."

For the "Theory and Practice" course in particular, this description is so broad that it tells us very little. Such courses were intended to cover a wide spectrum—nothing short of the etiology, diagnosis, and treatment of disease. (In some institutions, "Theory and Practice" also included pathology; until microscopes were commonly available, however, and the disciplines of histology and bacteriology emerged from infancy, little could be done in the way of scientific pathology.) As already hinted, and as will become clear later, both etiology and diagnosis typically relied on theories that were often only shallowly rooted in reality. The gradual move toward a more scientific medicine was hampered by "speculative and unempirical systems" that constituted "a serious detriment to medical education [by] turning the student's attention away from empirical observation toward rationalistic nosologies."[21] We shall also examine later the role these taxonomies of disease played. Often they were quite idiosyncratically conceived, and based more on speculation—even wishful thinking—than on observation.

What the Board of Trust expected or wanted under the title of "Chemistry and Materia Medica" is also unclear. By today's standards, there was little that could be taught. Even so, as defined by Daniel Drake, the great doctor of the American West (whose floruit came slightly later than Smith's), materia medica was the study of the "facts and principles which related to the operation of the various medicinal agents on the human body, both in health and disease; together with their natural history and pharmacological preparation."[22] Obviously, this had a lot to do with the practice of physic and thus overlapped with that course; equally obviously, there was room for a great deal of theorizing as the lecturer's time was apt to be spent describing and classifying treatments of all manner. In principle a useful course, with little laboratory or field work it was bound to be only as good as the experience of the instructor.[23] When that experience was limited, as it so often was, materia medica may have been the most difficult course to teach. The brilliant French physiologist and surgeon Marie-François-Xavier Bichat (1771–1802) once characterized it thus:

There have been no general systems in the materia medica; but this science has been alternately influenced by the prevailing theories of physic. From hence proceeds that indefiniteness and uncertainty which marks it even in the present day. It is an incoherent mass of incoherent opinions, and probably of all physiologic sciences, that in which the inconsistencies of the human mind are most glaring. . . . It is not a science for a methodical and philosophic mind; it is an incongruous combination of erroneous ideas, observations often puerile, means at the best fallacious, and formulae as fantastically conceived as they are preposterously combined. It is said that the practice of combined physic has something repelling in it. I will say more: in those principles which connect it with the materia medica it is absolutely revolting to a rational mind. Let us expunge from our classes those medicines that have been closely watched and accurately ascertained, . . . and what knowledge shall we be found to possess of the remaining functions?[24]

Bichat's concerns, however, were of little importance to Smith, since he did not seek a "rational" basis for what he taught. Rather, it was precisely the "closely watched and accurately ascertained" effects of medicaments and procedures that informed everything he did. Thus he was, happily, equally comfortable teaching materia medica as part of medicine and anatomy as part of surgery.

An examination of Smith's lectures by means of the notes taken by Dartmouth and Yale students (the notebooks date from between 1806 and 1826) shows that Smith was able to organize material clearly, and to balance an awareness of history with an appreciation of what could be learned from close observation. His detailed, practical hints for treatment were prefaced by straightforward and clear (if somewhat oversimplified) statements of his concept of disease.

"Health," William C. Ellsworth (in 1806) quoted Smith as saying in the opening lecture of one course, "is that state of the human Body wherein all the different functions perform their Powers regularly & cum ease . . . ."[25] At the outset of another course (probably in 1815), David Shelton Edwards took down the following statement: "[B]y diseased action we are to understand an action begun & carried on in some part of the human system which is opposed to healthy action & which tends either directly or indirectly to destroy life." Edwards tells us that as Smith went on to speak of the causes of disease, he distinguished—and stressed the importance of doing so—between the nature of the exciting cause and the nature of the part on which it falls. He further ensured his students were following him by using the lecturer's standard tools of emphasis ("I would have you mark this") and prolepsis ("This will be better understood when we come to the nosological arrangement").[26]

When Samuel Farnsworth sat in Smith's lectures at Dartmouth (in 1822), the distinction between "exciting cause" and "the part on which it falls" was put slightly differently; this time the stress was on the importance of realizing that this distinction was not an adequate way to study or understand disease: "*Classification of Diseases*. There are two circumstances to be considered in the classification of diseases. The cause of the disease & the part affected. These two general divisions would not lead us far in the investigation of diseases."[27]

In introductory lectures, Smith might go into some detail concerning the history of medicine, as we have learned;[28] he might also (or instead) take time to explain the relationship between the various branches of medicine, and to expound on why two courses were quite sensibly required for a medical degree and why attending lectures was more important than mere book learning, as Avery J. Skilton reported.[29] Smith was also wont to remind students that they must take responsibility for their own education, and Skilton wrote down just such a cautionary note from one of Smith's introductory lectures (in 1826): "Your advancement as physicians depends on yourselves, all that your teachers or books can do for you will be to little purpose unless you observe, & this will be of little use unless you reflect, resolve things, symptoms, effects, into principles. You have 5 witnesses, the 5 senses . . . ."[30]

No doubt Smith's teaching style was refined over the years, so perhaps he was a smoother lecturer by the time Skilton heard him at Yale than he had been at Dartmouth when Tully listened to him with such dismay; certainly the passage just quoted was coherent and sensible enough. And of course Smith added annually to his experience, giving him new (and perhaps ever more varied and interesting) cases he could cite to make his points. Notes taken by students during Smith's final years of teaching show a much fuller range of topics than were probably present in his first lectures at Dartmouth, and they therefore give the clearest picture we have of how and what he taught.

Of the many student notebooks safely tucked away in libraries (see the Bibliography of Student Notebooks, on page 339), among the most thorough and complete are Worham L. Fitch's, taken in Smith's lectures at Yale in 1824–26.[31] Fitch, a conscientious youth duly impressed with the importance of the lectures and great penman whose flourishes attest to his skills in these requisites, was registered in the medical school at Yale a year before Avery Skilton studied there. Eventually settling in Springfield, Massachusetts, where he practiced for years, Fitch joined the Massachusetts Medical Society in 1837 and died at the age of sixty-nine in Springfield, in 1872.[32]

Fitch's notes provide example after example of the main characteristics of Smith's teaching. These included reports on patients seen and cared for (in other words, Smith employed a case-study method of teaching remarkable for its modernity). Smith also gave clear indications when he was expressing a mere belief (as opposed to something he was certain of, from experience), and he exhibited a no-nonsense acknowledgment of unsolved problems. His independence showed up in bold challenges to those who stubbornly held outmoded views and criticism of standard procedures (he often named the individual whose principles and procedures he was taking issue with) when experience showed him another approach was preferable. Fitch's lecture notes run to nearly nine hundred pages; accordingly, excerpts of varying length must suffice here to illustrate these themes. The examples could be multiplied many times over for most of the points made, and parallels can be found in other student notebooks.[33]

Among the most striking features is the blunt way Smith criticized standard practices without being either rude or condescending. In a discussion of the treatment of puncture wounds in the joints and hands, "frequently . . . productive of bad consequences," for instance, he had this criticism to make:

When a puncture is made through [the tendinous fascia (fibrous tissue) that covers the muscles] into the soft parts beneath a swelling is produced [that] puts it upon the stretch; and when those membranes or ligaments are put on the stretch and are inflamed the most excruciating pain is produced. Matter [generally, fluid or pus] may form under the fascia and extend round the limb. It has been recommended to enlarge the wound by making a free incision through the fascia, but this is not always practicable, and I do not think it best.

It is better not to enlarge the wound till necessity call for it.[34]

When a limb cannot be saved, Smith said in a lecture on "Contused Wounds,"

amputation should be performed immediately.

It has been argued by some that persons sound and healthy cannot so safely bear the operation as they could after suppuration has taken place.

This principle if brought into practice would be productive of great injury. . . .

In contusion, suppuration may never take place if you wait for it. If you wait for suppuration you must wait for separation between the dead and living parts.

I have operated within 24 hours after the accident with perfect safety. The period during which amputation may be performed depend[s] on the circumstance of the cases.[35]

(The experience of a slightly younger contemporary of Smith's, Dr. Usher Parsons—a surgeon during the Battle of Lake Erie in 1813—is relevant. He wrote that one "cause of success worthy of special notice was *the delay of severe surgical operations until the system was entirely recovered from the shock of the injury*." In fact, "to wait or not to wait" was much under debate at the time.[36])

On gunshot wounds, which Smith said should be treated "as simple wounds only with this difference, that the wound should not be closed," he went on thus:

They will always suppurate. Nothing is better than the *Fermenting Poultice*. Some however recommend to lay open the wound, but this should not be done till necessity for it appears.

The same rule will apply as in puncture wounds. Merely opening the external parts will be of no benefit.[37]

What he saw to be plain error was matter-of-factly presented as such:

It was formerly supposed that the bones were first fluid and then became cartilaginous, then bones; or that they changed gradually from a fluid to a proper bone. I suppose there is nothing correct in this theory . . . .

Bones are not formed any more from the ends of the break than from the surrounding membranes. The erroneous opinion concerning bones and their union has led to incorrect practice. They supposed the ossific matter was able to shoot out in a variety of directions.[38]

Nor was Smith afraid to take on the giants of medicine—but even when he thought an idea completely wrong, he took issue without the hint of a sneer. In a discussion of "Hemorrhagia," he turned to the theory espoused by the oracle of Edinburgh, William Cullen:

Doct'r Cullen supposed that some cases of hemorrhage arose from an increased action of the capillaries. This he called active hemorrhage, and he said that others arose from *relaxation*. This he called passive hemorrhage. He supposed that a greater quantity of blood than usual was thrown upon a particular part with such force as to burst the vessels, integuments &c. and thus force its passage out of the system. This theory however does not appear very satisfactory. I do not think that hemorrhage ever depends on relaxation or general debility. I think it doubtful, too, whether it ever arises from increased action of the arteries, as the arterial action is often increased without hemorrhage. It more probably depends on the imperfect manner in which the blood is transmit[t]ed from the arteries into the veins.[39]

He was not always as thorough as one might have wished; at another point his attack on Cullen was simply a dismissive "Doct'r Cullen's Theory of the proximate cause of fever does not appear very satisfactory"[40] (a noncommittal phrase Smith frequently used in his criticisms). Nor was Smith always right. In what was presumably meant as a devastating attack (though made, again, more in passing than in detail) on Cullen's reliance on theory, Smith came out with the following curiously ambiguous observation of his own: "Dr. Cullen considered the Dysentery contagious but by facts we should not think that it is, because, if it was, it would attack all people alike."[41]

Smith's sense of humor frequently emerged, but it was seldom expressed broadly. Much more typical were wry remarks like these that appeared in a lecture on "Injuries of different Parts":

In some books published about the time I commenced practice, the authors took great pains to distinguish between suture [the natural line of junction between two bones, especially in the skull] and fracture. They inculcated the doctrine that wherever there was a fracture or even a pressure an operation was necessary. Much was said about the place where an operation might be performed. 1st They said an operation should not be performed over a suture, 2d over the frontal sinuses. They talked about it as if they could command the place where the injury should be inflicted. We must operate in the place where the injury occurs.[42]

In a similar tone, discussing "Tic Douloureux" (a "painful affection of the nerves of the face accompanied sometimes with spasmodic twitches and contractions of the muscles of the face"), Smith said it is "sometimes mistaken for pain in the teeth and several of the teeth are frequently extracted without producing any good effect. I would not recommend to extract a sound tooth for pain in the face."[43]

The sad truths that a physician does not always have a remedy and that there are some things the doctor simply does not know were part of Smith's regular teaching. Discussing possible treatments for cancer, Smith mentioned in passing, without expressing his own view, that the plant dock root "has been supposed to have some effect in the cure of cancer"; and he brought his auditors up to date ("Within a few years [past] Pyrola Latifolia has been introduced") before continuing as follows:

> Mercury I consider has no specific effect. In many cases it has failed. It commonly palliates but does not cure. There is no remedy known that will cure inveterate cancer. . . . An operation will undoubtedly in many cases save the patient.
> The difficulty is in ascertaining the rule to regulate the operation. No one has seen cases enough to give all the necessary rules. In many cases if the operation does not succeed it will do no injury, only by the pain it produces. Still we should not wish to operate unless there is a probability of success.[44]

Similarly, in many instances he preached the healing power of nature. The physician's role, he insisted, was simply to assist:

> All the application necessary for a simple incised wound is *Simple Cerate* in order to heal it. Time with these simple dressings is all that is necessary to affect a cure. It is very immaterial whether we make any other applications or not. . . . [W]hen the wound comes to heal the parts will again approach each other. We may assist the approach of the parts and thereby expedite the cure by pressure properly applied.[45]

The most prevalent feature by far of the lectures as taken down by Worham L. Fitch is Smith's repeated references to his own practice and his own experience: "I have never tied an artery in the amputation of fingers and toes." "A young lady had the tibia broken and the points of the bones extended through the external parts. I laid open the wound and replaced the bone and the patient recovered as soon as though it had been a simple fracture." "I have seen several cases where I think I was able to discover a fluctuation of water. In one case the ribs of one side were so much separated as to be distinctly perceived between them and in another case it pressed down the diaphragm . . . ." "I have known astringent injections useful." "I have observed that dyspeptics are very subject to cold particularly coldness of the feet. . . . They should therefore be kept warm."[46] No one reading these notes could doubt that Nathan Smith learned from his practice—and expected his students to do likewise when they had practices of their own.

Of course lectures on surgery and on the theory and practice of physic were not the only ones Smith gave; it just happens that the notes we have from Worham L. Fitch are on these topics. Another of Smith's Yale students who likewise dutifully took down what his professor had to say (though by no means so extensively) was, as we have seen, Avery J. Skilton. In his notebook, extracts from lectures given by Smith's Yale colleagues Eli Ives ("On Diseases of Children") and Jonathan Knight ("On Obstetrics") flank notes from Smith's "Medical Jurisprudence" lectures. These latter included—for example—discussions of wounds and contusions, malpractice, infanticide, abortion, concealed birth, rape, and poisoning.[47] Skilton also recorded Smith's "Directions to the Accoucheur"; the fact that what we find there is for the most part exactly what Fitch wrote a year later on that subject tells us Smith must have been writing out and reading at least some of his lectures.[48]

We see, then, that by the end of his career, Nathan Smith was lecturing on a wide variety of subjects. What we do not know is how many of the subtopics he attempted to include in his first lectures at Dartmouth. In one area we know he turned to another doctor for help.

Making Room for Chemistry

It was all very well for the Board of Trust to include chemistry in the materia medica course, but there was by no means agreement even about what chemistry was or could do, never mind about its usefulness to medicine. A quarter of a century after Nathan Smith was being enjoined to teach chemistry, John Ayrton Paris, in *The Elements of Medical Chemistry*, included an imaginary dialogue between himself and a practitioner, to explain why the latter should include chemistry in directing the medical studies of his son. The practitioner, in talking about the early days of his own career, is placed (fortuitously for us) precisely at the point in time when Nathan Smith was beginning to teach at Dartmouth. He argued as follows:

I need scarcely observe that in my younger days Chemistry was scarcely regarded as a branch of medical study; my knowledge on this subject is necessarily, therefore, extremely imperfect; but I feel no hesitation in declaring, that in no single instance do I remember ever having felt an embarrassment at the bed side, or in the Surgery, from my deficiency.

But when the practitioner (whose favorite word seems to have been "scarcely") went on to say, "You will scarcely venture to assert that the living power is . . . constantly opposed to chemical action," Paris responded thus:

[F]or that reason, it is essential to learn the nature of chemical action, before we can attempt to appreciate the extent of that force which modifies or resists it. But there are changes perpetually going on in the animal body that are beyond the control of the living principle, and therefore the Physiologist, who is not a Chemist, will be utterly at a loss to comprehend them.[49]

Just such a controversy had split the faculty at the Philadelphia School of Medicine, in 1818, a few years before this plea for chemistry was published;[50] the importance of the new science was by no means universally understood.

Smith did understand, but from the beginning of his professional career, as we saw, he counted on others to help. Ads placed in *The Medical Repository*, listing Nathan Smith and Lyman Spalding as "Officers of the Institution," help make this clear.[51] Making Spalding his colleague was a way for Smith to bring additional prestige to the school. Beyond the fact that Spalding had just received his M.B. degree from Harvard, he had received a thorough education prior to that: He was a graduate of Charlestown Academy, where he studied both Latin and English; while he was at Harvard, Paul Joseph Nancrede tutored him in French.[52] That in turn meant he would have been able to follow and teach the new chemistry being developed by Antoine Lavoisier (1743–94), Claude Berthollet (1748–1822), and others in France far better than could Smith, for whom French and the principles of the new experiments alike were quite foreign.

During that first year at Dartmouth, Spalding found that no available teaching materials fitted his pedagogical needs. He therefore wrote and published a twenty-page student manual, a nomenclature of chemistry based on the work of several of the French chemists. Although his booklet consisted mainly of a collation of the new technical terms, it was highly regarded and served its purpose in the classroom.[53] In later years Spalding used it as a sort of calling card and sent a copy to all the physicians with whom he wished to do business.

Smith no doubt would have been happy if Spalding could have been persuaded to become a permanent member of the faculty, but it was not to be. He was well liked at Dartmouth, but neither success nor approbation was enough to keep him there. He was an ambitious young man, with wide interests; he could not resist the chance to set up a practice of his own. When Spalding moved to Portsmouth, New Hampshire, in June 1799, Smith did everything he could to get his young assistant to return annually for the winter medical school classes. But Hanover was a hundred miles of hard riding northwest of Portsmouth, and after the session of 1799–1800 Spalding resigned.[54]

The resignation brought forth a letter of protest from Abraham Hedge, a student who had benefited from Spalding's teaching at Dartmouth: "Some who had attended your lectures, said that chemistry had dwindled in your absence, which I verily believe. Tho' I consider Dr. Smith as a great & universal genius, and possessed of more virtues than generally fall to the lot of one man, yet I think him wanting in accuracy as a public instruction [sic]."[55] That plea also failed to make Spalding change his mind. Nor did a letter from Smith several years later bring him back—though the tone of it is typical of Smith's teasing type of humor (at least it is difficult to believe Smith seriously thought what he was describing would solve his problems with the chemistry course). Written in 1809, the letter indicates Smith still regretted Spalding's departure:

I have found a plan for my future proceeding as relates to chemistry which is to procure sixty boxes & in those boxes to put all the preparations in complete readiness to perform 60 lectures, which shall comprise my next course on that branch. This I can cause to be done by my pupils, which will be a kindness to them & will abridge my labors very much.[56]

A bit of unpleasantness marred Lyman Spalding's last session at Dartmouth, which may have been another factor in his decision to resign. Daniel Adams, who earned his A.B. at Dartmouth in 1797 and his M.B. in 1799, dedicated his thesis to Smith—just as Spalding had dedicated his Harvard thesis to Smith in 1797.[57] More than the dedications were similar, however, and Spalding accused Adams of plagiarism.[58] Adams vehemently denied the charge: "I have made use of no man's arguments to support my subject for in truth I have seen none. And altho I have called into my assistance some experiments and sentiments of different authors they were made by them with different views than those for which I have used them.... My treating of the subject was on a plan entirely my own."[59] Adams's refusal to back down is no proof that he did not plagiarize (though he certainly was firm in insisting that he had not), and we cannot know at this distant remove why either of them was willing to let the matter drop. But in the end they apparently settled their differences, and an interesting and valuable correspondence developed between the two men. (Such epistolary exchanges were frequently then used by doctors as a form of continuing postgraduate education.)

Chemistry continued to be a problem for Smith, despite what William Tully (in an uncharacteristically generous mood) had to say about Smith's "Introduction to Chemistry" lecture in 1808: "What he laid down was done with great precision, and his divisions were lucid and satisfactory."[60] On another occasion a former student, Nathan Noyes, filled in by lecturing on chemistry when Smith was out of town "to attend a sick brother in medicine," eliciting from Tully the observation that "in the plain sailing of chemistry, he did as a lecturer quite as well as Doctor Smith."[61] Whether this remark was intended as praise of Noyes or as a criticism of Smith is unclear. Information of substance seemed generally to be lacking. Andrew Mack in his journal, kept "during a course of chemical Lectures" given by Smith at Dartmouth, for example, dutifully wrote down Smith's definition of chemistry from the first lecture: "Chemistry is that science which treats of the action of one body upon another." This action, Mack went on to say, "was explained in relation to mechanical action or power."[62] The teaching of science was no more sophisticated when chemistry was put into Rufus Graves's hands somewhat later; he "gave a few lectures on this subject, but not having any apparatus for experiments it did not amount to much," Isaac Patterson recalled years later.[63]

Yet at least some of the time it sounds as if Smith's efforts to teach chemistry were more rigorous; Ezekiel Dodge Cushing wrote home with the perennial student complaint of fatigue: "In attending the lectures I find more than sufficient to employ my whole time. I have been employed . . . with 5 others in performing chemical experiments till 3 o'clock in the morning two thirds of the time since the lectures have begun . . . ."[64] Though Smith made clear his belief that chemistry was important (he belabored the point in at least one end-of-course lecture[65]), it was—under the best of circumstances—never the jewel in his crown.

Genius and Driving Force

Nathan Smith's students may not have been aware at the time of what a rare teacher he was; there is little doubt that he customarily used ordinary language in a day when most professors cloaked their lectures in rhetorical excess. But with the wisdom of hindsight, almost a century after Smith's death, the great physician and teacher Harvey Cushing spoke of how "the genius and driving force" of Dartmouth Medical School's one-man faculty enhanced its reputation to the point that it began to overshadow Harvard's. Smith, Cushing went on to say "had the sound judgment of a great teacher."[66]

Even allowing for the sentimental hyperbole typical of eulogies, it is striking that Jonathan Knight, a fellow professor at Yale when Smith died, described Smith's teaching (which he presumably had ample opportunity to witness and which he surely heard students evaluating) as follows:

As an instructor, the reputation of Dr. Smith was high, from the time he began the business of instruction. . . . His mode of communicating instruction [while at Yale] has been simple, natural and unaffected. He sought no aid from an artificial style, but merely poured forth, in the plain language of enlightened conversation, the treasures of his wisdom and experience.[67]

Given this assessment of Smith's style, it is difficult to believe that his rhetoric was directly responsible for inspiring the extraordinary prayer Dartmouth's President Wheelock uttered on one occasion in 1810—though the subject matter does seem to have come straight from Smith's classroom. On the heels of one of Smith's lectures, evening prayers were held in the old chapel; there Wheelock prayed as follows: "Oh Lord! We thank Thee for the Oxygen gas; we thank Thee for the Hydrogen gas; and for all the gases. We thank Thee for the Cerebrum; we thank Thee for the Cerebellum, and for the Medulla Oblongata."[68] Perhaps Wheelock truly was impressed by Smith's lecture—or eager to show what he had learned! This flight of imaginative praying seems to have been characteristic of the president's own oratorical style, however. A couple of years earlier, William Tully had written in his diary on more than one occasion about Wheelock's prayers:

The President's Prayer did not correspond at all to my notions of supplication; for he seemed to be endeavoring to display his knowledge; and his phraseology was mere bombast.[69]

Smith's offerings to his students could by no means be dismissed as "mere bombast." In addition to instilling in his students a healthy skepticism toward empty theories, Smith indirectly performed another great service to patients in the way he taught his students. By word and example alike, Nathan Smith taught that it was all right to do nothing if symptoms were not urgent, that what we now call "watchful waiting" could also be good therapy.[70] There are times, he said, when it was better to

leave the disease to cure itself, as remedies, especially powerful ones, are more likely to do harm than good. In such cases, the patient gets along better without medicine than with; all that is required is to give him simple diluent drinks, a very small quantity of farinaceous food, and avoid as much as possible all causes of irritation.[71]

This is typical of the regimen that Smith taught to half a hundred students a year. Many of them became professors and taught their own half a hundred students annually. When Jacob Bigelow, in 1835, raised his voice in the first publicly acknowledged protest in the United States against "heroic" practice in medicine[72]—a euphemism for the violent purging and puking regimens mentioned earlier—a second generation of New England medical students was already learning a modern, cautious approach to therapeutics in a dozen medical schools where students of Nathan Smith were teaching.

The final, ceremonial step in turning students into colleagues was the annual valedictory speech Smith gave to the graduates—a grand send-off into the real world of medicine. One year he is reported to have reviewed the importance of the various branches of study the students had engaged in, before summing up (as William Tully wrote in his journal) with reminders on several points dear to his heart:

The Doctor next spoke of the immense sacrifices a good physician must make upon the altar of public good.

Indolence, ease, wealth, all, must be given up. The importance of physicians in society, the respect due to them, the necessity of their good behaviour, the indispensability of philosophy of medicine, etc., etc., were all ably touched upon.[73]

Another student, William C. Ellsworth, wrote down Smith's 1806 valedictory, apparently verbatim. The text was not altogether original; strong echoes of the farewell Dr. John Warren gave at the conclusion of the first course at Harvard Medical School reverberate in it[74]—and Smith had doubtless heard something very like it when he was there in 1790. Nonetheless, for all the derivative content and the nineteenth-century rhetorical flourishes, there is personal earnestness and a notable lack of pretension to give it distinction. Perhaps most important are the frequent and clear reminders to students that their education has just begun. We can reasonably imagine the scene: Appreciative students listen solemnly to words of advice from their medical professor; sobered by the realization that they are about to begin doctoring truly on their own, most of them sit quietly and seriously. They are likely to be deeply touched by his words of farewell.

Valedictory Charge by Nathan Smith

If the last sight of anything be attended with distressing emotions what must be the feelings of a Teacher when he takes a last and Farewell look at a number of his Pupils, endeared to him by Diligence in their studies, by their most amiable Deportment, and Numerous Instances of Personal Respect in his Intercourse with them. Under the influence of these affections, I feel, Gentlemen more than I am able to express, and were I permitted to obey the impulses of my Heart, I would only squeeze your hands and by an affectionate Silence convey to you my wishes for your future welfare. But as the custom of our University [sic] calls for a separation upon this public occasion, I shall endeavor to discharge this Duty by briefly suggesting to you a few directions intended to promote your improvement, & usefullness in your profession, and while my voice sounds in your ears, imagine you hear your other professors, inculting [sic] the same advice upon you. You have not finished your studies, you have only laid a Foundation for them on which to Build, [this] must be the business of your further Lives. To continue your application to Books Reading will be necessary, not only to increase your stock of Ideas, but to increase those you have acquired. For such is the nature of the Human Mind, that unless it be continually excited by Fresh accessions of Knowledge, it will soon loose [sic] all that it had acquired in early Life, hence it is no uncommon thing to find an old Physician more ignorant than he was when he first began the Practice of Medicine.

Improve, perfect, & perpetuate what has been so happily begun by the present Generation. We commit their unfinished Labors to your Care, and while we are descending into the Vale of Life, we shall be consoled in reflecting that the Science we have loved and taught Will be improved in your hands, more than it has been in ours. In your intercourse with your Patients, I have only to suggest to you to act towards them as you would [have] them act towards you on like Circumstances. Under the Direction of this heaven born precept, you will be prompt and Regular in your attendance Upon them, treat them at all times with Delicacy and Respect, sympathize in their sufferings. Forgive the changes in their Tempers and Conduct. Forbear to oppress the Unfortunate, be strictly just in your demands, by this Means you will endear yourselves to your Patients & impart a Dignity and Splendor to your Characters which they never can possess from exclusive display of Talents and Knowledge.

You have this day, Gentlemen, ceased to be our Pupils, but you have acquired a new and more intimate Connection to us. You have become our younger Brothers in the profession of Medicine and as such we invite you to Commend our Fraternal Services.

Proceed with Assiduity and Ardor in the course of your Studies. Hasten to perform the parts alloted to you in this Opening Scene of Usefulness & Glory. Remember how greatly your Preceptors have labored for you, and carry with you wherever you may go the Determined Resolution to be Useful to Yourselves, Your Country and the World, and be assured of my best wishes for your prosperity and Happiness.[75]

CHAPTER SIX

Trouble in the Anatomy Department

❦

The body-snatchers they have come
And made a snatch at me;
It's very hard them kind of men
Won't let a body be!
—THOMAS HOOD [1]

Teaching Anatomy and Surgery

FOR NATHAN SMITH, teaching always meant performing dissections and having students do them as well. In particular, dissections were crucial to the teaching of surgery; this, he believed, was how a doctor learned enough anatomy to do effective surgical work. He never said where his interest in dissections was first stimulated (we know Josiah Goodhue thought it began when he decided to put his dead horse to good use). Certainly Smith was exposed to the practice when he was at Harvard. John Warren would have been the perfect mentor.

Already when Warren entered Harvard in 1767—at age fourteen—"he exhibited a taste for the study of anatomy," we are told; "his anatomical acquirements excited interest . . . [and i]n 1780, he gave a course of dissections to his colleagues with success. . . . [N]one of them ever forgot the impression received from his lectures."[2] When John Warren was made a professor at Harvard, he was charged by the Corporation to " 'demonstrate the anatomy of a human body with physiological observations and explain and perform a complete system of surgical operations.' " His anatomy lectures, probably given in 1782, were the first in Boston to be accompanied by actual demonstrations. His 1790 lectures, focused more on anatomy than surgery, indicated an intense interest in the former.[3] We also know that Warren's son, John Collins Warren, began his own "adventures in body snatching" while still an undergraduate. At least one account the younger Warren gave of such an expedition included a remark about his father's distress at the son's involvement—coupled with admitted pleasure at the quality of the "subject" (a euphemism widely understood to mean "cadaver") acquired.[4]

Whether Warren was his model in this arena or not, Smith made explicit in his lectures the importance he attached to dissections: "It is of little consequence that a man read anatomy if he cannot have demonstrations. He must have demonstrations to have correct knowledge of the parts. It cannot be obtained from partings, drawings, or reading books."[5] Smith clearly believed that students needed opportunities to do their own dissections. For a prospective doctor, direct experience was the best way to fix the knowledge of anatomy essential to the work of diagnosis and treatment.

Furthermore, Smith insisted on performing autopsies whenever possible, because he understood that such postmortem examinations were the only way to ascertain confidently the cause of death. And just as students needed to do dissections to teach them the anatomy they needed to know for therapeutic purposes, they needed this knowledge of anatomy to enable them to perform autopsies for diagnostic purposes. Only in this manner would they be in a position to correlate autopsy findings with treatments prescribed, in turn the only way they could hope to "improve and perfect" their courses of therapy.[6]

Smith's experience at Harvard under Warren's tutelage would have been re-inforced by what he learned from Cullen (indirectly through Waterhouse) and then—while he was abroad—from Lettsom or some others of his English colleagues and instructors. Certainly A. P. Wilson Philip (whose book on fevers Smith later edited) everywhere showed an abiding interest in pathology. Behind all of this interest, of course, lay the publication in 1761 of Giovanni Battista Morgagni's *On the Seats and Causes of Diseases . . .* , a stunning piece of work that made vividly public for the first time the results of years of anatomical study. Not for nothing is Morgagni (1682–1771) generally considered the father of anatomic pathology.

We have no evidence, direct or indirect, that Nathan Smith read Morgagni. Nonetheless, in his teaching Smith consistently showed his agreement with Morgagni's statement that "[d]ogmatism is easy for the ignorant, but those who have dissected or inspected many bodies have at least learn'd to doubt when the others, who are ignorant of anatomy and do not take the trouble to attend to it are in no doubt at all."[7] Smith's affinity for Morgagni's approach shows him to have had more in common with some other great teachers of the past than he did with the great English physician Thomas Sydenham (1624–1689). For although Sydenham (a great hero of Smith's in other respects, as we shall see in chapter 9) was in many ways well ahead of his time, he was suspicious of the motives of those who insisted on doing autopsies:

Others have more pompously and speciously prosecuted the promoting of this art [Medicine] by searching into the bowels of dead and living creatures, as well sound and diseased, to find out the seeds of disease destroying them, but with how little success such endeavors have been and are likely to be attended, I shall in some measure make appear.[8]

Nathan Smith presented to his students a more modern attitude. Furthermore, he relied on postmortems and dissections for his own continuing education, as we can tell from the way he documented such experiences in his lectures and his writings. John P. Kimball—taking notes during Smith's lecture on his first operation for ovarian dropsy (about which more later)—quoted Smith's explanation of how he came by the necessary confidence to undertake the operation: "I had also had an opportunity to dissect the body of a patient who had died of Ovarian Dropsy after being tapped seven times."[9] Another example appears in a short article called "On Amputation of the Knee-joint." There Smith wrote, "I had often performed the operation on the dead subject, and found that it might be so accomplished as to leave a very good stump."[10]

Smith's anatomy courses were illustrated by as many dissections as circumstances permitted as we can see from the following examples out of Worham L. Fitch's notes:

I dissected an old man who had [osteomyelitis of the hip] from childhood. The joint contained near a pint of matter; near half of the head of the bone was destroyed and it was removed out of its socket and the ligaments much destroyed.

In one case where the lungs of a boy did not appear to be fully inflated I applied my ear to the chest and could hear the air make a hissing noise in the chest. I therefore thought there was an obstruction in the Bronchiae and a dissection confirmed the observation.

A boy had a severe wound of the thigh. The lower portion of the thigh bone turned obliquely outward and stuck through the flesh. . . . [S]ome weeks after this I amputated the limb. On dissection I found the bone partly united. The upper part had passed down nearly to the knee and it was firmly united to the other bone. There was no appearance of ossification only between the two bones where it could do some good.[11]

Thus Smith's students learned that dissections were a way to confirm diagnosis and thereby learn from experience.

Students responded with enthusiasm to the breadth of Smith's experience; one of them, for example, wrote home that he had "notes from the Lectures on the theory and practice . . . which I think will be of great service to me hereafter, as they contain the observations drawn from 20

Augustus Torrey's admission ticket to Nathan Smith's lectures, Dartmouth, 1800. Courtesy of Dartmouth College Library.

years of extensive practice. . . ."[12] Former students of Smith's also frequently attended his anatomy lectures for another round of instruction. Abraham Hedge was one such. Having received his M.B. degree from Dartmouth in 1799, he made a visit to Hanover in late 1800 and then wrote to Lyman Spalding of staying longer than expected to take advantage of an opportunity to witness a dissection: "Dr. Smith had just obtained a subject for dissection, and as I had no urgent business here, I tarried . . . a few days. His lecture rooms were much crowded, he having more, he told me, than ever attended before."[13] One incentive for reappearing at Smith's lectures was that those who had paid for two rounds were permitted to attend free.[14]

Physicians eager to expand their knowledge made such a practice fairly common; in other medical schools, too, for years to come, the audience that witnessed a dissection was as likely to include practicing physicians as students.[15] Likewise, in late 1812, a student wrote from Hanover to his cousin, a doctor in Keene who obviously was interested in observing some of Smith's anatomical lectures:

There are now I believe two subjects in the Anatomical room—The brain of one has been dissected & lectured upon. Nothing farther has been done. The other we have not as yet seen. . . . [N]ot much will probably be done before Friday next, which I think will give you plenty of time to come up, if you are so inclined.[16]

Every great anatomist of the sixteenth and seventeenth centuries was interested in both systematic and morbid anatomy. Thomas Bartholin (1655–1738) pointed to the contrast between the anatomist as natural philosopher, who can limit himself to the exploration of normal structure, and the anatomist as physician, who must derive information useful for his practice from the bodies of the sick.[17] Earlier, something of the key role autopsies could play in understanding disease processes was made evident when the extensive notes of surgical cases and follow-up post-mortem examinations done by the Florentine physician Antonio Beni-vieni (1443[?]–1502) were published posthumously in 1507 under the telling title *On the Hidden Causes of Diseases . . . .*[18] The publication of Morgagni's monumental work more than a century and a half later repre-sented the culmination of efforts at clinical-anatomic correlation, which had originated in casual observations and then had gradually become more deliberate and convincing. And herein lies the eternal contribution of Morgagni: He convinced at least some in the medical profession of the supreme value of morbid anatomy for the advancement of medicine.[19] But for a long time to come, it was left optional whether physicians would use the anatomic method for their investigations of disease.

The problem in Smith's day was that those who wanted to follow Mor-gagni's lead had to face considerable public opposition to the idea of cut-ting up bodies, which in turn led to the enactment of anti-dissection laws. As a result many medical schools did not make a course in practical anatomy a requirement, though most offered such a course even if the in-structors might have to acquire "subjects" for dissection surreptitiously. If necessary, when challenged they would resort to the ruse of claiming the bodies came from out of state—or at least from somewhere other than the local cemeteries.[20]

Historically, outrageous stratagems have at times been used by medical students to get the requisite cadavers. Andreas Vesalius (1514–1564), who revolutionized Western perceptions of human anatomy in 1543 when he published *On the Design of the Human Body*, had his own difficulties getting bodies for dissection, without which he could not have produced his elegant and accurate drawings:

As a medical student in Paris, Vesalius fought off savage dogs while collecting hu-man bones from the Cemetery of the Innocents. In Louvain he stole the remains of a robber chained to the gallows and brought the bones back into the city hidden under his coat. Grave-robbing incidents were reported wherever Vesalius con-ducted his famous lecture-demonstrations. One ingenious group of medical stu-dents obtained a corpse, dressed it, and "walked" their prize into the dissection room as if it were just another drunken student being dragged into class.[21]

That was centuries before Nathan Smith's time. Nonetheless, the general disapprobation for those engaged in "raising" or "snatching" bodies was still very pronounced in the late eighteenth and early nineteenth centuries; for a variety of reasons, the public generally loathed the very idea of anatomical dissection.[22] A peculiar tension existed between those like

Smith, who defended the need for teaching hands-on anatomy, and those whose traditional attitudes—often religiously based—toward death and the corpse, resulted in "an uncertain solicitude towards the corpse and fear of it."[23] By the nineteenth century it was also generally held that the "cemetery offers a celebration of life and death, hope for the dead, and repose for the living."[24] No wonder most people did not want buried bodies (or those awaiting burial) disturbed.[25]

At Dartmouth, it turned out that Smith was in some ways worse off than his colleagues at the other medical schools. Cadavers were more easily obtained in cities, where the unclaimed remains of paupers were available and where the large and numerous cemeteries made it relatively easy to find corpses that would not be missed. In contrast, Hanover was rural, isolated, and thinly populated; if a body were dug up anywhere in the vicinity, everybody would soon know. Consequently, as we shall see, Smith at times hired people to find bodies for him or attempted to get subjects sent to him from Boston. Yet even at Harvard, we are told, "[b]ody snatching was by no means rare. There are no helpful data to describe how bodies for dissection were procured, but some undoubtedly were brought into the state from outside."[26]

One standard method of circumventing the problem was to have cadavers shipped by water from a distant port "pickled" in whiskey barrels; they were less likely to be discovered than if they were brought into town by horse and cart. Details of how this might be done come down to us in an 1830 letter from a doctor who, having apparently solved the problem well enough to be of assistance to others, wrote to a medical colleague as follows:

It will give me pleasure to render you any assistance in regard to subjects. I think you may rely upon having them. I shall immediately *invoke* Frank, our body-snatcher (a better never lifted spade), and confer with him on the matter. We get them here without any difficulty at present but I would not [for] the world that any but ourselves should know that I have winked at their being sent out of [state?].

I will cause three to be put up in barrels [of] whiskey, I suppose they will require about half a barrel each, of whiskey. This at 35 cts a gallon will be about $16.80. The barrels a dollar each; the subjects, the putting up, etc. $10. each making in all $50.00.[27]

Nathan Smith does not appear ever to have been quite so open about his procurements, and he tried to keep as much out of the messy business as he could. Among those he relied on to help him were students, as we shall see; one who became especially adept, apparently, was Amos Twitchell. Henry I. Bowditch, in his memoir of Twitchell, reported that "Dr. Smith depended almost wholly . . . upon his young and ardent friend [Twitchell] for the procurement of subjects for dissection. . . . For many

ANOTHER GRAVE-YARD PLUNDERED. The burying ground in West Haven, was entered on Saturday evening last, and robbed of the corpse of a young lady of 19 years, who had been dead about ten days. The fact was soon discov-

Headline from the 15 January 1824 New Haven Pilot.
Courtesy of Beinecke Rare Book and Manuscript Library, Yale University.

years he labored thus a great deal for Dr. Smith."[28] The concern about finding cadavers for dissection was to remain with Smith from the beginning to the end of his career. Trouble with "anatomy riots" in Hanover (to be discussed shortly) and public attitudes toward "digging and dissecting"[29] would eventually prove to be a factor in Smith's decision to move to New Haven. He wrote pessimistically on one occasion to Lyman Spalding, saying: "I hope . . . I shall live to see the dearth of anatomical & surgical knowledge which has so long hung over our land done away & those who undertake the cure of diseases instead of being [called] the tormentors of the unfortunate & the afflictors of the afflicted become the benefactors of Mankind & justify the gratitude of succeeding generations."[30]

But the problem persisted, and Smith would continue to be agitated much of his time at Yale over what he saw as public misunderstanding of the issues. He expressed concern more than once about changes in the Connecticut laws that were being contemplated, as, for instance, when he wrote the following to Mills Olcott in mid-1819: "Our Legislature [Connecticut] did not quite pass the Law which was to hang all the Doctors but they came so near it, as to strike a death blow to the Institution by the prosecutions &c. which has lead [sic] me to contemplate a removal from this place . . . whether it will be to the east or south I am not determined."[31]

Whether Smith was worried primarily about the medical school or about his own reputation—and whether he was right to be so concerned—is difficult to assess fairly at this late date. It cannot have helped set his mind at ease when, in the aftermath of one grave-robbing episode a few years later, a search warrant was served on his Yale colleague Jonathan Knight. When a body was then found at the medical school, public outrage expressed itself in nightly rioting for much of a week.[32]

Smith was by no means alone in his concerns. In a circular letter prepared at the behest of the Massachusetts Medical Society and issued to

Fellows of the Society in 1829, Abel Lawrence Peirson and his colleagues on the appointed committee took a bold line: "It is time that the facts upon this subject be laid before the public—that the wants of the profession be fairly and distinctly stated,—and the science of Anatomy rescued from degradation and persecution."[33]

But support from fellow physicians neither sufficed to remove the stigma nor produced bodies. Smith does not appear ever to have developed so thick a skin or as blasé an attitude as some other doctor-anatomists. (Remarkable stories exist of physicians who bragged about their skill in getting hold of bodies—thanks largely to "resurrectionists" and "sack-'em-up men"—and were not embarrassed about the need to consort with and rely on such typically low-life characters.[34]) Things got much better (from Smith's point of view) in 1824, when—after the riot against doctors and medical students in New Haven just referred to—Connecticut passed a law that specifically allowed medical students to take possession of unclaimed corpses from its prisons.[35] But that all lay far in the future.

Smith was by no means the first or only physician in the new country to use autopsies and their results widely in his own teaching. Within five years of the appearance of Morgagni's masterpiece, Dr. Thomas Bond was explaining in his introductory lecture the uses of autopsies, among which were learning from one's own errors and saving others from the same.[36]

Like Bond, Smith autopsied every case he could, from early in his teaching career. In his day book for 1798, for instance, one entry shows a charge of $8.00 to a Mr. Roberts of Strafford "to visit attendance and dissecting the Body of his Daughter"[37] (unfortunately, he noted neither the reason for the autopsy nor the findings). To what extent his students appreciated the opportunities Smith put in their way we do not know. But in 1808 he took steps that would shift the focus of attention away from those who procured the cadavers to those who used them to teach. Nathan Smith hired a specialist in anatomy to join him at Dartmouth Medical School.

Visiting Anatomist: Alexander Ramsay

When his school of medicine was barely a decade old, Smith arranged to bring to Dartmouth a famous but extremely controversial Scottish anatomist, Alexander Ramsay (1754–1824). As it turned out, Ramsay—who had first come to the United States around 1805—lasted only one term at Dartmouth (and no longer in most of the several other places where he taught from South Carolina to Maine[38]). His presence can hardly have done much to reassure the general public about what was going on at the medical school. Though anatomy might be regarded as "the queen of the medical sciences, the subject around which much medical education revolved," it also continued to be "a source of considerable conflict between doctors and the public" and was "popularly considered slightly disreputable."[39]

Against this background, Smith's move to add a full-time anatomist to the medical faculty in Hanover made a dramatic statement. Furthermore, there were features of Ramsay's reputation, quite apart from his being an anatomist, that would hardly make him an appealing addition to the community. For starters, there was his physical appearance. Not only was he extremely short (accounts vary, but he probably was barely five feet tall); he had a great humped back, and—according to one writer—"the whole man seemed thrown together by nature in a fit or whim of negligence." He was widely considered a strange character. To "the mass of those who met him in life," he was remembered as "a sort of monstrous compound of personal deformity, immense learning . . . ferocious insolence and ill-temper, and inordinate vanity."[40]

Furthermore, he had a notoriously egocentric style. James Rush, son of the eminent Benjamin Rush, was among those who heard Ramsay lecture in Philadelphia in the term before the Scotsman went to Hanover. Years later, young Rush scribbled a few trenchant remarks about his teachers at the University of Pennsylvania during 1807–08 on the back of the lecture admission tickets he had saved. He described his experience of Ramsay as a teacher thus:

This Alexander Ramsay was a little, big headed—crookspined—ham bo[ne] shin[n]ed short legged—abortive, rickett spoiled quack of a philosopher who, as a painter's boy was employed to paint the anatomic theatre at Edinburgh, and thinking himself cut out for an anatomist, took up the study; came to Philadelphia in 1807 and delivered a course of foolishness. He was a good specimen of bodily, mental and moral distortion.[41]

Given the insulting way young Rush characterized a whole array of his instructors (only his father escaped his biting criticism), one has to balance his description of Ramsay against what others said. At Dartmouth, William Tully's observations (both before and after he heard the visitor's first lecture), though by no means unqualifiedly complimentary—we know Tully!—were more measured. "Doctor Ramsay has arrived, and I have this day had a view of him," Tully wrote in his journal:

He is a rickety fellow, not four feet high, but with a face large enough, and a body big enough-round, for a man of 7 feet. The hump on his back is as large as a Pedlar's-Wallet, and his legs are semi-circles. He has a mighty commanding air, however, and his looks seem to say, "stand off, for I am holier than Thou." Tomorrow evening, as a pompous advertisement in the Dartmouth Gazette says, he is to deliver "hints, on Medical Education at Rowley's Assembly-Hall." The ladies, and what not, are all invited. I hope none of them that calculate to attend are in a way of being like to "Tumble to pieces"; for if they are, I tremble for the consequence. I do not do right, however, to run on this way, for Dr. Ramsay, I suppose, is one of the first anatomists and physiologists in the world, though I am told a petulant disposition nearly spoils his usefulness. Dr. Smith will, undoubtedly, manage well enough with him, but most people think the wilderness of Fryburgh, [Maine,] where he has actually pitched his tent, is the most proper place for him.[42]

Many of those who studied under Ramsay considered him, unequivocally, "a human anatomist, second to none of his time, . . . a teacher never to be excelled."[43] The fact that he was said, when at a patient's bedside, never to have missed a chance "to speak of fellow practitioners as 'murderers and vile Hottentots'"[44] cannot have endeared him to colleagues. But Smith, who had a fine relationship with other physicians, seems not to have been at all fazed by reports that Ramsay was a curmudgeon who had set the medical faculties in several British cities on edge. In fact, one source on Ramsay goes out of his way to say that the "only man I ever knew who managed Ramsay properly, was Dr. Nathan Smith . . . . When he was waspish, Smith laughed at him, and when good-natured recounted what he had done to others, and approved all approvable things in and about him."[45]

Another side to Ramsay's character and temperament is exhibited in his response to a request in 1818 from Lyman Spalding. In what we would call a letter of recommendation, Ramsay wrote a detailed (even excessively gracious) "Certificate" on Spalding's behalf, which included the following:

[At] Dartmouth College, Dr. Spalding acted as my assistant & friend, with that ability which claimed my confidence & respect. He filled the same responsible office when I taught the Institute in New York 1817 with that increased ability, which drew from the pupils the warmest acknowledgements and my unbounded approbation. . . . Dr Spaldings character in my estimation, unites every property which lay[s] claim to the confidence & encouragement of his country.[46]

Why this eccentric anatomist should have chosen to teach in the frontier "wilderness"is unclear; he must have been "more than visionary, to believe that from a country village like Fryeburg . . . he could exercise any permanent influence upon American medicine."[47] Though all seem to have agreed about both his talent and his irascibility, he was beyond doubt an inspiration to some. Usher Parsons, a Maine boy destined to become one of the leading lights of Rhode Island medicine, went out of his way to take Ramsay's course in 1809, having been encouraged to do so in turn by another enthusiastic medical student, Abiel Hall, who studied anatomy under Ramsay in 1808.[48]

Ramsay was famous for his collection of anatomical specimens (his "museum") as well as for his knowledge of anatomy, which came at least in part from the work done preparing the museum specimens. Smith was eager to expand the faculty at Dartmouth; he was bound to regard having persuaded Ramsay to come to Hanover to teach anatomy as a coup, not least because it meant he could share the responsibility for the procurement of "subjects." He continued to work on the issue himself, however. Just prior to the beginning of Ramsay's course, Smith wrote to Lyman Spalding to inquire about the possibility of his providing certain very particular specimens.[49] A month later, after Ramsay had arrived at Dartmouth, Smith wrote Spalding again: "If you want to contrive it as to bring with you a subject it would be very important to us, at this time."[50] Obviously, he was not turning his back completely on the nasty business of worrying about the supply of cadavers.

It was between the two courses in Fryeburg attended by Abiel Hall and Usher Parsons that Ramsay went to Dartmouth. He was scheduled to give a course on natural theology as well as his anatomical lectures, according to Tully. (This might seem odd except that Ramsay, a deeply religious man, is said to have seen it as his mission in life to " 'justify the ways of God to man' by means of anatomy and the allied sciences."[51] This got him into trouble later, when he taught briefly at Fairfield Medical College. There "he was soon detested for introducing religious discussions into his medical lectures."[52])

Ramsay's opening public lecture at Dartmouth on a nonmedical topic was where Tully was initially exposed to Ramsay's style, and where his impressions of the visiting anatomist were acquired. The next day, after hearing the first of the anatomy lectures, he confided the following to his journal:

I am convinced, from Ramsay's lecture last evening and that of to day, that the little man is an original. He has advanced a great many old ideas, but in a strange dress, and a great many as strange as the form in which they were presented. . . . I can't possibly find fault with the two specimens that we have had of this Edinburgh man, on the ground of his diction's being too colloquial. He is so full of his technics, his *non Pareils*, his *fauxpas*, and the like that, together with his Scotch dialect and accent which he sometimes uses, I question whether two thirds of his Class understand him fully.

For my part, I rejoice that I understand Latin and Greek and have a smattering of French, else I should be quite in the dark.[53]

Once again, we learn almost as much from the journal about its self-satisfied author and his character as we do about his ostensible subject. A month later, although conceding that "Ramsay gives us information by his very extensive Anatomical-Museum and his lectures," Tully could not resist adding that "we have found he is a pettulant, conceited, ranting fellow." Summing up his views of the moment on his instructors, he says, "One [Smith] I like much, and the other [Ramsay] is by no means deficient in powers of mind, or scholarship, but he makes a fool of himself."[54] Thus, we see two students—James Rush and William Tully—from two different medical schools and at different times essentially agreeing about Ramsay's unpleasantness, and only one of the two granting (somewhat grudgingly) that there was much to be learned from the man.

Why would Smith have taken the trouble to bring such a character to Dartmouth? (This was, incidentally, very much Smith's own project, not Dartmouth's. He paid Ramsay's salary of $1,000 himself, borrowing money from Mills Olcott to do so.[55]) In Ramsay, Smith had a colleague of prodigious energy and enthusiasm when it came to doing anatomy, and he was apparently more impressed by reports of Ramsay's skill as an anatomist than he was put off by the potential difficulties of dealing with an eccentric. He may also have welcomed the prospect of having on hand someone known to be a lightning rod for controversy. If Ramsay could not only teach anatomy but absorb whatever ill will lingered in the community on the sensitive matter of the "cutting up of bodies," Smith would be relieved of considerable pressure.

Smith's first thought was to arouse the interest (and assistance) of his first apprentice and colleague, long since in practice for himself. In September 1808, he wrote to Lyman Spalding:

You will see by the advertisement with which I am troubling you, what I am doing for Dartmouth College. I have, at great expense, engaged Dr. Ramsay the greatest anatomist in the world to give a complete Course of Lectures on Anatomy and Physiology, to instruct in the art of dissecting, making anatomical preparations, etc. I am very confident that our ensuing course will far exceed anything of the kind before attempted in New England. Therefore, if you have any young friends in the medical line be so kind as to send them as soon as possible. I wish you to [have] the following advertisement published two weeks in your Portsmouth paper:

"Medical Lectures at Dartmouth College. The course of Chemistry will commence as usual by Doct. Smith, on the first wednesday in October.

Doct. Ramsay, from Edinburgh, has consented to give one course of Anatomy & Physiology, as given by him, at his Theatre, in Edinburgh, at Columbia College in New York, and his present school in Fryeburgh.—In this second course, Doct Ramsay will commence his Anatomical demonstrations & doctrines of Physiology, Pathology, &c. on the second week of November next—and will continue his course two months.

Doct. Ramsay's Anatomical Museum will be transported from Fryeburgh, to Dartmouth College, for the benefit of those who may attend; and will not be returned to Fryeburgh until the expiration of this course of Anatomical Lectures.—Gentlemen will be permitted to study the subjects of the Museum & demonstrate them to each other, on saturdays, as at Doct. R's school in Fryeburgh; on paying an additional fee of ten dollars. [S]uch Gentlemen, as evince a thirst for knowledge, will be admitted to the private closet of Doctors Smith & Ramsay, as Assistants in composing a Museum for Doct. Smith. Doct. Smith will give a compleat course of practical surgery, founded on the principles of Anatomy & Physiology; and will close his course with Lectures on the practice of Physic.

On the Gentleman, who shall produce the best dissections and demonstrations of the Organs of Vision, Hearing, Brain & Heart, at Dartmouth College; Doct. Ramsay will bestow a gold medal, as given to his pupils in Edinburgh; and as proposed to his pupils, in Fryeburgh, to be adjudged by Doct. Smith."[56]

Spalding dutifully made the arrangements, and the notice appeared in the *Portsmouth Oracle* for 1 October 1808.[57] Spalding also apparently located a prospective pupil, for a week later Nathan Smith wrote him again:

You may inform Mr. Taft that Dr. Ramsay is in my opinion the best anatomist in the United States.[58] I have seen his anatomical preparations & have heard him lecture;[59] . . . The plan we have chalked out [is] to make me a complete museum & will require a number of subjects. Therefore wish if possible that you would lay by a few for me. An infant with the Placenta [attached] would be very agreeable. I think [one] from six to ten or from ten to 18 would be very usefull or an adult subject would not be amiss. If any of this kind of gentry can be obtained you can preserve them very easily by opening the cavities & injecting a few veins. Just turn down the scalp & saw out a piece of the skull on one side so as to admit the spirit & so with the other cavities.[60]

Shortly after Ramsay arrived in Hanover, Smith wrote Spalding yet again, urging him to consider taking direct advantage of the fantastic opportunity about to unfold in Hanover:

Dr. Ramsay has a very extensive & useful collection of anatomical preparations which will exceed your expectations. You will also be highly pleased with his mode of teaching. . . . We shall commence a new era of anatomy at this time & after being instructed in the best method of dissecting & preserving preparations shall go on improving our stock, & if you will contribute raw material we will when ever we have duplicates give you them in preference to any other person.[61]

Smith was apparently pleased at the way things were going. With mounting excitement, he wrote to George Shattuck later in the same month: "I have a prospect of procuring a very handsome set of anatomical preparations, in season to use them [in] the ensuing course of lectures; if I succeed I shall have a better collection than there is this side of Philadelphia."[62]

Shattuck probably did not go to Hanover, but Spalding did. A letter he wrote to a friend includes a wonderfully detailed description of Ramsay's teaching methods:

Doct. Ramsay, the present lecturer on Anatomy is from Edinburgh, and undoubtedly the best [anatomist] in America, certainly the best I have ever seen. He is perfectly master of his art, never at a loss either in his lecture or in his dissecting rooms. He obliges us all to attend to the minutia of Anatomy, to dissect and demonstrate for ourselves and this is the only way to learn the art and not be hearing dismal psalm tune lectures of what has been seen. The Doctor's mode of lecturing is impressing and at the same time persuasive, he is all fire and animation while speaking, chaining down your attention, and carrying you along with him convincing you of the truth of his doctrines by demonstrative facts.

Doct. R. is now engaged in making an Anatomical museum for Mr. Professor Smith; this gives us an advantage over those who shall follow us, for we are all obliged to labour with our own hands at these preparations; in fact the rooms are an immense workshop, you see every kind of anatomical manufacturing going on, & can work on such preparations as you think most for your improvement. Then you know we learn more by doing ourselves than by seeing others do, or simply viewing the work after it is done. We to be sure have the advantage of inspecting and studying Doct. Ramsay's museum which consists of more than one hundred choice anatomical preparations. I hope Sir to be able to bring home with me a specimen of my work, to convince you that I have not been idle & mispent my time.[63]

On the same day Spalding was writing the above, Smith was writing to Shattuck with obvious satisfaction over the whole arrangement: "Dr. Ramsay has commenced his lectures with much applause and I think him a very able anatomist. Being relieved from anatomy I shall be able to do better justice to the other branches so that Dartmouth will not sink this year."[64]

This happy note notwithstanding, and despite a promise from Smith that he would engage Ramsay for a second round of lectures if more students would sign up,[65] Ramsay did not teach at Hanover again. Smith's ability to get along amicably with Ramsay was not enough to hold the restless and annoying Scot; he clearly really wanted an "Institute" of his own.[66] He never stayed—or repeated a course of lectures—anywhere except at his own school in Fryeburg, and thus his abandonment of the scene in Hanover is no discredit to either Smith or Dartmouth. What it did mean, however, was that the challenges and problems of teaching anatomy were fully back in Smith's lap in 1809.

Ramsay spent his last years lecturing (for the most part privately) in Maine, and trying to dispose of his museum. No one wanted to pay what he thought it was worth. If he did not die a broken and forgotten man, he was at least disappointed; history remembers him in part for the beauty of his anatomical drawings,[67] to be sure, but perhaps equally for his eccentric manner and the oft-repeated esteem in which Nathan Smith held him. His brief career at Dartmouth is perhaps best summed up by the remark one student made in a letter in the spring following Ramsay's teaching stint at Dartmouth. "You wished to know how Dr. Ramsay is esteemed in this place," John Bontell wrote to Andrew Mack. "Tho' it is generally difficult to give general opinions, perhaps, I may say he was esteemed a *good* Anatomist, but vain, petulent, and a despiser of everything that was American."[68] Yet this is not the way Ramsay saw himself. In an address he gave in New York in 1818, reminiscing about his experience there in 1807, he observed, "I ranked the ingenious practitioner as my attendant, and the learned host of lovers of their country as my friends."[69] More than one way to take Ramsay's measure exists; he remains something of an enigma.

Nonetheless, Smith seems to have been well pleased with the way things went at Dartmouth during Ramsay's one term there. In a letter to Shattuck urging him (unsuccessfully, as it turned out) to do what he could to get Ramsay a position at Harvard, Smith spoke happily of the benefits— to Dartmouth and to him personally—of Ramsay's short stay.

Dr. Ramsay has just closed his course of lectures in this College which have been delivered much to the satisfaction of all concerned. Dr. Ramsay has begun a new era in our College in relation to Anatomy and Physiology and has put it in my power to do more in that science than I knew how to do before.[70]

Anatomy Riots

That anyone would want to steal bodies from their newly dug graves is an idea difficult to take seriously today; the very thought of "body snatching" or "resurrecting" bodies seems grotesque. But two centuries ago, the whole business of the "resurrectionists" made more apparent sense. Physicians everywhere, despite the risks, were beginning to study systematic pathology as the basis for their treatments. The professor of anatomy "in almost every medical school in 18th- and early 19th-century America had to face charges, usually verbal but sometimes delivered by armed mobs, that he engaged in grave-robbing to get materials for classroom dissections."[71]

In this hostile environment, after Ramsay had left, Smith resumed teaching the anatomy course in 1809. Thanks to a young student—Ezekiel Dodge Cushing—an avid letter-writer who arrived in Hanover that term, we have an account of how the teaching of anatomy proceeded in the months following Ramsay's departure. From a wealthy Salem (Massachusetts) shipping family, Cushing followed his experience at Dartmouth Medical School with study in Philadelphia under Dr. Rush and Dr. Physick (it was Cushing who wrote home praising Smith in comparison to those two famous teachers); later he studied in England under Sir Astley Cooper, making him more widely educated than many of his contemporaries. Cushing's early death deprived him of the opportunity to make much of a name for himself, but enough of his correspondence remains to give insights into his character and to hint at what he might have become.[72]

Cushing's correspondence includes a letter to his father vividly describing an "anatomy riot" in Hanover in which he played a central role (rather against his will and better judgment, it appears), and subsequent letters contain numerous references to the subject. If it is true, as seems probable, that this case helped stimulate the action of John Collins Warren and the Massachusetts Medical Society that led to passage (in 1831) of the model Massachusetts law making human dissection legal (a similar law was enacted in New Hampshire in 1833), there is added historical significance to this episode in Hanover.

Young Cushing's description of what transpired is graphic, and worth quoting at length because it shows so well what prospective doctors and their instructors faced:

I wrote you concerning the advice which I presumed you would think I wanted for my conduct in the medical lectures or in that part of them which treated of Anatomy. As you did not take the hint which I was afraid to give openly for fear my letter should be opened at the Post Office here, I was forced to act according to the best of judgement. In this part of the country the people are so enraged to the distance of fifty miles around that it is as much as one's life is worth to attempt getting a subject for dissection. Under these circumstances, and considering that the law was much more severe here than in Massachusetts, the penalty being $2000. fine, two years imprisonment, setting on the gallows, 50 lashes; from what I considered prudence but some called cowardice, I declined being engaged in any undertaking of the kind. And to get clear honorably, I proposed to the medical class for each one to contribute so much as would be sufficient to undertake this business, this was accordingly done, and a subject procured about a week ago. The very night it was procured [the undergraduates hired by the medical students] were by the suspicion of a woman at the tollgate so far put off their gard [sic], by her close questions that they lost their senses almost and the one that paid the toll in making change took out his pocketbook and left it at the toll-house, it contained a letter without a signature addressed to the students who left the pocketbook. [The authorities] instantly began searching the grave yard pointed out in the letter, and yesterday found that a boy of 10 years of age was gone. This morning they arrived at about 6 and with a sheriff demanded leave to search for the body, they had in the night set a guard to every window and every door leading to the lecture room. Dr. Smith wished me to attend the sheriff in the search and saying that to my prudence he committed the conducting of the whole affair, he was scared almost to death. The body was thrown into a closet which was rather concealed a little in the wall as we could not remove it. I had as lives [sic] be at home as undertake the office, Sylvester and I attended the sheriff in his search, he was an intelligent man and would not have searched much if he had been alone but there was two with him, he had to do his business thoroughly, to make short of a long story after a long search they found it. During the search I had, to conceal my feelings, been reading. When they had found it . . . the men threatened to destroy the anatomical museum and to open the door and let in their companions for that purpose. I refused to do it and one of them took up an ax and threatened to knock me over. I told him that if he valued his own life to be quiet for the students without if they made the least disturbance would tear them limb from limb and deliberately unbuttoned my coat to let them see the doctor's pistols in my jacket pocket, that stilled them.[73]

Smith also wrote at least one letter (a few months later) with a passing reference to the same "riot," to Lyman Spalding, giving us another perspective on it. Apologizing for dilatoriness in his correspondence with a comment about "much business together with a little bad luck," Smith added that he had "obtained a Truce for a time." He went on to explain:

Towards the close of our last course of Lectures I contracted with a certain person to go to Boston to procure, if possible, a Cadaver. But instead of going to Boston he went to Enfield [about ten miles from Hanover], as it appears, & procured a subject, which was taken by an Officer when about half dissected. The circumstances made a prodigious bustle for a time & gave me great inquietude but I believe we shall survive the accident without material injury either personal or to the Institution.[74]

Smith thus acknowledged having hired someone to get a "subject" for him, but he did not bother to point out how he relied on a student to handle "the whole affair" once the sheriff arrived on the scene.

Yet another view of the situation comes from a letter that Ebenezer Adams (of the Dartmouth College faculty) wrote to George Shattuck, a friend of his as well as of Smith:

But for the present the Medical department occupies all our attention. The public mind is extremely agitated, and with sufficient reason, with regard to a subject taken up for dissection. Fortunately Dr. Smith is, in this instance, in a great measure free from the imputation of blame. He had contracted with one of his pupils, and given him a letter to you upon the subject [recall that Smith told Spalding he intended the student to get a "subject" in Boston—apparently he was counting on Shattuck to help]. The pupil to save expense, took [one] up in a nearby town, kept it 3 or 4 days, and then brought it forward for dissection. The body was missed from the grave, search was made, and [it was] the body of a lad 9 years of age, of a very reputable family. Some abuse and insult offered by the students to those, who came in search of the body, irritated to a high degree the public resentment already justly very great. What will be the issue I know not, but I think it must either overset the institution, or at any rate work as an effectual cure for the evil.[75]

By the middle of December, Cushing could write to his mother that all was well for the present:

We have had quiet times here lately. The scholars of College have mostly gone off and we find it easy to pacify the enraged people [for the dissection of the local boy]. One of the Medical Students has had a trial and is bound over to the Supreme Court in May in bonds of 1000$ and there are nine men gone different routs to apprehend another who has fled for his life.[76]

Smith at least rallied round to help the students. In the case of Ruggles Sylvester (the student responsible for digging up the body of the boy in Enfield in the first place, Cushing's companion in the search instigated by the sheriff, and the one Cushing told his mother was bound over to the court), this meant paying Mills Olcott to go to court with the accused. A $10 charge against Nathan Smith appears in Olcott's personal ledger "to attending at the examination of Ruggles Sylvester for digging up a dead body at your request . . . and arguing same."[77]

In Cushing's case, Smith wrote to George Shattuck to advise the young man in this business, which dragged on for months. Indeed, more than a year after the near-riot described above, Ezekiel Dodge Cushing "made solemn oath" on November 18, 1810, before Benjamin Gilbert, Justice of the Peace for Grafton County (New Hampshire), protesting his absolute innocence, and in January of 1811 he added a note to the end of a letter home, "How does my law suit come?"[78] Since his deposition (see below) utterly fails to discuss what happened in the lecture room or the role he admitted to his father that he had played in proposing how the medical students should obtain a "subject" at the end of the previous autumn's course of lectures, it is possible he was being deposed in connection with a second (more recent) charge. That seems unlikely, however; surely he would have gone out of his way to avoid a second encounter with the law so soon after the first. On the other hand, if his statement was occasioned by the earlier event, there is—to put it mildly—considerable room to question the veracity of what he did say to the Justice of the Peace, particularly in light of a letter he had written to his sister in mid-February 1810 (that is, between the time of the raid and the time he was deposed). To her he wrote as follows:

I have been very much engaged in anatomical studies and believe that I have proved that I was not concerned in vain in digging up the body of Daniel Doyle, I am now making some anatomical preparations which it is impossible to tell what I shall do with, when done, as our mother would have a "pigeon fit" if she but saw them once. . . . I have this moment returned from the dissecting room, where there are at present the remains of fifteen of our fellow creatures in every stage of decay, and of all ages, sexes and colours, to ease myself from the labors and fatigues of the day by writing to you.[79]

Even if some of that letter was composed with the intention of shocking, even offending, his sister, it is hard to square its contents with the deposition he supplied the court nine months later. There he swore as follows:

I did not during this journey [neither the time nor the place of the journey is mentioned, unfortunately], nor have I ever at any other time, procured any human body for dissection nor have I caused or known it to be done by others either in Boston or its vicinity; that Doctor Nathan Smith, or any other person have not at any time either directly or indirectly requested me to procure a subject or subjects for dissection either from Boston or any other place; that no one has ever given me money, or in any way engaged to give me money to obtain any subject whatever; and that I do not recollect that Doctor Smith did ever speak to me relative thereto.[80]

The ever-helpful and supportive Shattuck wrote directly to Cushing, two weeks after he had been thus deposed:

I have not been idle in relation to the contents of your letter, though in despite of all my efforts to prevent it you are indicted by the Grand Jury for an attempt to raise the dead. I have consulted Mr. Blake about what you ought to do in relation to appearing in Boston for trial. He thinks it advisable that you come into town: otherwise a warrant will be issued . . . . It is true you may avoid being taken by concealing [yourself] at Hanover or going into Vermont — but it will make more noise, and the rumors will be the most unpleasant part of the business. Mr. Blake says the probable extent of punishment will not exceed a fine of twenty dollars . . . . Both the Board of Health and the Grand Jury now believe Dr. Smith entirely free from implication in the late attacks on the nights of September.[81]

Regarding further details on the case and its outcome, Smith remained silent. We have only Cushing's allusion to Smith's having said he behaved admirably; no evidence of any written word of thanks from Smith to Cushing appears to have survived.

In view of the controversy the whole issue of body procurement in Hanover tended to arouse, Cushing seems surprisingly unconcerned in the weeks following the "riot." Perhaps he was merely naive, assuming he would not be called to legal account. Just after Christmas of that year (1809), he wrote to his father, reporting "I received yours of the tenth instant, and am happy to inform you that at present we are tolerably quiet, about digging up people. The anatomical lectures have been rather dry, from our misfortune with regard to subjects."[82] A few months later he again wrote home, saying, "If I should die I should make an excellent subject for I have fed so much on salt meat that I should be sufficiently preserved."[83]

The next autumn, not yet having had to testify, Cushing was optimistic and upbeat: "All things go on well as yet and from appearances it is probable that we shall have no difficulty from the lectures this year."[84] Only a few weeks later, however—ten days after he had given his deposition— Cushing's mood had turned somewhat more defiant: "The lectures have been peaceable entirely so here, and the rumbling of distant thunder is all we have had to disturb us, whether it will burst on our heads I cannot tell, and only inform you that armed with conscious innocence, we feel ready to meet its vengeance. . . ."[85]

In the aftermath of the unsavory reputation that attached to the medical school after the body-snatching episode in which Cushing was involved, President John Wheelock undertook to exercise his authority (with the help of his Board of Trust) over student discipline in the medical school. How effective this was is unclear: "[T]he Medical Department continued to function more or less independently," not least because "relations between the two faculties were often strained."[86] Certainly a degree of notoriety attached to Nathan Smith's school. In early 1810, when Smith was seeking public monies to build a "Medical House" (see chapter 8), an extract of an angry letter "from Grafton County [where Hanover is located]," was published in the *Concord [N.H.] Gazette*. The portion of the letter that appeared in the paper began bluntly enough: "Ever since the dead bodies were found in the lecture hall [at Dartmouth] . . ."; it ended in outraged opposition to having state funds support Smith and the medical school. "What say they," cried the irate letter-writer, "are we to be taxed for the purpose of giving Dr. Smith 3 or 4000 dollars to build a slaughter house?"[87]

The strain of obtaining cadavers by dangerous and illegal methods weighed heavily on Smith. By a little later that same year—1810—he was sputtering about wanting to leave Hanover (as we shall see in chapter 11). One reason was his fear that the New Hampshire legislature might "enact laws which will inflict corporeal punishment on any person who is concerned in digging or dissecting."[88] Yet life in the anatomy department was not always problematic. On some occasions, things went well, as a letter Smith wrote to Shattuck eighteen months after his outburst about possibly leaving testifies: "We were very fortunate in obtaining subjects and have dissected three [in our present anatomy course] who were all pretty good."[89]

Even so, when Nathan Smith moved to Yale Medical School in 1813, one of the first difficulties to bother the new faculty there was the dearth of "subjects." At Yale, procurement and the attendant problems should have been the concern of Dr. Jonathan Knight, to whom Smith had turned over the teaching of anatomy. But Smith himself, as professor of surgery, was of course also very much concerned with the problem and could not altogether escape responsibility for finding bodies. He was promptly called upon for help:

We have had a little of the old Hanover spirit [i.e., "resurrections"] here this winter but having seen a little service & not being so immediately concerned, I did not feel quite so much as I had done before. But Dr. Knight and myself were both summoned to give in evidence what we knew on the subject. I told Dr. Knight to go on and as I had patients on the way I would be there soon, but he had so much reliance on my former experience in such cases that I could not prevail on him to go an inch without me. So I had to go on & meet the mob in town meeting who treated us with great civility and as it so happened, that I knew nothing of the matter & having bowed very respectfully to those we hate they [suffered?] me [to] depart &

appeared very well satisfied. . . . The business . . . has terminated without any serious injury only we had to meet a Committy on the subject.[90]

This was not the only incident. Another occurred in 1818, for example; Nathan Smith wrote to Lyman Spalding that "of late owing to some headstrong & unforesighted young men in procuring subjects we have been brought into much trouble & perplexity . . . ."[91] And in 1824, there was trouble again. Smith wrote to Olcott at the end of January:

Just at the commencement of the vacation another affair took place which has given us as much trouble. Some foolish & rash fellow went to West Haven about 20 miles from this [place] & took a female subject from the ground it was discovered & found in the deep cellar of the medical building where it had been placed by the person who got it . . . without the knowledge of the Faculty. This raised a mob who broke more than 100 panes of glass in the building before they could be dispersed.

Within a month, however, he could begin to relax, writing reassuringly to Olcott that "the storm seems to be past [sic] by & all is now quiet."[92]

If Smith himself (instead of Ezekiel Cushing) had been indicted in 1809, it is possible that he would have been in sufficient trouble with both college and law-enforcement authorities to destroy his effectiveness as a teacher (even if not as a physician). On the other hand, an indictment might also have left us with information that would have helped us understand better how he managed to accomplish so much as a teacher of anatomy despite the stumbling blocks. As it was, so-called anatomy riots were few and far between in Hanover, perhaps because Nathan Smith's contacts in Boston and elsewhere enabled him most of the time to arrange for shipments of cadavers from "away." Perhaps his students learned to avoid collecting bodies too close to home even when they (or their hired accomplices) did resort to grave-robbing. Or perhaps he was unusually adept at getting others (Twitchell and Cushing as students, Ramsay and Knight as colleagues) to handle the necrological, resurrectionist activities found in every anatomy department of that day. Though public attitudes were changing, the problems persisted for a very long time.[93] Teaching the subject involved too much detailed study for a few varnished exhibits to help much, and the best "Anatomical Museum" in the world—even when coupled with brilliant lectures—was not a solution.

CHAPTER SEVEN

Students, Colleagues, and Friends

I went to Dartmouth College and there pursued the study of medicine under Dr Smith in whose praise as a man of genius and science too much cannot be said. —SAMUEL ELDER [1]

N ATHAN SMITH stands out among the pioneers of American medicine as a doctor with a knack for accurately appraising prevailing ideas, correctly advocating treatments of diverse ailments, and emphasizing the importance of uncovering new truths. Another special quality was his ability to capture the devotion of students and to impart a zeal for improving both the lot of the patient and the state of the profession. Even a partial roster of Smith's students makes his success as a teacher manifest.

One factor in the affection for and loyalty to Nathan Smith of many of his students may have been that he was not so busy, distracted, and over-involved as another of the period's outstanding physicians: Benjamin Rush. Often portrayed as the very paradigm of early American medical educators, Rush was a person of great talent, and he had the advantage over Smith of practicing and teaching in the thriving metropolis of Philadelphia (a very public figure, Rush was a signer of the Declaration of Independence). He taught classes of up to five hundred well-prepared young men from all over the country, in the country's first and—by every measure—premier medical school.

Smith, in contrast, even at the height of his Dartmouth career, was lecturing to only sixty to one hundred largely unlettered, backwoods students; nor when he moved to New Haven was he much closer to the center of national affairs. Still, he had distinct advantages of his own. Raised in a farming community on the fringes of civilization, he was very much a student of nature; his insistence on learning from direct observation saved him from Rush's rigid dogmatism. Smith was also able to sift and synthesize what he read in the great thinkers of the past, what he was taught at Harvard, and what he heard from the theorists in Edinburgh during his study abroad. He had an unmatched ability to extract from the words of these authorities what was applicable to contemporary life and rural medicine.

In some important ways, studying medicine was not markedly easier two hundred years ago than it is now, even if there was much less to learn. Surgery, which followed anatomy, exposed students to a kind of suffering they were unlikely to have anticipated, suffering often caused as much by the physician with his knife and saw as by disease; the consequent infection, "laudable pus," and secondary healing also caused pain. Iatrogenic misery in Nathan Smith's day was as often as not the result of actions based on wild surmise. The septicemia (colloquially called "blood poisoning") that followed amputation or lithotomy (a common but risky operation to remove bladder stones), for instance, was not always recognized as caused by the surgeon; neither was it hidden from students that many patients grew worse or died under the care of surgeons and physicians.

In addition to the periodic disturbances and distresses connected with the procurement of bodies needed to teach anatomy, there were occasional spirited outbursts of criticism among the students. William Tully mentioned one episode, in 1808, when hard words rashly spoken by disaffected students reduced Smith to tears. Having intervened to keep the peace between two groups of students, Nathan Smith's feelings were badly hurt when "his exertions for the good of the Class" were misunderstood.[2] Two other instances of minor trouble are mentioned in a letter from another student, Alexander Boyd, in 1810:

[O]ne medical Student [was expelled] for using some tough language to the tutors of this College. There was another medical Student who borrowed money and bought a horse & things out of the store to the amount of about Ninety or one hundred Dollars besides fifty Dollars to Doct. Smith who [i.e., the student] went away a week ago and has not been heard of since neither is he expected to return (nor pay his tuition either).[3]

Naturally, Nathan Smith's students varied in their responses both to him and to the opportunity to study medicine under him. Their notebooks and letters give some insights into Smith as a professor of medicine. A brief sketch of the careers of a few students—those whose names have come down to us quite independent of their study under Smith—will tell us more. Overall, the evidence indicates that Nathan Smith had an enormous influence on the way medicine was practiced and taught in New England.

Skeptics: William Tully and Jo Gallup

William Tully we have already met; the journal he kept during his first term at Dartmouth, in 1808, is one of the most valuable resources we have on life for early students of medicine at Dartmouth, even though Tully never took a Dartmouth degree and had remarkably little to say about the actual content of the medical lectures. But his description of a typical day for a student is informative: Breakfast at 8:00 preceded the lecture from 9:00 to 10:30. Reading until noon was followed by an hour's exercise and dinner from 1:00 to 2:00; another hour-and-a-half lecture came after dinner, with time for study until tea and exercise again until 6:00. Yet another lecture period of ninety minutes was on the schedule before the rest of the evening was free to be spent with friends. Wednesdays were a bit different: Public speaking in the chapel delayed the afternoon lecture by an hour, and meetings of the special student society (the "Boulenterion," or "High Court") replaced the evening lecture. On Saturdays, also, there were only two lectures.[4]

Beyond such details about the daily schedule, the main value of Tully's journal is the blunt honesty with which he expressed his misgivings—about Hanover in general, and about Dartmouth and Smith in particular. In Dewey's Tavern, where he first sought accommodations upon arrival in Hanover, he found "a sour landlord, and a very dirty bar room full of persons of all descriptions," and his initial impression of Smith was of a man whose dress was "quite plain, very heedlessly chosen and carelessly put on. He received us in a blunt but civil way . . . very much like a Connecticut farmer."[5] In other regards, too, Tully appears to have been unenthusiastic; when the opportunity arose to ride with Smith on home visits to patients, as an entry in his journal soon after he arrived in Hanover in early October of 1808 illustrates, he was not at all sure he wanted to be part of it:

This morning, Dr. Smith was to perform the operation for an aneurism, but at sixteen, or seventeen miles distance from Hanover. I felt desirous of seeing it; but to go so far for the purpose, would have been literally skinning a flint for threepence, and spoiling a knife that cost six-pence. Had the patient, however, been within half a mile, I should have felt somewhat sheepish at attending, with such a concourse of students as the good Doctor commonly has with him. . . . Many of the medical students, in this instance, were unwise enough to be at much pains and expence to hire horses and to post off, breakfastless, to the patient's house, not to return, probably, till midnight, a dollar or two expended, a day's study lost, themselves fatigued, and six-cents worth gained.[6]

When Tully finally did write, at the end of the course, that the "Lectures have gone on in their old round. Dr. Smith we admire and revere, more and more as we know him better,"[7] we see that Smith's teaching must have been truly outstanding to have overcome Tully's initial negative mind-set. His summary judgment, in fact, was that Dartmouth's medical school was excellent, but that the only hope for the future of the institution was to move it out of Hanover:

At Dartmouth it is said that the students have come to years of discretion and if they do not do as they ought, the loss is their own. . . . A student may become an excellent scholar, but he is never obliged to study. . . .

Such a system as this cannot be very excellent, but it is far better than none. The example of the other New-England Colleges, if nothing else, will, in time, lead to improvements, and in case it is ever removed from Hanover, it will undoubtedly be stationed in a place ten times more advantageously situated for a Literary Institution. Of Dr. Smith's School . . . I cannot speak too highly, but I have my doubts whether after Dr. Smith any deserving man will take charge of it, under so many inconveniences.[8]

Given Tully's skepticism about schools in what he thought of as the wilderness, it is curious that he spent a number of years teaching in Castleton, Vermont, hardly a bustling urban center. His most distinguished appointment took him back to Yale, where he taught from 1829 to 1842, having joined that faculty after Smith's death.[9]

Many of Nathan Smith's students were at pains to credit him for what he taught them, and to praise his skill as a teacher; William Tully stands out as a considerable exception to this pattern. Despite having as much exposure to Smith as many other young medical students, despite becoming a distinguished physician and educator in his own right, and despite writing extensively on a wide variety of medical subjects in later years, Tully never cited or quoted Smith. Why Tully failed so utterly to give credit where one might reasonably assume credit was due may have had something to do with his fondness for "heroic" measures in medicine. In this he was very unlike Smith. Even so, it is difficult to believe that the younger man's success in later life—quite apart from his teaching appointments, he was author of an outstanding book on materia medica,[10] and other physicians often called upon him as a consultant in difficult cases—was not at least indirectly a result of what he learned from Smith. Between Nathan Smith early and Sir William Osler late in the nineteenth century, Tully was perhaps more effective than any other American physician in improving therapeutics. He was, in his own way, a worthy disciple of Smith.

Also worthy and less skeptical—but in the end even less like Smith in his approach to therapeutics—was Joadam Gallup (originally named "Joseph Adam," he consolidated his two names, much as an ancestor—Benjamin Adam, called "Benadam"—had done; he nonetheless continued for the most part to be called "Jo").[11] As one of the first two students to earn a medical degree from Dartmouth—an M.B. in 1798 (he was awarded an M.D. in 1814)—he stands in a critically important place in the story of Dartmouth Medical School, as we saw earlier. His willingness to put himself under Smith's wing as an apprentice shows an admirable degree of interest in self-improvement, as does his studying later under Rush at Pennsylvania.

There Gallup was confronted with approaches to medical treatment that were diametrically opposed to what he had just learned from Smith. And although a number of students studied under both Smith and Rush, Gallup remains a prime example of those who were drawn more to Rush's bold self-assurance than to Smith's methodical caution. The manifest differences between Rush and Smith were not only superficial matters of personality, however. Therapeutically speaking, the contrast was fundamental. These two Edinburgh-trained professors were no doubt in agreement on some points. But Rush, ever eager to harness nature's destructive power by bleeding and then bleeding again, had little in common with Smith, who believed firmly in letting nature take its course wherever possible. Where one of Smith's chief precepts was that the physician should do nothing until he was certain he was right—which implied a willingness to observe, to watch and wait—Rush simply took for granted that he was right. He saw no need for delay. Gallup, with the best will in the world, outrushed Rush—to his patients' ultimate detriment.

There is some irony in this, for Gallup was among those students of Smith who were most active not only in teaching but in founding and otherwise playing central roles in the life of more than one medical school. Appointed as professor of "Theory and Practice" at the Vermont Academy of Medicine in Castleton, he was president of that institution at the crucial point when it merged with the University of Vermont, where he taught for one session in 1825. He then founded the Clinical School of Medicine in Woodstock, Vermont, where he taught for twenty-four years. Ambitious and hard-working, he made important early contributions to epidemiology: Like Smith, he was among the first in northern New England to vaccinate with the cowpox; he collected and published clinical records and autopsy findings both from his own practice and from others' reports; he wrote the locally popular *Sketches of Epidemic Diseases in the State of Vermont*.[12] Although many of the concepts in this treatise are woefully misguided, the monograph had its merits. Buried beneath the turgid prose and sometimes baffling ideas was evidence that cooperative efforts among physicians from a wide geographical area could yield valuable information about disease entities and their progress. And unlike Tully, Gallup did at least mention Smith as a reliable source about epidemics (he never referred to Smith when it came to etiology or treatment).

His book would be of greater interest today if he had not devoted himself to theorizing on celestial phenomena (influenced no doubt by Noah Webster's similar efforts[13]) and trying to explain what perplexed him by reference to effluvia and miasmata and the like—all catch-words of the then-current European theories about disease etiology.

Gallup was also active in more general professional affairs. He founded the Windsor County [Vermont] Medical Society, and he helped promote the Vermont Medical Society (he was its president for roughly a decade). The infirmary he established in Woodstock in 1827 not only served the local populace, but gave him a place to demonstrate his belief in the importance of bedside instruction for medical students.[14] That principle—which showed him kin to Nathan Smith after all—may have been his greatest contribution, even if his Rushian therapeutics were such that none of us today would wish to be his patient.

True Disciples: Ezekiel Dodge Cushing and Amos Twitchell

A sharp contrast to Tully's skeptical independence from Smith and to Gallup's therapeutic opposition to his mentor is found in the sadly brief career of Ezekiel Dodge Cushing (who earned his M.B. in 1811). We met him caught in the unsettling business of defending Dartmouth's medical establishment in the face of an incipient anatomy riot. Cushing's willingness to follow Smith's instructions, coupled with his undeniable enthusiasm for anatomical activity, allies him more with Smith than either Tully or Gallup. Indeed, his eagerness to be out and about is reminiscent of Smith's when he was apprenticing with Goodhue.[15]

Early in his time at Dartmouth, in October 1809, Cushing wrote his parents about what he had already been able to see and learn by accompanying Smith on distant rounds:

Last Monday afternoon the Dr was sent for to [visit] a man that had a burst [a hernia] in which the intestine had broke through the muscles on the belly and a portion of it was confined there in such a manner that nothing could pass through him. The Dr opened the tumour and enlarged the opening through which the gut had passed that it could be pushed back into the belly. This was at Barre 50 miles from Hanover. Nineteen students with the Dr at their head set out from Hanover about 4 o'clock in the afternoon [Monday], we stopt twice and arrived at Barre about 4 o'clock Tuesday morning the operation was performed about twelve we started from Barre at 1 and arrived at Hanover just at 3 [the next morning].[16]

And in February 1810, Cushing wrote again with great excitement:

I have been continually riding since I returned with the Dr. . . . Alden [a fellow student] went with the doctor 70 miles down the river and was gone 5 days . . . I went with the Dr. to Corinth [about 30 miles away] to see a man who had the rheumatism and was gone 2 days . . . [on another occasion] a man came after the doctor to go to a woman that had broke her leg. The doctor was gone and I went. I found the doctor that belonged to the place there but he said that he did not pretend to set bones. I looked at it and told the woman that I could set. I tried and put it exactly right in about a minute bandaged it up, told the woman when it got out of place to send for me, she said she would, and asked me how much I charged, they were pretty rich folks I told them about 5$ the man paid me in Vermont money and I went home, gave the doctor the money, and he ran all over the village to blazen forth my marvellous exploit.[17]

Trips out of Hanover were sometimes long and presumably arduous, but Cushing characteristically emphasized their benefits. In August 1810, he wrote to his sister while "confined altogether in the house from the violent fall of rain which is . . . pouring into the sides of my *superb* apartment," reporting that he had been on

a journey of 95 miles up Connecticut River in which I saw four operations successfully employed, three of them were the removing a portion of the bones which had perished in the limb [this would become a specialty of Smith's, as we shall see], other which was the most difficult one that ever I saw . . . . It took Doctor Smith above an hour to perform it.—have likewise been to Walpole to see an important operation.[18]

Perhaps Cushing's upbringing in a seafaring family was what endowed him with a desire to go everywhere, do everything, and make the most of every opportunity.

Students often boarded with Smith, just as anyone who had already read with a doctor would probably have lived in the household of his preceptor. Of course not all of them could, and thus Cushing had reason to be pleased at being chosen:

Dr. Smith yesterday told me that after the lectures were finished that I should board with him which I think is good news, not only as it gives me a greater chance of improvement from enjoying more of his company but shows that I have so behaved myself as to gain his goodwill and confidence, as he made me the offer without any solicitation on my part.[19]

A few weeks earlier, sounding honestly weary, Cushing had written his father, saying "I am tired almost to death and have seen more real service since I have been here than ever I did before."[20] But perhaps he confided such complaints only to the family; there is plenty of evidence, as we have seen, that Smith considered him a reliable and unusually competent student. His early death in 1828 must have saddened his mentor as much as anyone. As one historian put it, "His sickness and death . . . shrouded in gloom his whole neighborhood."[21]

Another student quite prepared to express his gratitude and indebtedness to Smith was Amos Twitchell, who earned his Dartmouth M.B. in 1805. An outstanding young scholar—an 1802 Phi Beta Kappa graduate of the College—he was a Dartmouth man more or less by default. Having ridden his horse to Cambridge, confident that Harvard would welcome his matriculation, he was at a loss for but a moment when told he didn't measure up (he had no Latin). He promptly remounted and headed for Hanover, saying—in effect—that he never really wanted to go to Harvard in the first place and that he had stopped only to take a look as long as he was passing through.[22]

A more congenial pairing of teacher and student than Nathan Smith and Amos Twitchell is difficult to imagine. For one thing, it put Smith—who had ably donned the master surgeon's mantle that had long been worn by his mentor, Josiah Goodhue—in a position to pass on the honorific of "premier surgeon of northern New England"; it is generally agreed that Twitchell became the next in line.[23] Twitchell in turn is among those said to have attested to Goodhue's having been "for many years the most celebrated surgeon in this upper portion of the valley of the Connecticut"[24]—but one should recall that, as if to close the circle on this triumvirate, Twitchell had married Josiah Goodhue's daughter. By the end of his career, Amos Twitchell stood "pre-eminent among his fellows of the medical profession," according to physician Henry I. Bowditch (no mean judge of such matters). "He was autocrat in surgery for all the country round."[25] The three men were linked in more ways than one.

In addition to studying two years with Smith and earning a degree from Dartmouth, Twitchell was another in the long line of assistants to Smith in chemistry. When he settled into his own practice, across the river in Norwich, he also occasionally filled in for Smith when the latter was out of town, lecturing on anatomy and surgery.[26]

Loyal to the principles of rural practice learned from Smith, Twitchell moved in 1810 to Keene (no more a major city then than now), where he settled into a long and distinguished career as a surgeon that ended with his death in 1850. Twitchell was much sought after as a general surgeon; today his fame rests largely on his having successfully spliced the carotid artery for a patient. If he was not the first to do so—it has been argued that he was the second, the first having been none other than William Tully's early mentor, Mason F. Cogswell[27]—he certainly did it a year before the same operation was performed by Sir Astley Cooper (1768–1841), the eminent English surgeon. (Cooper commonly gets the credit that belongs either to Twitchell or Cogswell for pioneering this procedure.)

Further evidence of Twitchell's position as a leading physician in nineteenth-century New England can be found in the records of several medical schools. He was repeatedly invited to apply for a position as medical

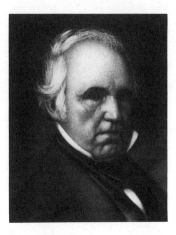

Amos Twitchell, 1781–1850.
Used with permission of the Francis A.
Countway Library of Medicine.

school professor or, indeed, to accept a position; also repeatedly, he declined. (Exactly how many times he did so is unclear.[28]) Most relevant for our story is what Twitchell said in a letter to Dartmouth President Francis Brown, in 1819. He listed several reasons for declining the offer of a professorship at his alma mater, while diplomatically saying he would have liked to be associated with a "literary institution." The likely income was too low and too uncertain, he insisted—not least because prospective students would be drawn off by Ramsay's latest educational endeavor (he was proposing to open his anatomical museum in Concord, New Hampshire) and by Smith (then in New Haven). Twitchell also believed he needed to devote his "time & talents to the pursuit of such objects as will be most beneficial to my fellow creatures."[29] Twitchell may have taken pleasure in turning down appointments at educational institutions just as Harvard has once turned him down, but it is also possible he sincerely believed he could do more for his "fellow creatures" by continuing his practice in Keene.

Certainly he knew from personal experience what the solicitous care of a physician could mean. Bowditch, in the memoir of Amos Twitchell already cited, tells in detail the story of how Nathan Smith's devoted attention helped cure the young man's crippling bout of despondency during the early years of his practice in Norwich.[30] One can imagine Twitchell deciding that care of patients mattered above all else. His reputation was assured, in any case. President of the New Hampshire Medical Society from 1827 to 1830, he was later chosen as representative to the American

Medical Association convention in Philadelphia;[31] the papers were full of his praise when he died in 1850.[32]

Fellow Teachers: Lyman Spalding and
Reuben Dimond Mussey

Lyman Spalding, although he received his M.B. degree from Harvard (his Dartmouth degree was honorary) surely counts as a student of Nathan Smith, having been one of his earliest apprentices. As we saw, he probably attended Smith's lectures at Dartmouth during the period he was chemistry instructor; he was also elected to Phi Beta Kappa at Dartmouth on May 23, 1799[33] (perhaps at Smith's instigation), further making him a Dartmouth man.

He was, as considerable evidence shows, one of Smith's closest friends.[34] Moreover, when he came to his mentor's rescue by joining him as an "officer of the institution" at Dartmouth, he was truly—however unofficially from the trustees' point of view—Smith's first colleague. Spalding's usefulness to Smith and reasonable success as a colleague in chemistry has already been touched on. But Spalding, restless and ambitious, was not destined to be a mere assistant in someone else's institution. Furthermore, pecuniary and political considerations[35] made continuing at Dartmouth unsatisfactory from Spalding's point of view, and after teaching two or three terms[36] under Smith's aegis, he left. His formal letter of resignation ended thus: "Therefore, Be it known that I Lyman Spalding on this 14th day of October A.D. 1800, resign the Office of Lecturer, on Chemistry and Materia Medica in Dartmouth University."[37]

This must have been a blow to Smith, but the fallout from Spalding's resignation does not seem to have had any negative effect on their friendship.[38] Even after Spalding had opened his own busy practice in Portsmouth, New Hampshire, the two men stayed in close touch. Letters from Smith to Spalding (alas, Smith seems to have destroyed virtually all letters written to him) show an extensive correspondence covering a wide range of topics.[39] We have already seen, for instance, Smith's reliance on the younger man to help him find "subjects" for his anatomy classes and to publicize the arrival of Alexander Ramsay.

Spalding, though not a born teacher like Smith, was nonetheless installed, in December 1813, as the first president of the College of Physicians and Surgeons in Fairfield, New York.[40] The tentative, almost apologetic, note on which he opened his inaugural address ("I cannot but wish that the presidency of this college had been conferred on one better qualified . . . ."[41]) was no doubt meant to demonstrate a becoming modesty; it may, however, have been a harbinger. The six years Spalding spent there were by no means the years of his greatest success. During that time, he made plans to publish a textbook, but the friends (including Smith) to whom he sent drafts dissuaded him. Smith, in particular, went on at some length to let Spalding know that his proposed *Institutes and Practice of Medicine*, as announced in an ad in the *New England Journal of Medicine and Surgery*,[42] diverged significantly from Smith's own views and was therefore a work to which he could not give his full endorsement.[43] The book was never published. Neither teaching nor educational administration nor textbook authorship was to make Lyman Spalding famous.

He did far better as a practitioner. The twelve years Spalding spent in Portsmouth (before going to Fairfield) were busy and active. In 1801 he helped found the Eastern District of the New Hampshire Medical Society; by the time he left for New York in 1812, he had held every possible office in the Society. Once he moved to New York he was immediately active in similar circles there.[44]

Lyman Spalding's place in American medical history was secured by his work on the first United States pharmacopoeia. (The significance of that publication is easy to underestimate today, when national and international pharmaceutical agreements and standards are largely taken for granted; in the first decades of the nineteenth century, the significance of consolidating and standardizing epidemiological or therapeutic information had not yet been grasped.) Within five years of moving to New York, in January of 1817, Spalding had proposed to the County Medical Society "a project for the formation of a National Pharmacopoeia."[45] Out of that grew plans for a national convention, which met on January 1, 1820. The chairman, S. L. Mitchell, was a friend of Spalding's, which no doubt had something to do with Spalding being appointed head of the publications committee. The choice proved to be a good one.

The purpose of the project was clearly stated in the preface:

It is the object of a Pharmacopoeia to select from among substances which possess medicinal power, those, the utility of which is most fully established and best understood; and to form from them preparations and compositions, in which their powers may be exerted to the greatest advantage. It should likewise distinguish those articles by convenient and definite names, such as may prevent trouble or uncertainty in the intercourse of physicians and apothecaries.[46]

So well were the contents of the whole project organized that for more than a century little needed to be changed. Furthermore, so vigorously did Spalding press the work forward that the book was printed in less than a year after the convention. Letters written by Spalding to Jacob Bigelow (another member of the project team) midway into the project make clear that many niggling questions about size and scope and format, politics, science, and art, conspired to complicate the undertaking.[47] The speed with which such difficulties were met and the excellence of the finished project speak for Spalding's great ability.

Publication of the volume on schedule must have been all the more gratifying to Spalding when one takes into account the freak accident that laid him low while the work was still very much in progress. One day late in 1820, the forty-five-year-old Spalding was walking down Pearl Street in New York City. Pearl was a long, busy road that led into the heart of the East River dock area in lower Manhattan, where some three dozen cases of yellow fever had occurred in 1819.[48] (This may well be why Spalding was in the area—following up the investigative work he had done on yellow fever the previous year.[49]) By the 1820s this densely populated part of the city was a neighborhood where "[f]ashionably dressed gentlemen and racially mixed crowds mingled with prostitutes and pigs."[50] The box of rubbish that fell (or was thrown) from a second-story window[51] as Spalding walked along would have been difficult to dodge, given the crowded street—and Spalding had no time to do so. Hit on the head, he incurred an injury that left him struggling "in search of health" until his death nearly a year later, on October 21, 1821, from chronic traumatic meningitis.[52]

A number of Nathan Smith's Dartmouth medical students joined the Dartmouth faculty at one time or another; among them was Reuben Dimond Mussey (A.B. 1803; M.B. 1806). Mussey was destined to follow Nathan Smith's steps as a successful teacher more closely than perhaps any of his other students. Not only did he join the Dartmouth faculty in 1814, shortly after Smith had left; he later succeeded to Smith's chair at Bowdoin, and he was also one of several Dartmouth-educated doctors who taught at the medical school in Fairfield.[53]

Smith's influence is therefore easier to see on Mussey's career than on the careers of some of his other students. Yet here was a man who had not originally planned to be a doctor at all, a prime example of those who turned to medicine only after discovering they did not have the character or—equally important—the stamina for studying divinity. (Ashbel Smith, who later studied under Nathan Smith—no relation—at Yale, was another who took up medicine only when poor health forced him to abandon a career in law.[54]) College was, after all, primarily a place for training ministers (Dartmouth had been founded for that purpose); for many, turning to medicine was a second-best choice. Thus even though Mussey's father was himself a physician, the young man needed to justify his change of plan when he decided to become a doctor rather than a minister. As he was finishing work for his A.B. in 1803, he wrote to his father to explain himself:

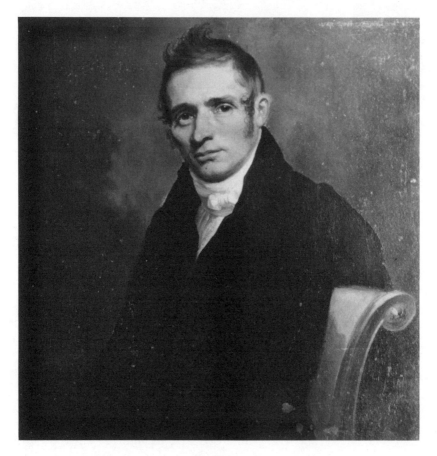

Reuben Dimond Mussey, 1780–1866. Private Collection, reproduced with permission.

Having long deliberated, with respect to the course I am to take, after leaving College, I have, at length made some determinations, which, I shall now communicate to you.

The profession of divinity, of all others, is the best calculated to give satisfaction of mind and domestic enjoyment. But few are so happy as to possess all the qualifications requisite for the important calling of a Minister of the gospel. . . . Consistently with my ideas of this profession, and its requisites, I can not think it my duty to engage in it at present.—

My intentions are to study physic. The following is the plan which [I] have fixed upon.—To tarry here after Commencement and *read*, thro' the vacation, and, during the fall term, to pay strict attention to Dr. Smith's Lectures.— Then to go home, and study with you a year and an half, or two years. . . . I shall stand in need of *your* assistance, to carry this plan into effect. If you *can* afford me any aid in this way, and do not think proper to do it by way of gift, I will, if I am ever able, refund all I shall receive from you. If you *cannot* assist me, I must relinquish the idea of studying physic at present.[55]

Mussey not only completed his medical studies; he later became Dartmouth's professor of theory and practice and of materia medica—though he had misgivings about whether being a colleague of Cyrus Perkins would be lending too much support to what he regarded as the wrong side in the political controversies arising at the College (see chapter 8). Subsequently, Mussey achieved renown for experiments in physiology, disproving Benjamin Rush's theory that substances could not be absorbed through the skin.[56] In 1838, a letter from one New Hampshire man to another tells us of Mussey's professional esteem: "It is a humiliating confession, but it is no less true, if you remove from the [New Hampshire] Medical Society the present Professors [Reuben D. Mussey and Daniel K. Oliver] . . . no one remains whose professional attainments has made him known beyond the limits of the state." (This was excepting Amos Twitchell, who "does not . . . attend our meetings.)"[57] Smith—had he still been alive at that point—would have been pleased by Mussey's participation in affairs of the state medical society as well as by his standing in the profession. More than three decades earlier, Smith had written to Daniel Webster that "Respecting Mr. Mussey I can with confidence recommend him as a gentleman & scholar. . . . His genius & industry are such as convince me that he will arrive at eminence in his profession."[58]

Smith was presumably pleased and proud that when Bowdoin needed to replace him, they could turn to one of his former students—though he recommended another student ahead of Mussey (see chapter 13). In the end, Mussey was offered the post; he accepted and served both Bowdoin and the profession well.

Friend Beyond Compare: George Cheyne Shattuck

A medical school classmate of Mussey's was destined to make the most difference in Smith's life in the medical world. George Cheyne Shattuck (A.B. 1803; M.B. 1806) was far more than a student and a colleague. He was a friend of the sort only a fortunate few ever have—companion, colleague, confidant—always ready to give whatever aid was needed (including frequent financial support, both to Smith and to family members long after Smith's death).

George Shattuck looms large in American medical history quite apart from his friendship with Nathan Smith. Of all Smith's students, he was probably the most influential in the most areas of early New England life. A good doctor (though he early gave up private practice and devoted himself to hospital work), he was also the progenitor of a line of outstanding New England physicians. As William Osler put it, he was "the father, grandfather, and great-grandfather of the Shattucks who . . . helped to make the profession of Boston famous during the nineteenth century."[59] He was a medical educator as well; he, too, taught at Fairfield, and at Harvard he was successively professor of clinical medicine and (for nearly two decades) "Hersey Professor of the Theory and Practice of Physic," and later (for five years) dean of the faculty. Shattuck additionally supported several medical schools with advice and help. He gave Dartmouth an astronomical observatory, a large library, and several oil paintings— gifts that added visible prestige to the College.[60] In 1854, he endowed the professorship of morbid (later pathological) anatomy at Harvard and provided that school with many scholarships. He was president of the Massachusetts Medical Society from 1836 to 1840, and he established the Shattuck Lectures for the Society.[61]

He took further medical training in both Boston and Philadelphia, and seems to have fared better with the contradictory features of such a composite education than Jo Gallup did, having the wit and perception to choose the best and reject the rest. When Shattuck finished his education, he asked Smith to write a certificate of proficiency for him, which he could submit to the Massachusetts Medical Society. Even allowing for some exaggeration, Smith's description of the young physician is striking:

I do hereby certify that the Bearer George C. Shattuck has studied the medical profession under my instruction, that he has been a faithful & intelligent student exhibiting a good genius & pure moral character. I do further certify that he is a man of sincerity love & action and as one who promises to do much good to society & honor to the profession.[62]

Smith's assessment proved accurate indeed.

Although they came from very different backgrounds, the two men took to each other immediately. The friendship must have been firmly established as early as 1806, when Shattuck had just earned his M.B. degree at Dartmouth. Smith wrote a long letter in June of that year to the twenty-three-year-old student, expounding his own philosophical approach to diseases and their classification, and his hope that none of his pupils would so far forget the practical problems of treatment as to rely on the theories of the day (and particularly not on Rush's outlandish ones). He addressed the letter, simply enough, to "Dr. George C. Shattuck, Medical Student, Philadelphia."[63]

Perhaps because Shattuck had won the Massachusetts Medical Society's medical essay contest (the Boylston Prize) several times,[64] or perhaps because he hoped Shattuck would join him as co-author, Smith wrote him a detailed explanation of his views on cancer. With an eye on writing a pa-

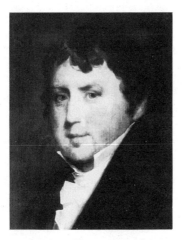

George Cheyne Shattuck,
1783–1854. Used with permission
of the Francis A. Countway Library
of Medicine.

per on "scirrhus" (a common medical term of the day for some forms of cancer), he was eager for Shattuck's advice, and quite prepared to share personal information about his own mood and health:

> If you have time to make any alterations in what I have written in either of the points above pointed out I wish you to do it. . . . I wrote it under very great disadvantages. I had to struggle with a weight of business and with very ill health . . . this is the first evening which I have felt like myself for more than two months.[65]

Editorial advice was the least of Smith's requests of Shattuck. Late in December 1808, Smith wrote him to introduce Alexander Ramsay to "Mr. Boylestone" in Boston.[66] He also used Shattuck as his agent in procuring supplies of various sorts. In September and October of 1809 he wrote several times:

> I wish now that you would be so kind as to procure for me two tin reflectors and two cannisters which you will find described in Henry's Chemistry in his chapter on Calorics . . . .

> [O]ne quarter of a hundred of red lead, sixteen pounds of mercury and about fourteen pounds of winter strained linseed oil . . . . If opium is less than $1.50 an ounce ask the apothecary to put up four ounces for me.

> [A] pound of each of the following acids in as great a degree of purity as they can be obtained:
> Nitric Acid
> Muriatic Acid
> Sulphiric acid
> . . . some earth and glass retorts.[67]

Once when unpleasant rumors about Smith (of precisely what nature is unclear) were apparently circulating around New England, he wrote with more feeling and vehemence than was typical, asking Shattuck to

have some person inform Dr. Warren that if he has taken it upon him to report to his class what he supposes to be facts about his fellow professors on the credit of Dr. Mac Kinstry he may be apprised that Dr. Mac Kinstry is a liar, a man of no credit and a most consummate scoundrel, and that what you stated as coming from him has no foundation in truth and that the whole of it is a fabrication of Mac Kinstry's. I will write you soon on the subject.[68]

Smith surely would have loved to induce Shattuck to teach in Hanover, though there is no evidence that he tried very hard. Perhaps he respected Shattuck's independence too much or understood too well his ties to Boston (where he eventually became consulting physician to the city[69]). Shattuck's Hanover friends hoped that when Ebenezer Adams joined the Dartmouth faculty, Shattuck, too, would accept a Dartmouth professorship. Adams himself wrote Shattuck on the point:

Could you not acquire a higher, a much more extensive, and more durable reputation, than in any other situation, which can be offered you? Come then, and be the Boerhaave,[70] the Hippocrates, the anybody you please of New England. Can you hesitate one moment? If you do not, I do not care how soon I receive your answer. If you do, though I shall be glad to hear from you upon other subjects, I insist, that you shall not give me a negative within six months. . . . Come then, and help to raise your Alma Mater to a proud eminence above her sister seminaries.[71]

The attempt to lure Shattuck to Dartmouth ended only with Cyrus Perkins's appointment in 1810.

During this period Smith was operating on the eyes of his patient John Derby. In the course of attending to Derby (after whom he would name his youngest son), he also met other members of the family, including a niece, Eliza Cheever Davis. In mid-July of 1810, Nathan Smith wrote Shattuck, performing the most delicate service one man can provide for another:

On our way home [I was] informed . . . that . . . your addresses would be very well received by Miss Davis . . . . Miss Davis is in my opinion a lady of superior understanding, possessing a most affectionate heart, in short, she possesses all that would be requisite to make a sensible man happy.

Perhaps you will think it strange that my pen should be so ready in bestowing praises on a young lady, but I assure you I should think myself guilty in my duty to you if I did not urge you to urge your suit in such a case with all the management you are master of.[72]

Eliza Davis did, indeed, subsequently marry George Shattuck. When she died, eighteen years later, the letter Smith wrote to Shattuck—in sincere grief—is one of the most intimate communications we have from his hand:

Your letter announcing the melancholy death of Mrs. Shattuck has been received. My sympathies for you are very great, nor do I know what consolation to offer. Your loss is irreparable. I have felt the same, but the circumstances were not similar. My [first] wife [when she died] left me no children and I can readily conceive that the thought of your motherless children will add much to the poignancy of your grief for the loss of their excellent mother.[73]

Shattuck seems always to have directed particular generosity to the Smith family. Most touching of all, perhaps, he came to Smith's bedside as the older man lay dying and eased his friend's mind by promising (with Mrs. John Derby) to take over the education of Smith's son John Derby Smith. He arranged this with his customary skill and kindness (as we shall see in chapter 14). Given that Smith's estate consisted of little more than a small unmortgaged house, this was valuable assistance indeed. Shattuck was, in every sense of the phrase, a friend to the end.

Other Lives, Other Careers

The influence Smith had on the medical profession by no means ended with the students profiled above. Among the medical schools where his protégés taught—beyond Dartmouth, Yale, Bowdoin, the University of Vermont (UVM), Fairfield, and Castleton—were others, like Western Reserve and the Medical College in Memphis. His own son, Nathan Ryno Smith, after starting at UVM, taught successively at Jefferson Medical College, Transylvania University in Kentucky, and the University of Maryland.

Although some of those who did not teach went far afield, a high percentage of the earliest Dartmouth graduates practiced in small towns and rural areas.[74] Smith's dream of populating northern New England in particular with doctors trained there was well on its way toward fulfillment.

Assuring the Medical School's Future

Life in Hanover

WITHOUT LYMAN SPALDING to assist in the teaching, Nathan Smith was truly on his own in the medical school he had founded: He was teaching the whole curriculum to all the medical students. And—maybe as an acknowledgement of the magnitude of this effort—the Board of Trustees at Dartmouth voted in 1801 to award an M.D. degree to Nathan Smith.

Holding the composite and difficult position of sole medical school faculty member had its stresses. Sally chose to stay in Cornish with the children and did not settle in Hanover until 1805, which almost certainly meant a good deal of travel between Hanover and home for the doctor. His wife's roots were deep in Cornish—and, consequently, so were his. Already in 1792–93, he had been a member of the Cornish School Committee,[2] and as late as 1803 he was still sufficiently at home in Cornish to be appointed by Trinity Church as one of three deputies to represent the Cornish congregation at a convention in Concord.[3] Furthermore, although he was spending time in Hanover, his medical practice in Cornish continued to be busy, as the crowded pages of his day books and ledgers attest.

Not until after the death of her father, General Jonathan Chase, in January of 1801 did Sally apparently give serious thought to moving. Domestic economics may have been a factor, though in the previous year Sally had made some substantial purchases from David Curtis in Hanover.[4] The feather beds, looking glasses, desk, tables, chest of drawers, chairs, curtains, cutlery, and dishes—along with numerous other household items—lead us to guess she was planning to establish residence in Hanover, where Chase family furnishings would not so easily be available to her. The legacy that Nathan Smith received from his father-in-law was rather substantial, but it cannot have made much difference in the quotidian finances of the family since most of it was in real estate. In addition to property in Cornish and "four rights in Cornish Bridge valued at $533.32," there were "four disputable lots" in Vermont. The result was that the young Smiths were suddenly relatively wealthy, rich at least in land.[5]

Exactly when Sally moved to Hanover is unclear. She may have come for a while in 1801 and 1802; a hint that something of the sort happened is Nathan Smith's lease early in February 1801, from President John Wheelock ("for one ear of Indian corn"), of the house and barn on the west side of the road at the southwest corner of the College Plain, "and fifteen acres to Girl Brook."[6] Thus Nathan Smith's first home in Hanover seems to have been between the house of the Reverend John Smith and that of Mr. Jedediah Baldwin. On December 1, 1802, Smith paid $95.00 rent to Wheelock for this property "which when paid will be (in addition to all repairs made by him) in full for the rent . . . ."[7]

Neither impeccable neighbors nor whatever repairs her husband had undertaken were enough to keep Sally and the family in Hanover, however—if in fact they were there with Dr. Smith. We know that at some time after General Chase's death and prior to 1804, the family moved (for about three years) to Windsor, Vermont, a larger community across the Connecticut River from the farm fields of Cornish. More household purchases were made there, from William Leverett and the Hale Brothers of Windsor, and Smith bought live chickens (for $1.00), and two bushels of seed wheat, a cow and calf, and a milk pail (all for $51.63). Some less obviously practical acquisitions were also made; on July 2, 1804 (perhaps anticipating a Fourth of July gala), Sally bought a pair of extra long English silk gloves ($2.40) and one pair of best English kid shoes ($2.92).[8]

Smith wrote to George Shattuck that same July, with apparent satisfaction, "I am now situated in Windsor, Vt., have perhaps as good accommodations for students [he had nine at the time] in the neighborhood as I had at Hanover." The house itself must have offered "good accommodations" as well. By 1803 the Smith brood numbered five children, and more were to come; we know, too, that students and others like Smith's brother Nicholas and an occasional seriously ill patient often boarded with the family. Smith planned, he continued, that summer and thereafter, to give a special set of private lectures on the theory and practice of physic in Windsor, in addition to the College-mandated "public" lectures in Hanover.[9] How much of that scheme was carried out is not known, but even after seven years of teaching at Dartmouth—during at least part of which time he was commuting from Cornish or Windsor— Smith was not living near the College. (He may on occasion have stayed over or even have rented short-term for himself in Hanover.)

The College authorities were understandably eager to have their man on the scene, as well as on the job. Perhaps they were concerned about those private lectures. Perhaps they just wanted to be certain that Dartmouth's professor of medicine, with his growing reputation, was unmistakably attached to Dartmouth—which meant he should be in Hanover. Available housing in Hanover may not have been so spacious and comfortable as either the Chase-owned houses in Cornish or the house he had found for his family in Windsor, and Sally may have dragged her feet. Or Smith may have been testing the Board's commitment. If so, he got what he wanted; members of the Board soon took actions that showed they really did want him. In a series of votes, they slowly increased the amount of money they would pay him (most of his professorial income, it will be recalled, came directly from student fees). In August of 1801, they granted him $50 for the year past and another $50 for the year to come (part would be used to pay off the loan Smith owed the Board; a year later he was again voted $50 for the ensuing year and $50 for expenses past and future.[10] Then, in August of 1803, it was

Voted that there be allowed and granted to D^r. Nathan Smith the sum of one hundred dollars a year for the purpose of accommodating him with a house in the vicinity of this College in Hanover provided he return to reside here as Professor and also the use of not exceeding ten acres of land to be assigned him by the Financier for pasturage, both grants to continue during such his residence in this place and his continuance in office as Professor of Medicine at this College.[11]

Still he did not move, but the Board was persistent. In 1804 they granted him $60 for the past year (despite his failure to move, they clearly believed he was entitled to some compensation) and then voted an annual salary of $200—provided, again, that he would make his permanent residence at the College and move the next winter or spring.[12]

Smith finally acquiesced. This time the move apparently proved satisfactory; we will see that by the time Nathan was ready to leave Dartmouth for Yale, Sally was so well settled that she was reluctant to go, and indeed delayed following him to New Haven. Whether she was stubborn or just a practical woman who did not want to move until she was confident her peripatetic husband's next endeavor was likely to endure, we cannot, alas, ascertain now. We do have at least one bit of evidence that Nathan—far from being annoyed at Sally's dilatoriness—appreciated his wife and what she did to make his life's work possible. As one student wrote home in 1809, "Mrs. Smith, the doctor says, is the best woman the world affords and he always asks her advice in things of importance and appears very fond of her."[13]

Both before and after the family settled in Hanover, Nathan Smith was engaged in local life—in College and town affairs, as well as in matters that had to do directly with his own business or the medical school. And even while he was thinking about the medical school's future (which involved him in college politics, as we shall shortly see), Smith still had his own practice to consider: the care of his patients, and his need for equipment.

He found help with some of these matters from Richard Lang, a merchant in town. The running account he had with Smith indicates Lang was not only selling him food, fabrics, and building supplies, but was also paying bills for him. An entry for September 8, 1800, shows he paid Lemuel Davenport on Smith's behalf; on October 3, 1800, he similarly paid Major Lines, charging items bought by some of Smith's students (twice in November 1800, Elijah Curtis—identified as one of Smith's students— bought and charged something), and loaning money (on October 27, 1800, he noted a payment to "Doct.ʳ Spaulding [sic]"), and so on. He also on one earlier occasion, in December of 1799, received for Smith the munificent sum of $27.00 from the selectmen of Chester, Vermont, "for medicine & attendance" (presumably for an indigent ward of that town).[14]

Jedediah Baldwin, the local silversmith who was also Smith's neighbor, likewise provided services to Smith. In October 1797, he charged the doctor $1.25 to mend tooth instruments; in December he charged 10¢ for "making an instrument" (Baldwin apparently did not care to learn technical terms even though he had been in the chemistry course taught by Nathan Smith and Lyman Spalding). In June of the next year he charged 12½¢ for "setting a couching needle" (for the removal of cataracts) and in December he made "a double cannula" (tube for wound drainage) for 83¢ and "another thing" for 58¢. In April 1799 there was a charge of 8¢ for "setting a needle" (perhaps it was not so elaborate as the couching needle, or perhaps he set it more easily thanks to prior experience).[15]

Baldwin also appears in Smith's accounts as watchmaker and clockmaker, and as what may have been a partner in selling medicine. In April 1804, he received a long letter from Thomas Stokes & Co. accompanying a "small box of our medicines" together with some advertisements and directions on how to display the medicine.[16] Goods such as this (billed at $106.80) would have another dollar or two in freight charges added for shipping up the Connecticut River, the easiest means of transport.[17]

Smith may have been involved in controversies over issues of public

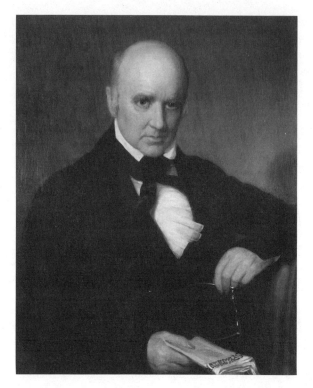

Mills Olcott, 1774–1845. Oil portrait by Francis Alexander.
Hood Museum of Art, Dartmouth College, Hanover, New Hampshire;
gift of Katherine B. Thompson; photo © 1997, Trustees of
Dartmouth College.

health; we know he was in later years. A certificate dated November 1808, signed by Nathan Smith, bluntly asserts: "This may certify that I am fully of opinion that a stove is better for warming school houses than an open fireplace both on account of oeconomy and the health of Scholars."[18]

By far the most important development concerning Nathan Smith's life in Hanover, however, was the very durable friendship that began with the influential lawyer in town, Mills Olcott (1774–1845). Already in 1801 there had been a letter to Olcott from Asa Porter, a relative of his in Haverhill, asking him to get Smith "to explain the Business" of a treatment, which one of Olcott's relatives had been unable to understand.[19] The first record of Smith's own communication with Olcott is a letter from Cornish (dated March 16, 1802) that shows Olcott and Smith were then reasonably well acquainted—hardly surprising, given that Olcott

had opened a law office in Hanover in 1800. Whether Smith was anticipating moving his family to Hanover or merely wanted a place for himself, he wrote as follows:

I wish you to send over to Constant Morduck's & inform him that if he has not
rented his house on the plain I wish him to reserve it for me . . . . As you have a
good name for buying wood I wish if you have an opportunity without much
trouble that you would engage some person to bring about 10 or 12 cord of wood
& put [it] in the woodhouse at the house of Morduck's, if I can have it & I will account with you for your trouble etc.[20]

Smith's jocular "as you have a good name at buying wood" suggests that
a close relationship between the two men already existed. But one wonders whether Mills Olcott had any idea what this casual piece of business
with the local professor of medicine would lead to. By the summer of
1803, fifteen months later, Nathan Smith was authorizing Mills Olcott to
act for him in collecting several bad debts that "Mr. Hutchinson has not
collected . . . & you may pursue such measures in the collection as you
please. I have delayed the suits till I have no remorse of conscience in com-
pelling my debtors to pay me . . . ."[21]

From then on Smith searched no further for a lawyer to represent him;
he could hardly have made a better choice. Olcott would become a justice
of the peace, a bank director and later president of the Grafton Bank. He
repeatedly represented Hanover in the state legislature, and he was much
in demand to preside on public occasions—"Being of a commanding appearance, and understanding the proprieties of large public meetings." In
1816, he would be appointed secretary and treasurer of the College, and
in 1821 he became a trustee (a position he held until his death).[22] Mills
Olcott did all Smith's legal work in Hanover, whether Smith was resident
there or elsewhere. Overall, the Olcott correspondence throws relatively
frequent and brilliant shafts of light on Nathan Smith's business dealings
and family affairs, and shows Mills Olcott to have been a patient and
meticulous manager, willing to deal with small details of unpaid bills and
large matters of financial and personal concern alike.

Olcott and Smith remained friendly throughout their lives. Their letters crackled with good feeling and understanding. One of the best examples is in a long letter written to Olcott late in Smith's life. Tacked on to a
discussion of several serious matters—as usual, both personal and financial—was the following paragraph:

The White Mountains I believe have gone to sea as we have not heard from them
of late. Perhaps they may fall in with the baptist Meeting House which went to see
[sic] from New London some years since. We have nothing very interesting in the
newspapers of late excepting that dead men talk & Jonah, wife & son have been
found, & certain idiots on the north river have second sight, & see wonders—[23]

From the earliest entry in Mills Olcott's accounts having to do with Nathan Smith (August 7, 1802), through the numerous notations of fees sought and paid in legal cases, up to Olcott's handling of the family's legal affairs after Nathan's death, there is never a hint of discord between the two men. Olcott seems to have done a prodigious amount of work for Smith; more than once, he charged nothing. Smith and Olcott also kept an eye on (and even boarded) one or another of each other's offspring. Clearly they were professionals with mutual respect and tolerance for the foibles and difficulties that attend any family.[24]

State Politics and the New Medical House

As early as 1790, when he was still just beginning his medical practice in Cornish, Smith began thinking about the possibility of getting help from the state to further his dream of teaching medical students. He wrote to John Warren, one of his professors at Harvard, that he was "determined to petition the General Court [Legislature] of this State for a small Lottery, for the purpose of purchasing a Medical Library." A barely disguised ulterior motive for sharing this information with Warren is evident in the same letter; Smith went on to point out that "if they should not grant it, I shall be under the necessity of purchasing [my] own property, which [may delay] my payment to you [of tuition fees still due]." Perhaps in an attempt to make Warren see the delay in payment as nothing to be concerned about, Smith further remarked that there were "several young men waiting for me to procure a Library, when they purpose to commence the study of Physic with me, & to finish their Education at Cambridge . . . ."[25] Smith did make application to the New Hampshire General Court for a medical library, but the petition, perhaps not surprisingly, appears to have been refused; no record exists of it having been granted. He was, after all, only a private citizen—a young physician who had only the year before earned his M.B. degree and who was not known much beyond the fifty-mile diameter of his practice.

Once the medical school had been established, Smith still had work to do if the institution was to survive. His plans for strengthening the medical school took many forms beyond efforts to raise funds for a library. Starting at least in 1801, he used the newspapers to ensure that word of the lectures was spread, for example. Already while he was living in Windsor, receipts that have survived show Smith annually advertised his medical lectures in the local Windsor paper, the *Reporter*; later he paid for ads in the *New Hampshire Gazette* and the *New Hampshire Patriot* as well. Students were, in one instance, notified that the medical lectures would "commence upon the first Wednesday of October next."[26] He of course bought books and supplies for himself and his teaching. On February 10, 1803, for example, his accounts indicate he bought books—"1 Hewson on blood" for $1.50, and "1 Cruickshank on absorbents" for $4.50— among other items.[27]

Meanwhile, Smith was by no means ready to give up on the legislature, especially considering that by the time he was ready to try again, he was in a position to make a more substantive argument. No longer a mere private physician, he was professor of anatomy, surgery, and chemistry at Dartmouth Medical School, a growing institution; furthermore, he had added two academic degrees and an imposing string of letters to his name. Thus emboldened, in the June session of 1803 Smith applied for a $600 grant to purchase apparatus that was to remain the property of the state (a shrewd move on his part that may have helped sway the legislature), and the petition was voted on favorably.[28]

In 1805, he made a third application—this one jointly with President John Wheelock—that succeeded in securing $900 for Dartmouth for general college use. The Board of Trust went so far as to thank Nathan Smith and President Wheelock officially for their exertions on behalf of the College (and to urge them to keep it up).[29]

Obtaining benefits for the College (or her medical school) was not Smith's only interest in the legislature. Over the years he was also periodically involved in attempting to fight quackery. Early in 1808, Smith wrote Lyman Spalding asking when and where the next annual meeting of the New Hampshire Medical Society was to be held. "I have an intention to attend if possible," he wrote; "I intend to renew the effort to obtain an Act of Legislature to discourage quackery. . . . The business was not properly managed this year. I was out of town when the question was tried, . . . Several of the members have solicited me to renew the application."[30]

Smith amassed an impressive record in his political maneuverings.[31] It may very well be that the successful applications he had made in the past helped put the legislature in a receptive frame of mind for his most important appeal, in 1809. This time he petitioned for $6,000—a huge sum in those days—to erect a new medical school building; bricks and mortar as well as students and books were part of his dream. The "New Medical House," as it came to be called, was the capstone of Smith's bold plans for a true medical school. He was already excited about the prospect when he wrote to George Shattuck at the end of December 1808, mentioning it for the first time: "I am now projecting a scheme to procure a building for medical purposes at Hanover. I expect to be in Boston in the course of next month, and will then acquaint you with all my plans relating to the advancement of our infant but somewhat thrifty medical institution."[32]

Nowhere in New England were there truly adequate facilities for students interested in medicine. Harvard's medical department was still crowded into Holden Chapel; nowhere was there an operating theater where a roomful of students could observe surgery and dissections. Smith's plans for an enlarged faculty made the need for additional space even more pressing. Moreover, lecture audiences had grown to number a hundred or more, typically, making the double classroom in Dartmouth Hall wholly inadequate as a lecture hall.

Ten weeks after sharing his idea with Shattuck, Smith announced his intentions to Lyman Spalding. He followed up with further details three months later:

I have received your letter respecting my intended application to the Legislature. I propose to make it in this manner, viz: that I will procure a Deed to the State of a parcel of land sufficient to place the building on, to be the property of the State forever, for that purpose: that the Building shall be built at the expense of the State, and remain the property of the same forever, under the inspection and control of some Board, whom the Legislature may appoint, to be used and employed for Medical and Experimental Philosophy. I suppose that about ten thousand dollars would be sufficient to build the House and furnish the necessary Library, Apparatus, etc. I have high expectations that something will be done for me, which will be important to the interest of Medical Science, as I have the assurance of many members of the House of Representatives in my favor.[33]

Thus Smith set about finding money to turn his latest idea into reality.

In June, he wrote to Spalding again; by that time, he was fairly bubbling over with optimism: "I have proffered my petition, and have leave to bring in a Bill, which we have no doubt will pass. The Bill will provide for the building of a Building 60 by 35, 2 stories high, which will answer our purposes very well."[34] The petition to the General Court on June 14, 1809 ran as follows:

Your petitioner begs leave to represent, that in the year 1798 a Medical School was established at Hanover [sic: 1798 was the date the Board of Trust officially approved of the institution; as will be recalled, Smith had begun teaching medical courses in Hanover already in 1797], that there being no building erected exclusively for the use of the establishment, the Trustees of Dartmouth College ordered several rooms to be fitted up for that purpose—one for public instruction, others for a laboratory, apparatus &c., which have since been improved for the benefit of said school—

Your petitioner also begs leave to represent, that the said rooms are found very inadequate to the wants and conveniences of said school, that the hall appropriated for public instruction is not sufficient to accommodate the number of students, who usually attend the Medical Lectures, and that the other apartments are not capable of holding the apparatus and other things belonging to the Institution—Wherefore your petitioner humbly prays, that this Honorable Legislature would in their wisdom devise some means for erecting a suitable building for the use of a Medical School at Hanover—and furthermore, your petitioner proposes,

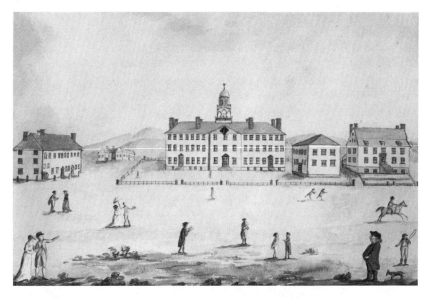

Old Dartmouth Hall in 1803, site of early Dartmouth Medical School classes.
Watercolor by eleven-year-old student George Ticknor.
Courtesy of the Hood Museum of Art, Dartmouth College, Hanover, New Hampshire.

that if means are granted for the purpose before mentioned, he will deed to the State of Newhampshire a suitable tract of land on which a building may be placed —the building to remain the property of the State and at their control forever— and furthermore your petitioner proposes that he will covenant to give into the possession of the State all the apparatus, anatomical museum and other appendages of the School, being now his own private property, for the benefit of said School and of those who may succeed him in the Institution—

From a thorough conviction of the utility of a Medical School in this State, and having, as he thinks, at his own risk and expense, established its practicability, your petitioner humbly hopes that this honorable body will not hazard the existence of an Institution, which has for its object the highest and most important interests of society, by refusing the means necessary for the erection of a building, that may give it perpetuity and extend its influence—and your petitioner as in duty bound will ever pray,

Nathan Smith[35]

A petition was one thing; several more steps would be required before final action in Smith's favor was taken.[36] First, the matter was referred to a bipartisan committee of six, who reported back immediately that Smith should be granted $6,000 and bicameral "leave to bring in a bill"; this was what Smith had triumphantly reported to Spalding. The permission was stated simply enough:

On hearing and considering the petition of Nathan Smith, and the report of a committee thereon: *Voted*, That the prayer be granted and that the petitioner have leave to bring in a bill.

Likewise in the Senate, on the same day:

A vote, granting the prayer of the petition of Nathan Smith, with leave to bring in a bill, was brought up, read, and concurred:

Presented and approved.[37]

But when the bill was in fact brought to the House, numerous objections were raised, particularly with respect to the amount of money; it was sent back to a separate committee of three, who amended it by reducing the sum more than 40 percent, to $3,450. Back to the House it went for further debate; the roll-call vote was taken, and the bill passed, on June 20. Debate was again the order of the day, however, when the bill went to the Senate. But a motion to postpone was defeated 7 to 5, whereupon one of those on the losing side switched his vote, and the bill passed on a roll-call vote of 8 to 4 in the second chamber on June 22. Finally, on June 23, 1809, the act became law, by a vote of 102 to 59, in the following form:

AN ACT APPROPRIATING THREE THOUSAND FOUR HUNDRED AND FIFTY DOLLARS, FOR CERTAIN PURPOSES THEREIN MENTIONED.—

Whereas Nathan Smith Professor of Medicine at Dartmouth College, hath represented to the Legislature, that a building for the use of the Medical School is much wanted, and hath offered gratuitously to convey and assign to the State a suitable lot of land whereon to erect a building for that purpose, together with such parts of the anatomical museum, and chemical apparatus as are his private property; and whereas it behoves an enlightened Community to foster and encourage those institutions which are devoted to the promotion of scientific and useful knowledge—
 Therefore
 Sec. 1. Be it enacted by the Senate and House of Representatives in General Court convened, that the sum of Three Thousand, four hundred and fifty dollars, be, and the same is hereby appropriated, for the purpose of erecting a building of brick or stone, for a medical School, sixty five feet in length, thirty two feet in width, and two stories in height.
 Provided the said Nathan Smith before the said money, or any part thereof be paid out of the Treasury, convey to the State of New Hampshire, by a good and valid title, one half acre of Land, contiguous to Dartmouth College, whereon to erect said building; and provided the said Nathan assigns to the State aforesaid, such parts of the anatomical museum, and chemical apparatus, as are his private property—
 Sec. 2. And be it further enacted, that David Hough Esq'r of Lebanon, Daniel Kimball Esq'r of Plainfield, and Mills Olcott Esquire of Hanover, or either two of them, be a Committee to erect said building . . . .
 Sec. 3. And be it further enacted, that the said Nathan Smith shall have the occupancy and use of the said building and apparatus, while he continues a teacher of said Medical School, and no longer.[38]

Though Smith wrote to Shattuck in annoyance in October complaining that "some of our people are making a political affair" of the "late grant for a medical building,"[39] it is not clear that the heat the bill generated really was partisan. Democrats and Federalists alike had apparently been somewhat loath to support it.[40]

In light of the political hesitation, what Smith had managed to do is nothing short of stunning: He persuaded a state legislative body to give money for a building to be used for a medical school but essentially privately run by an individual for Dartmouth College. Already in 1751, to be sure, Benjamin Franklin had accelerated the establishment of the Pennsylvania Hospital by persuading the colonial legislature there to match the funds raised by private subscription; the promise of matching funds turned out to be critical in loosening the strings of private pocketbooks where donations had previously been sought in vain.[41] But Smith's successful application is historically important as the second such attempt to have public monies allocated for a private medical institution—and this was not just matching funds. Others would pursue the same strategy later, but years would pass before states began supporting publicly financed medical schools on a routine basis.[42]

The satisfaction with which Smith wrote to Shattuck "I obtained both grants by my petitions alone"—referring to the legislature's 1803 grant of money for chemical apparatus and the grant in 1809 of $3,450 for the medical building—is therefore understandable.[43] He had achieved a great deal for Dartmouth—even if it was not entirely of his own doing. In sharp contrast, a few years later he disclaimed credit—with more becoming modesty—for the grant the Connecticut legislature gave to the Medical Institute of Yale, saying "tho, I went myself I think it was principally owing to the good disposition of the members of the Court towards that institution . . . ."[44]

Smith's success resulted from a kind of formula he had devised. He deeded land he owned to the state, convinced the legislature to acknowledge the need for college-trained medical graduates, and managed to keep control of the school for himself. (In the years ahead, Smith would use the same approach to get grants from the legislatures of Connecticut, Maine, and Vermont to help the Yale, Bowdoin, and University of Vermont medical schools respectively; he had impressively little trouble in each instance.) Smith guarded his medical school jealously and wisely, while allowing the legislature to bask in a sense of control; members of the legislature did not seem to notice that the only supervisory committee appointed by their body was a building committee. This was triumph, indeed, for Smith.

The original estimate Smith made of what would be needed turned out to be accurate, and he proceeded to spend the money he did not have. As usual, he remained optimistic that the legislature would eventually see things his way and come up with the balance. In a letter of April 1811 to George Shattuck, Smith declared he was "about to petition the Legislature of New Hampshire at their next session for an additional grant to cover one thousand dollars over and above what the State granted for that purpose and for another thousand to begin a botanical garden."[45] Fourteen months later Smith wrote Shattuck again (for reasons that are unclear, his optimism continued): "Our Legislature did not see fit to allow me the 1,217 dollars I expended in building the medical house at Hanover over and above the grant made by the Legislature for that purpose but I have no doubt but they will at their next meeting."[46] Financial problems having to do with the building and repair of the Medical House persisted. Five years later, in January 1817, Smith (by then settled in New Haven) wrote to Mills Olcott that he was still troubled by money issues connected with the medical building at Dartmouth.[47] Finally, however, a month after that, New Hampshire's Governor William Plumer—directed by the General Court—ordered the state treasurer to pay $1,449.55 for Dr. Nathan Smith's Medical House.[48]

In the meantime, however, the erection of the building had gone forward. In May of 1811, Smith wrote cheerfully to Shattuck that "every part of the business toward the completion of the building is in happy progress,"[49] though a couple of months earlier there was evidence that some were not pleased with the site: "The new Medical house is to be set about twenty rods directly above the chair I now set in [at Nathan Smith's home]," one student wrote a friend and former student; "I think it a foolish plan to mount it on the top of those rocks in solitary gloom. I hope Dr. Perkins will effect to bring it down to the road when he returns."[50] Dr. Perkins did not succeed, and generations of medical students who worked there in the hot and humid months familiar to New Hampshire residents thanked Smith for its breezy perch.

Lemuel Cook was hired to do the preparatory work essential for laying a firm foundation. One receipt bearing the date June 29, 1811, read "Rec'd twenty-two dollars of Nathan Smith . . . today & [somewhat confusingly] twelve sometime since towards the Job of digging cellar & drawing stone."[51] Another, ten days later, acknowledged receipt "of Dr N. Smith Eleven Dollars on acct. of our contract for digging & stoning the cellar of yr Medical house."[52] Whether this $11.00 was in fact the vaguely put "twelve sometime since" is unclear.

The complete financial records for the building no longer exist, but the accounts of another workman, Lemuel Davenport, tell an important story. Nathan Smith's discontent with the original plans precipitated his decision to insist on an extra course of brick:[53]

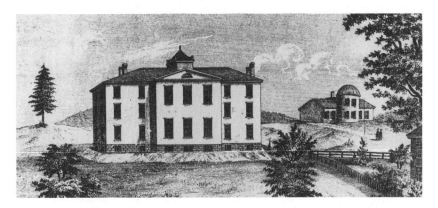

Nathan Smith's "New Medical House" at Dartmouth, pictured in 1855.
Photo courtesy of Dartmouth College Library.

July 4ᵗʰ 1811	Dr. Nathan Smith Dr.	
	to digging sellar, for Laying stone in the medical sellar	$12.00
17	to drawing water three weeks	14.80
	12M̶ bricks for basement story at 30/	60.00
	Laying 12M̶ brick at 18/ per M̶	36.00
	Lim[e] for Laying 12 M̶ brick, [?]	25.00
	to making 12 window frames sound stuff	12.00
	to making sashes for 12 windows in basement story and setting glass at 10 cts per square	14.40
	making doar frame and casing	1.75
	making doar and han[g]ing	2.00
	hinges & screws	.28
	50M̶ bricks put into the walls more than what was agreed to by sd. Davenport which Dr. Smith said he would pay being the width of one brick all over the walls of the Medical house bricks at 30 / per M̶	250.00
	Lim[e] for Laying the same 20 [?]	100.00
	Laying the above bricks at 3 per M̶	150.00
	paid for drawing water for plastering	5.75
		689.68
	painting house	103.26
		786.94
	oil for painting	38.00
	white Lead	27.00
	three weaks [?] at 9/ per day	27.00
	Spanish brown	11.26
		103.26
October	700 ft. clear bords	8.00
	7 days work making shelves and other work	9.33
		120.59

		689.68
		804.27
Cr. for Leaving out middle walls		25.00
		779.27
paid masons for going after storm sills		2.25
		781.52
	[credit]	50.00
		731.52

Despite Smith's care in adding strength to the structure, the bill from Long & Clement shows that repairs were already necessary by 1815. Possibly the result of damage during an anatomy riot, the wear and tear could also have come simply from rough usage:[54]

Oct. 4	To 21 sq^{rs} glass for the Medical House	$2.94
	3 lb. putty for d[itt]o	.50
	Work repairing windows for d[itt]o	1.56
	To making & painting Grave fence	15.00
Nov. 17	To 2 days work by Clement Jewett	.50
	1 lb. putty	.17
Nov. 25	To repairing, hanging & painting Door	4.00

The New Medical House of which Nathan Smith was justifiably so proud in 1811 came to an ignominious end in a pile of rubble a century and a half later. The demolition of the old building in 1963 removed the most visible tie that remained between Dartmouth Medical School and its founder. At the time it was torn down, it was the country's oldest[55] edifice designed and used continually for medical school teaching. The decision to raze the Medical House was based on structural problems—not a weak foundation or weak timbers, but crumbling brick walls. If Nathan Smith had not discovered the flaw in the original plans and insisted at great personal expense on the extra course of brick, the building might well have failed by collapsing in his own lifetime.

College Politics and the First Colleague: Cyrus Perkins

In addition to Mills Olcott, Nathan Smith had another good friend in Hanover—a friendship that, though personally less rewarding, had enormous political significance for him. John Wheelock, president of the College, rented Smith a home. Earlier we saw how he wrote a letter of introduction and support for Smith to take with him when he traveled to Scotland and England.

For all we know, Wheelock may have been looking out primarily for his own interests. Being president put him in a lonely spot; it did not help

that everyone knew he had been the third choice (after two of his brothers) of his father Eleazar Wheelock—founding president of Dartmouth—
and no one else's choice at all. Still, he was genuinely interested in seeing
the College grow and deserves credit for realizing that a "medical department" would be an asset. He dreamed of turning the College into a university and no doubt believed having a medical faculty would push Dartmouth in that direction in fact if not in word.

Whatever the reason, Wheelock seems to have had a warm feeling for
his professor of medicine, which was largely reciprocated. But being
friends with Wheelock was not an unmitigated blessing;[56] the classic division between town and gown in this case took the form of a great divide
between the Wheelocks and just about everyone else. For one thing, as the
quarrel between those who wanted the College to remain just that and
those who fancied a future for it as a university heated up, the faculty and
members of the Board of Trust grew steadily more vocal in their opposition to Wheelock; by 1815, they had in fact removed him from the presidency. Already during the first years of the nineteenth century, the forces
were at play in Hanover that led eventually to what would come to be
called the "Dartmouth College Case." Partisans lined up on the two sides,
opponents were maneuvered into embarrassing situations, the all-too-
scanty appropriations of money were saved for the use by the "right"
side, and so on. Even the social atmosphere in Hanover was affected, and
the mood was at times tense.[57]

If these were among the reasons Smith preferred to live twenty miles
out of town, it would be understandable. That he managed, in the midst
of all this, to stay friendly with both sides is remarkable—further evidence of his ability to get along with difficult people. It may also have had
to do with the reluctance of any of the contestants to give him up as their
physician; general respect for his shrewdness and common sense, and the
way he exercised these qualities, are possible additional factors. Nevertheless, local politics made the first decade of the century a trying time for
Smith, at a period when his hands were especially full with epidemics of
typhoid fever and meningococcic meningitis—to say nothing of anatomy
riots, increasing demands from across New England for the services of
one of her best surgeons, and recurring personal money problems on top
of medical school debts.

Regardless of distractions and tensions, Smith's relations at Dartmouth
continued amicably over a period of many years. One action of the College that took place early on must have pleased him enormously. He, who
had never been nearer to a college than Holden Chapel in Cambridge and
never pretended to be a traditionally trained academician with a classical
education, was proposed by Dartmouth undergraduates for membership

in Phi Beta Kappa on April 4, 1799.[58] Some of those who put his name forward were his students in natural philosophy (the basic science course); Smith's election served as a public affirmation of their esteem, which could not always be taken for granted. Dartmouth students could be very hard on a teacher whom they disliked.[59] At the time Smith was voted into Phi Beta Kappa it was a social fraternity, but considerable academic significance attached to its meetings nonetheless; on both grounds, he should have been pleased to be inducted. Then, eight years later, Smith was elected president of the local chapter,[60] another sign of the good will generally directed at him. (By 1807 Smith's thoughts were elsewhere, however, and we have no record of his ever having presided over a Phi Beta Kappa meeting.)

Nathan Smith got on well with the Board of Trust, too, his recalcitrance in the matter of settling permanently in Hanover notwithstanding. In August 1800, the Board voted to provide him—interest free—with $81.00 to purchase chemical apparatus (probably paraphernalia Spalding had left behind).[61] They appointed a committee to confer with him concerning both his compensation as professor of medicine—as we have seen, fifty dollars was granted for salary for the previous year and another fifty dollars for the ensuing year—and alterations to the medical school.

By 1809 it was clear that neither expanded publicity for his lectures, nor more books and equipment, nor even a new building, was enough for Nathan Smith. He made a proposal that the Board voted to defer; it was recorded in the minutes of the following year's meeting, when the Board did take it up:

Your memorialist represents that finding the labors required of him as a teacher of Medical Science too great and more than he can perform with convenience to himself and advantage to the public, he prays that some other person may be associated with him in that department and that such associate be appointed Professor of Anatomy, and that he himself be excused from teaching in that branch.[62]

It was, one could argue, high time. For thirteen years, Smith had been carrying the weight of the school almost entirely on his shoulders. Despite periodic help from Spalding, Twitchell, and others in chemistry—and the brief but dramatic assist from Ramsay in anatomy—Smith had officially been the whole faculty for well more than a decade. This unprecedented performance has inspired numerous commentators over the years to make Smith the object of a quip by Oliver Wendell Holmes (who himself held Smith's chair as professor of anatomy at Dartmouth 1838–41). Holmes's remark about a professor holding not a chair, but "a whole settee" was not a reference to Smith, at Dartmouth, however; in fact, Holmes said it about Albrecht von Haller (1708–1777), the great Swiss professor of anatomy, botany, and medicine at Göttingen.[63]

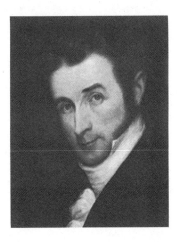

Cyrus Perkins, 1778–1849.
Used with permission of the Francis A.
Countway Library of Medicine.

The Board of Trust's action in August of 1810 included appointing Nathan Smith's former pupil Cyrus Perkins professor of anatomy.[64] Rufus Graves, who had been proprietor of the general store, landlord to Smith, and (like the silversmith Jedediah Baldwin) a quondam student in one series of chemistry lectures, was at the same time—astonishingly—appointed professor of chemistry.[64] A little more than a year later, a notice in the *Dartmouth Gazette* announced that Nathan Smith, Cyrus Perkins, and Rufus Graves would continue in the new medical building at Dartmouth College.[65] Finally the medical school had something approaching a full-fledged faculty, leaving aside how singularly unqualified Graves, at least, must have been. Apart from attending one chemistry course, Graves's only claim to academic preferment—his only academic involvement heretofore—seems to have been that it was he who had found Smith his first lecture room in 1797. Fortunately, perhaps, it appears that Graves may not have been called upon to teach the chemistry course very often; Nathan Noyes (A.B. 1796; M.B. 1799) and then Reuben D. Mussey took it over in the years ahead. Graves does seem to have participated at one point (perhaps as an apothecary) in some kind of business partnership with Smith and Perkins as well (again, like Baldwin), as an undated letter from Perkins to Smith about how the fees collected should be distributed makes clear.[66]

Less is known about Perkins than we could wish.[67] Moreover, the relationship between Smith and Perkins seems to have been more complicated—certainly less warm—than that between Smith and Spalding, or

Smith and Shattuck. We can infer that Perkins was a good undergraduate student from the fact that he gave one of the commencement orations the year he graduated. That he received his M.B. two years after his A.B. indicates he almost certainly began his medical studies immediately and progressed without problems. With Smith as his only instructor in medicine, there is no surprise in his having dedicated his inaugural dissertation for the M.B. degree to Smith; his reference in that dedication to himself as an "Obliged and Grateful Pupil" (though it verges on boilerplate language) hints that he had also done his apprenticeship under Smith.[68] Conceivably, this expressed admiration for and deference to his professor was a factor in his being chosen as the second professor in Dartmouth's medical department in 1810, thus turning the "pupil" into a colleague, though Smith seems unlikely to have been easily swayed by flattery alone (and Perkins was hardly unique in dedicating his graduation paper to Smith). But presumably Smith played at least some role in choosing who should receive the important appointment as professor of anatomy, and from this we can also infer that Perkins was more than competent (or that Smith at least considered him so).

The partnership that Smith set up with Perkins must have worked satisfactorily, because the arrangement lasted until Smith left for Yale in 1813.[69] Student assessment of Perkins, however, was somewhat mixed. A year after Smith had left Dartmouth, one student wrote home to his preceptor that "Professor Perkins . . . is to be absent next week . . . . It will be a great disappointment to the students." At the same time, another student expressed himself more cautiously to the same preceptor: "I conceive that Dr Perkins discovers a complete knowledge of his subject, is very perspicuous in his manner of demonstration and is sufficiently minute in his descriptions, which last I am sorry to say is to some tedious."[70] This latter student was, on the other hand, unstinting in his praise of Perkins as a surgeon, reporting (in the same letter)—after watching one delicate procedure—that he had "never seen surgical instruments handled with more skill and adroitness."

We should perhaps not be too hard on Perkins, remembering that his entire medical training seems to have been under Smith. Even with eight years of private practice to his credit by the time he joined the Dartmouth faculty, his education was not so well rounded as those of Smith's students who had spent time in Philadelphia or who had gone abroad. He was not alone. After Noyes and Mussey had joined Perkins (and Graves, still the chemistry lecturer) in the aftermath of Smith's rather abrupt departure from Dartmouth in 1813, the faculty remained even by the "comparatively low standards of that day . . . inbred and of limited academic experience."[71]

Perkins's fame, such as it is, comes less from his reputation as a medical man than from his involvement in the political controversy over whether Dartmouth should remain a college or become a university. How much overt tension there was between Smith and Perkins on this matter we do not know; it was in any case not sufficient to prevent Smith from being invited back to Dartmouth, after he had gone to Yale, to give a course of lectures in the fall of 1816. He agreed to do so, alongside Perkins and Mussey. Though the "medical department escaped the division into two separate halves which overtook the rest of the College and . . . continued a unified but uneasy existence during this period,"[72] there is no question that Perkins, in particular, was thoroughly committed to the university cause. Smith, too, we know was sympathetic to Wheelock, and thus it is not surprising he was willing to teach with Perkins under the aegis of the university. It was moreover clear that the land on which the medical school building stood belonged not to the College, but to the state, which supported the university cause; as we have seen, this was Smith's own doing, and he was thus hardly in a position to object. Mussey is reported to have had misgivings about getting involved with "university" doings, and he succeeded a year later in getting the medical lectures announced as being at Dartmouth *College*. By that time, Smith had decided he was best out of the whole situation.

How different the history of Dartmouth Medical School and Nathan Smith's relationship with it would have been if it had not been for the peculiar contemporary politics of the College, we can of course not even begin to guess. Nor can we know how much Cyrus Perkins's adamant support of the university cause affected Smith's position, let alone what would have become of Perkins himself if he had not worked so vigorously for what turned out to be the losing side. In the end, once the College cause had prevailed, Perkins was in an untenable position; he resigned in June of 1819, worked on settling his affairs in Hanover and Boston, and then moved to New York City. There he practiced for many years, but he never taught again; he died on April 23, 1849.[73]

At the time of his death, Perkins had long been out of the picture at Dartmouth. He and those other students of Smith's who taught at the College immediately following the founder's departure and during the politically difficult period deserve credit, however, for helping ensure that their mentor's first-planted medical institution continued in operation. Without them, history might well have been very different.

PART III

PHYSICIAN AND SURGEON

CHAPTER NINE

Nathan Smith's Medical Practice

Replacing Dogmatism with Patient Inquiry

[T]he clever, skilled physician who is versed in the fundamentals of medicine
thinks twice before he decides how to bring about a patient's relief, and . . . always relies on the work of nature . . . . In dubious cases, when the best course
is to do nothing, he would deliberate with himself if it were not better to leave
medicines alone and wait for nature to take its beneficial course.
—MOSES MAIMONIDES [1]

Theories and Nosologies

MEDICAL TREATMENTS and therapies in general were in a most
unsatisfactory state in Nathan Smith's day. Until at least 1800,
medicine in the new country "tended to be dominated by quackery, mystical and superstitious beliefs, [and] home remedies"; medical
care was as likely to be in the hands of ministers and schoolmasters as of
physicians—and the majority of those who did lay claim to being doctors
were ill trained.[2] Experts often advocated disease treatments without any
factual basis for their recommendations. Ignorance of the causes of disease frequently confused the issue further. Physicians unfamiliar with the
natural history of disease—particularly when they were not certain of
their diagnoses—were liable to urge aggressive interventions for every patient, regardless of the symptoms. Indeed, vigorous therapy has been
called "the hallmark of medical practice of the period."[3] The more dramatic the effect of the treatment, the better. Or so most patients and practitioners (quacks, irregulars, and regulars alike) seemed to believe.

Underlying many of the practices of early nineteenth-century medicine
were the still-popular rationalist teachings of Professor William Cullen of
Edinburgh. The irony is that what looks completely irrational to us today
was precisely what most people at the time considered highly rational.

That is, treatments were based on carefully thought out (and to that extent rational) theories and organizing principles, and "[n]o medical centre was so firmly linked . . . with rationalist systems as Edinburgh."[4]

The contrast was, above all, with the empiricism of French doctors who were making "free access to experiential knowledge of the body" central to medical teaching and practice.[5] Such physicians were slowly beginning to use systematic pathology as a basis for their treatments.[6] The result of paying more attention to what actually transpired in patients' bodies was that the contradictory (and sometimes harmful) therapies, unquestioningly followed for years, were finally being challenged.

In 1809—in the middle of Nathan Smith's career—an emphasis on experience rather than theory was very unusual. The same Edward Augustus Holyoke with whom John Warren had apprenticed was a sufficiently strong proponent of such an approach to have made a lasting impression on Boston physician James Jackson (1777–1867). Jackson, as a result, felt constrained to inscribe his Harvard thesis to Holyoke as follows: "By you I was taught to pay a sacred regard to experience as the source of all medical knowledge and by you I was forbidden to resort to speculative principles as guides to practice except where experience failed."[7]

Later, Jackson found himself opposing Oliver Wendell Holmes's rather different reading of experience. Holmes (1809–1894) argued that experience showed medicinal remedies were frequently injurious, and that doing less, or even nothing, was often the better course—a relatively radical approach that sounds like pure Nathan Smith. Jackson, in *Another Letter to a Young Physician* (written for and distributed to members of the Massachusetts Medical Society in 1861 in response to Holmes), insisted on the other hand that experience showed available medicines did more good than harm and that Holmes's skepticism went too far.

Smith would have liked the way Jackson emphasized that no system of medicine can be useful until facts in anatomy, pathology, physiology, and therapeutics put flesh on the bare bones of theory (though he would probably have been distressed that anyone still saw a need to argue about theory versus experience one hundred years after Cullen). He surely would have been more comfortable with—and would have applauded—Holmes's "do no harm" policy.

To understand Nathan Smith's contributions to the practice as well as the teaching of medicine one must also understand the great struggle among doctors both here and abroad who advocated rival systems of medicine. Roughly, the tension was between those who believed in a system where nature had to be controlled and those who sought to take all their cues by following nature's lead. Where most physicians subscribed to the theory that disease was due to nature's mischief and that strong drugs were necessary to punish and correct her in some mysterious way, Smith was one of the relatively few who believed in giving the body a chance to heal itself.

Some physicians, weaned on the old humoral theories, believed that what was needed was bleeding and purging—anything to correct the imbalance of the humors they saw as the universal cause of illness. Many of the more "modern" physicians, influenced above all by Cullen, had advanced new theories based somewhat loosely on what they understood of the physiology of vascular (particularly capillary) spasm; these theories in turn were thought to explain the origin of disease and to justify a variety of treatment procedures. For the most part, however, these amounted to the same old depletion regimens (bleeding, purging, etc.); only the arguments for their use were new.

One particularly dramatic story of depletion therapy is told by Captain Thomas Dover (1660–1742), later famous for one of the most popular patent medicines ever—"Dover's Powders"—of how he proceeded when disease struck his ship at sea. Having found that 180 of his men were suffering from the plague, he "ordered the surgeons to bleed them in both arms, and to go round to them all, with command to leave them bleeding till all were blooded, and then come and tie them up in their turns. Thus they lay bleeding, and fainting so long, that I could not conceive they could lose less than an hundred ounces each man." One imagines the deck awash in blood. Yet all but seven or eight of the 180 survived this treatment (plus oil and spirit of vitriol mixed with water to the acidity of a lemon, of which the afflicted were made to "drink very freely")—an astonishingly low mortality for plague or any other serious disease, considering what the patients endured.[8]

Other physicians eschewed depleting therapies in favor of "stimulating" treatments. They concluded (correctly enough) that Cayenne pepper, arsenic, and cantharides (Spanish fly) were stimulants, along with (more debatably) opium, wine, brandy, and cinchona (often called "Peruvian") bark.[9] Alas, those who supported such conclusions could not always say how or what these substances stimulated. Nathan Smith once wrote that he had heard a doctor boasting of having forced a patient to drink three pints of brandy accompanied by large doses of laudanum and cantharides, and that he had himself "seen a written prescription, in which opium, wine, alcohol, cantharides and arsenic, were all directed to be taken several times in the course of twenty-four hours."[10]

Smith did not belong to either of the extremist schools of therapy. He understood that if well-intentioned doctors with different philosophies could prescribe diametrically opposed treatment for the same disease with comparable results, then neither theory could be uniquely correct.

Hence Smith's inclination to challenge Cullen's teachings when he believed the older man was wrong. We have seen in the notes Smith's students took in his lectures how Smith used Cullen as his lecture-room adversary, mentioning the Scot's position frequently, almost always only to reject it. A specific example of how they differed may be helpful; what follows is a comparison of the regimens for typhoid fever propounded by Cullen and by Smith.[11]

Cullen's Antiphlogistic Regimen	*Smith's Treatment*
Good ventilation	The same
Keep cool or produce sweating	Keep cool; no sweating
Keep quiet	The same
Don't let patient think [Cullen believed "exercise of the mind" was stimulating and thus to be shunned]	Not mentioned
Don't let patient eat (until crisis)	The same
Eat least stimulating foods (after crisis)	Give patient choice of food, limit quantity
Drink freely except spiritous liquors	The same ("simple diluent drinks")
Vomit out stomach's crudities	No
Give Tartar Emetic	No
Purge, or use laxative glysters	No purging; use only occasional (mild) laxatives
Use antiseptic liquors	There is no such thing
Cool patient by air or water	The same
Cool patient by refrigerants	No
Cool patient by neutral salts	No
Cool patient by sugar of lead or other metallic salts	No
Diminish tension by venesection	Rarely (only if there is "a sense of fullness in the head")
Use antispasmodics (opium, camphor)	Use rarely, but with ipecacuanha in diarrhea
Use sudorifics	No
Blister	No
Vomit	No
Use tonic ens veneris	Not mentioned
Use copper preparations	Not mentioned
Use arsenic and alum	Not mentioned
Use Peruvian bark (always)	Rarely
Use wine	No; small beer or brisk cider
Allow no animal food	The same
Use antiseptics	No
Use acids	Muriatic, rarely; lemonade, freely
Neutral fats	Not mentioned
Fixed air	Not mentioned

Cullen of course had a theory to back up all these recommendations: Treatment was to be determined by paying proper attention to the proximate cause of the fever. The first task, then, was to moderate the violence of the reaction, after which steps should be taken to remove the cause of the debility and to correct what he saw as the tendency of the fluids to putrefaction. Smith, on the other hand, argued that unless specific symptoms demanded treatments known to be effective, the physician should do nothing at all.

Not that Smith lacked interest in or knowledge of the medical theories of his day. On the contrary, he was well enough informed to criticize those with whom he disagreed (like Cullen, Rush, and other "dogmatists"). He was also prepared to elaborate on the sound ideas of those with whom he mostly agreed (such as his older contemporary, the Scotsman Benjamin Bell [1749–1806]).[12] One of the authorities for whom Smith seems to have had the most affinity was the great seventeenth-century physician Thomas Sydenham, often called "the English Hippocrates."[13] (Although we do not find Sydenham explicitly quoted or cited by Smith, we can reasonably assume he was well acquainted with the English doctor, given that he used Sydenham's principles in his teaching and that his own approach to therapy so closely echoed Sydenham's.) Through Sydenham, Smith also had a direct line back to Hippocrates. Centuries earlier the "Father of Medicine" had pointed out that the healing forces of nature, if left alone, would often be adequate. "Nature is the physician of illnesses,"[14] was the central Hippocratic teaching Nathan Smith had in common with Sydenham. That Smith had been exposed to classical writers is clear; in his "Introductory Lecture on the Progress of Medical Science" given at Yale,[15] for example, he cited Hippocrates (among others) and discussed precisely this *vis medicatrix naturae* (healing power of nature).

Like Hippocrates, Sydenham generally argued that simpler was likely to be better, saying on one occasion that "it is the business of the physician to assist nature." Though great physicians might be tempted to disdain simple treatments, Sydenham went on to state his position humbly:

Nor do I think it beneath me to acknowledge, with respect to the cure of fevers, that when no manifest indication pointed out to me what was to be done, I have consulted the safety of my patient, and my own reputation, most effectively, by doing nothing at all.[16]

Smith frequently gave similar advice. Despite the influence of Cullen (through Waterhouse) on his Harvard education, Smith already in his dissertation—also on the subject of fevers, it will be recalled—showed a readiness to rely on the healing power of nature. "There is a phenomenon in fevers," he had written, that is itself "an operation" of the *vis medicatrix naturae*:

a preternatural quantity of bile, secreted and poured into the alimentary canal:

this has by some been looked upon as a part of the disease; and consequently they have prescribed methods to dislodge it: but I am so far from thinking it an aggravating occurrence in fevers, that I believe it has a considerable share in the cure.[17]

But despite the cautious approach Smith and a few others advised, variations on Cullen's theories (especially as put forward by Rush) were powerfully at work. Rush, as we have seen, was a prominent public figure. He had marched onto the scene in the 1790s burning with apocalyptic zeal for a new system of treatments, based on a "revelation" that came to him during the yellow fever epidemic of 1793 in Philadelphia. He became convinced that the proper way to treat disease—he believed that all illnesses really were only one disease, a position Smith explicitly challenged[18]— was to bleed and purge until all vestige of undue excitement of the central nervous system (including, in Cullen's interpretation, thought itself!) was abolished. Smith prudently refrained from arguing directly with Rush; the bombastic Rush was both popular and influential. Though he angered many people with his condescending and self-righteous manner, he was "a brilliant propagandist"; much of the responsibility for making Cullen such a hero and inspiration in American medical circles goes to him.[19]

Nathan Smith was among the relatively few who remained unpersuaded. In attempting to replace the Cullen-Rush "heroic" (for which, read "violent, dramatic") practice of medicine with treatments based on questioning patients about their symptoms, Smith was struggling against a well-established body of misconceptions. His apparent reliance on Sydenham to confirm basic principles he had discovered for himself is of particular interest, because Rush also considered himself indebted to Sydenham—going so far as to publish in 1809 a new edition of the 105-year-old textbook, *The Works of Thomas Sydenham, M.D., on Acute and Chronic Diseases, with Their Histories and Modes of Cure.* Only by torturing the text and amending Sydenham with his footnote-commentary, however, could Rush bend the old master's work to serve his own ideological purposes.

Sydenham carefully cautioned that a doctor should refrain from bleeding, for example, when the blood was anemic, as it generally was in children, in declining age, or even in young adults worn out by a lingering illness. But Rush did not refrain. In his footnotes he specifically denied these contra-indications in a magnificent example of his passion for bloodletting: "Our author means in this place by 'weak blood,' that which coheres but feebly [Rush chose to take Sydenham to be referring to poor coagulation], but this is sometimes a mark of preternatural strength in the blood vessels, instead of weakness, and is an indication of the necessity of bleeding." And when Sydenham proposed a moderate approach to therapy in cases of exanthemata (acute, probably viral, diseases that typically produce high fever), Rush responded indignantly.[20]

Rush, Cullen, and the other dogmatists were generally unwilling to curb their heroic practices. Although Cullen was honest enough to confess that he knew his system of medicine was incomplete and necessarily somewhat erroneous ("I have, myself, been jealous of my being sometimes imperfect . . . "[21]), he clung to the idea that his system was nonetheless better than those of others. With a mixture of condescension and mockery, he criticized those who trust

much to the constant attention and wisdom of nature . . . [and] have proposed the *Art of curing by expectation*; have therefore, for the most part, proposed only very inert and frivolous remedies; have zealously opposed the use of some of the most efficacious, such as opium and the Peruvian bark; and are extremely reserved in the use of general remedies, such as bleeding, vomiting, &c. . . . [T]he general doctrine of *Nature curing diseases*, the so much vaunted Hippocratic method of curing, has often had a very baneful influence on the practice of physic; as either leading physicians into, or continuing them in, a weak and feeble practice.[22]

Today, we can easily agree with Cullen that patients would have been worse off without opium or quinine correctly used as specifics for pain and (some) fever. But opium and quinine surely would have eventually earned their places in the physicians' armamentarium without the theorizing. And what a lot of misery would have been spared if Cullen had taught about the strong contra-indications to bleeding and vomiting, instead of insisting that whenever "the *vis medicatrix naturae* . . . is admitted it throws an obscurity upon our system [of medicine]."[23] No "watchful waiting" for Cullen.

Smith's practice showed he failed to see why it was necessary to trim observed facts to fit a priori theory. In 1794 S. Griffin had written to Levi Bartlett from the bottom of his exasperated, locally educated, country-doctor heart, criticizing

those selfswolen sons of pedantic absurdity, fresh & raw from that universal asylum of medical perfection, Edinburgh, . . . [who] enter with obstinate assurance upon the old round of obsolete prescription, which their infallible masters taught them, &, like the mule that turns aside for no man, push on in their bloody career till the surrounding mortality, but more especially the danger of their own thick skulls, brings them to a pause, & works in them a new conviction.[24]

Smith surely agreed. Confronted with the imposing edifice of "pedantic absurdity," which contrasted so sharply with his own experience, it is small wonder that he set about dismantling it.

The key to many of the preposterous treatments of the day was the fallacious reasoning of those determined to classify diseases as if they were so many plants and animals. A carefully constructed "nosology"—a tax-onomy for diseases modeled after what Linnaeus had done for botany—such as the one Cullen put forward, was, as has been pointed out, gener-ally "useless for medicine because [it was] founded on conjecture."[25]

Some physicians, even then, partially recognized this. A. P. Wilson Philip (1770–1847), whose massive work on fevers Smith would later edit and publish in an American edition, devoted the first part of his introduc-tion to explaining Cullen's nosology of disease. He then followed it with a detailed discussion of the ways (and the reasons) his version deviated from Cullen's arrangement; it seems to have been expected that every medical professor would have his own nosology. Smith in turn, feeling free like any good editor of the time to correct and expand on his author, inserted a nosology of *his* own after Wilson Philip's introduction (which ended with a complete "Arrangement of Febrile Diseases," classified into species and families). This second "Introduction," by Smith, was titled "A Nosological Arrangement of Diseases." Smith was apparently not troubled that the result was a book that had three complete nosologies, each of which differed from the others significantly.

Smith had reasons for wanting to include his version. "Nosological writers," he wrote to open his essay,

have generally adopted the plan of natural historians. This method, though it may have some advantages in arrangement, is defective in many respects. Natural his-tory, treats of things which have permanent characters, remaining the same under all varieties of circumstances, and is chiefly employed about obvious qualities. No-sology, treats of the changes which take place in organized bodies; always varying and never remaining the same for any length of time. The difference in the objects, in these two departments of science, is so great, that we should hardly expect the same scheme of arrangement would be equally applicable to both.[26]

These criticisms are trenchant. Throughout, Smith used his editing of Wilson Philip's text as an occasion to criticize Cullen in print:

If we look into Dr. Cullen's Nosology, we shall find, that some of the orders have *no affinity* with others belonging to the same class, either in their exciting causes, the part of the body on which they are seated, or in the remedies which are em-ployed in curing them, and that the similitude, which brought them together in the same class, depends on some circumstances trifling in its nature, affording no data, from which we can deduce the nature of the disease, or the proper mode of treating it.[27]

Even when Smith praised Cullen or commented positively on some as-pect of his work, it was—as in his lectures—only to demolish him. In the same introduction, he continued:

In justice to Dr. Cullen, it should be observed, that he has left us some important hints, respecting the similarity of diseases; in his preface to his nosology, he has these words, "I wish two things might be particularly attended to, which may greatly assist in indicating the similitude of diseases. The one is, that similitude of cause, argues a similarity in disease. The other thing, which shews the similarity of diseases, is the similarity of medicines by which they are cured." — Respecting the similarity of diseases, which are excited by the same cause, applied to different persons, there can be no doubt, but that the same cause, will produce similar diseases, on different persons. In proof of this we refer to the causes of epidemics and the effects of contagious and morbid poisons. But as to the similitude of diseases being indicated by the similarity of remedies by which they are cured, this must be very vague and uncertain, as it is an indisputable fact that some medicines will cure several diseases which are very dissimilar. Mercury is a remedy in several diseases which have never been considered as having any relations to each other, such as affections of the liver, lues veneria and dropsy. Dr. Cullen has hinted at the scheme of indicating the similitude of diseases from their being seated in the same part of the body, but he does it in a manner totally different from the plan I propose.[28]

Smith saw his nosology as merely introductory to "the first step towards a rational practice," which for him meant "investigat[ing] the disease" itself. "We do this," he insisted, "by carefully attending to all the functions of the body, to ascertain whether they are well or ill performed, and are governed in making our prescriptions, by the part of the body affected."[29] That Smith was consistent in his criticisms is clear from lecture notes taken by David Shelton Edwards when he studied "Theory and Practice" under Smith at Yale. Under the heading "Doct. N. Smith Nosological Arrangements of diseases," Edwards quotes Smith using language almost identical to that of his introduction to Wilson Philip's work (published the following year). Anticipating what he was to put into print, Smith said that if "we examine Dr. Cullen's Nosology (which is perhaps as good as any hitherto published) we shall find that some of the orders have no affinity with others of the same class . . . ." Smith summed up thus: "I have introduced these observations to show that diseases cannot with propriety be arranged in the same manner as objects of natural history."[30]

Further evidence of Smith's views about the relative merits of nosologies appears in an 1806 letter to his former student George Shattuck, then studying under Benjamin Rush. Again Smith's critical stance is hardly confrontational; he praises, where he can, before making his stab. "Dr. Rush must be a very interesting lecturer," he wrote:

As to his classification of diseases, I do not think it very material; however we may class diseases, we must study them in detail. I have observed that men of genius having accustomed themselves to view objects in a certain relation to each other for some time, consider their relations so obvious as not to escape the notice of the most inattentive observer, when in reality their reasoning is too arbitrary to be followed without much study and attention. This has generally been the case with nosologists, and perhaps Dr. Rush's method of classing diseases is not wholly exempt from arbitrary reasoning. . . . As to the unity of diseases, you know it is my opinion that we have in medical science of late generalized too much, and that the progress of medicine has been checked by it. This mode of proceeding tends to substitute idleness for industry, and dogmatism for patient inquiry.[31]

When Lyman Spalding tried his hand at preparing a nosology, Smith tried to dissuade him with gentle humor:

As for your plan of nosological arrangement, I have mislaid your letter on that subject but if I recollect rightly it was to take up the subject alphabetically. This will make [it] like the arrangement in a Dictionary, if I comprehend it. I have not given the subject such attention as to enable me to decide positively on it, but I had thought, that to arrange diseases according to the part of the body in which they were seated, or in such order that those in the same class should have some points of similarity between them was best. I recollect that when I read your letter a whimsical idea came into my head which was that if we arranged the diseases alphabetically we might arrange the materia medica in the same order & taking two columns, place all the names of diseases beginning with A on one side & for their remedies, all medicines beginning with the same letter on [the other]

Cancer	Cut out
Hydrophobia	Hydrargyrum

But this is all stuff. I do not pretend to condemn the plan till I have it more fully explained, perhaps there may be reasons for it & advantages that have not yet occurred to me.[32]

Five years later, Smith was still—or again—trying to convince Lyman Spalding of the merits of his (Smith's) views on nosology:

As to what Dr. Rush & others have said of Nosology & the general disrepute into which it has fallen it is to be attributed to the errors in those who attempted it rarther [sic] than the impossibility of classing diseases in a way which will assist the learner. Now I do not know how to define disease other than the deficiency or wrong performance of some of the functions of the body. Therefore if we know which of the several functions is deranged primarily by a disease such disease may therefore be considered as belonging essentially to that organ whose functions are changed. Now as anatomy & physiology have led us to a knowledge of the several organs of the body & their respective functions, if we class diseases accordingly as they affect the different functions we shall not have a great many classes of diseases not enough to burden the memory, while by thus confining our enquiries to this circumstance it will lead us one step toward the true character of such disease & its remedies.[33]

Perhaps the briefest and most explicit indication of Smith's position, late in his career, is found in notes taken by the student Worham L. Fitch. Under the heading "Nosological Arrangement," Fitch quoted Smith's proposal for how to "divide the body" preparatory to studying disease:

We divide the body in the following manner:
1st The Nervous system, including the brain, medulla spinalis, the nerves [issuing] from them, and the extremities of these nerves which are the immediate organs of sense.

2d The Sanguiferous System, including the heart arteries and veins.
3d Bronchial System.
4th The Chylopoietic Viscera, including all the organs concerned in Chylification and contained in the abdomen.
5th The Urinary Organs.
6th The Genital Organs.
7th The Lymphatic System, including the lacteals and lymphatic vessels with their common trunk.
8th The Skin or Cutaneous Diseases.[34]

Fevers

Among the reasons Smith was troubled by Cullen's nosology was that it resulted in such complete nonsense—in Smith's view—when it came to fevers. This was an area of medical practice in which Smith had had considerable experience, having labored long and hard on the subject. In addition to editing Wilson Philip's *Febrile Diseases*, Smith made his single greatest contribution to medical literature with his *Practical Essay on Typhous Fever.*[35]

Thus Smith's hackles would have been raised when Cullen wrote that other physicians had never been able to divide continued fevers into "sensible" categories—but that he had. Pompously using the first-person plural, Cullen pronounced:

[W]e think it agreeable . . . to distinguish continued fevers according as they show either an inflammatory irritation, or a weaker reaction. . . . But the most common form of continued fevers, in this climate, seems to be a combination of these two genera; and I have therefore given such a genus a place on our Nosology, under the title of SYNOCHUS. At the same time, I think that the limits between the Synochus and Typhus will be with difficulty assigned; and I am disposed to believe that the Synochus arises from the same causes as the Typhus, and is therefore only a variety of it.[36]

In other words, according to Cullen's nosology, although fevers might *seem* to differ, the apparent differences were all due to local external factors acting on a single disease (this may have been one source of Rush's "revelation" about the unity of disease, mentioned above). Smith concluded otherwise. His essay on typhous fever—what we know today as typhoid—reflected his experience with the disease ("I have practised physic and surgery for thirty-five years pretty extensively in all the New England states, except Rhode-Island"[37]). The essay, which included both a discursive analysis of the disease and case reports based on careful observation, was sound in principle and full of good sense. When the treatise was already seventy-five years old, Sir William Osler paid it a great tribute: "Try," he said, "to have a copy of Nathan Smith's *A Practical Essay on Typhous Fever* (1824) to hand any young physician who asks for something good & fresh on typhoid fever."[38] Two decades later, in 1913, the great Johns Hopkins clinician William H. Welch wrote that "[o]nly a later generation could appreciate fully how original and great was the contribution to medicine which he made in his essay on 'Typhus [sic] Fever,' now a medical classic." (Welch had earlier rhapsodized that Nathan Smith's essay was "like a fresh breeze from the sea amid the dreary and stifling writing of most of his contemporaries . . . never before had the symptoms been so clearly and accurately pictured."[39])

What Smith wrote in that much-praised essay tells us a good deal about the way he practiced medicine:

The Typhous Fever, as far as my experience, which has been considerable, enables me to judge, is a disease *sui generis*, exhibiting a little variety in the different individuals affected by it as some of the diseases which are acknowledged always to arise from contagion. . . .

Some late writers, have described a fever beginning inflammatory, and ending typhous, and vice versa. Upon this point, I would observe, that in many if not all acute diseases, there is a marked difference in appearance between the rise and decline of the same disease, whether it terminates in death or recovery, and generally, the early part of all febrile affections is attended with more symptoms of inflammation than the latter. This is undoubtedly the case with Typhus; but such difference of symptoms in its different stages, should not induce us to give the disease different names.

As I consider Typhous Fever as arising from a specific cause, if it begins Typhus, or arises from such specific cause, I believe it to continue Typhus through its whole course. Variations, in severity or mildness, can make no specific difference in the disease. . . .

The diseases with which it is liable to be confounded, and for which it is often mistaken, are pure unmixed catarrhal fever, the acute stomach complaints above referred to, and those bilious affections, which take place in the latter part of summer, and the commencement of autumn.[40]

Turning to treatment, Smith also spoke out plainly. Here it is that we get one of the clearest statements of the *primum non nocere* (first, do no harm) principle to be found in Nathan Smith's writing—a principle that he adhered to and taught, consistently, within the limits of his knowledge:

If the pathology of Typhous Fever we have just laid down, be correct, if it arise from a specific cause and has a natural termination, it may be a question, how far we are to attempt a cure of it, or if we possess the power, whether we can with propriety cut it off in its commencement and by art prevent its running its course. . . .

It does not follow, because we have no expectation of arresting the disease, that we are to neglect doing anything. In cases of the other contagious diseases, which are destined to run a certain course, as the small-pox, we often prescribe early in the disease, and with evident good effect, but not with a view to stop, or cut off the disorder; for whatever we do, we expect it will pass through all its regular stages, and our prescriptions are calculated only to render it milder and safer, and enable the patient to live through it. . . .

On the other hand, it does not follow of course, that this disease in all cases requires remedies, or that a patient should necessarily take medicines because he has the disease. In other specific diseases, we proceed on the principle of withholding our remedies unless they are called for by particular circumstances, and thus many cases of measles, hooping-cough, and other contagious diseases, go through their course to their natural termination without medicine.

In cases where the disease is going on regularly in its course, without any symptom denoting danger, and without any local distress, it is presumable that medicines, especially powerful ones, would be more likely to do harm than good. Although Typhous Fever is a more formidable disease than measles or hoopingcough, yet there are many mild cases, and in such cases, I apprehend that the use of powerful means, with a view of curing the disease, is liable to do great mischief.

I have seen in many cases, in which persons in the early stages of this disease were moping about, not very sick, but far from being well, who, upon taking a dose of tartrite of antimony, with the intention of breaking up the disease, have been immediately confined to their bed.

In fact, I feel well convinced, that all powerful remedies or measures, adopted in the early stage of Typhous Fever are very liable to do harm, and that those patients, who are treated with them in the beginning, do not hold out so well in the latter stages of the disease. . . .

From the time Dr. Cullen published his "First lines of the theory and practice of Physic," till very lately, students were generally taught to believe, that Typhous Fever was produced by some weakening power, and was, in effect, a disease of debility. . . .

The practitioners of medicine in New-England, have been divided on this subject; and while one part have become converts to the doctrine of blood-letting to a high degree in this affection, the other has condemned it *in toto*, and, as though opposition has produced a kind of re-action on their part, they have had recourse to the most powerful stimulants both internally and externally, such as opium, wine, alcohol, and the most acrid stimulants, as Cayenne pepper, arsenic, &c. . . .

In the autumn of 1812, Professor Perkins, now of New-York, and myself, attended between fifty and sixty cases of Typhus in the vicinity of Dartmouth College . . . .

Of the whole number, which came under our care, one only was bled, and that on account of a sense of fulness in the head.[41]

Venesection

The last several paragraphs of the preceding excerpt from Smith's essay on typhous fever help illustrate how easily any discussion of therapy could turn into talk about whether and when to engage in venesection. Technically speaking, venesection belonged to surgery rather than medicine (after all, it entailed cutting—in this case, of the veins). The definition of surgery given by the early French surgeon Ambroise Paré (1510–1590) makes clear why. Saying that there are "five duties in surgery," the first he lists is "to remove what is superfluous." Certainly the primary motivation behind the gallons of blood spilled by medics of one sort or another was "to remove what [was thought to be] superfluous."[42] Nonetheless, because bleeding was a common therapy for such a wide range of ills, most of which themselves had nothing to do with surgery, we will look at what Smith said and did about bleeding in the context of his medical practice.

The general attitude of the day toward bleeding (indeed, toward "depleting therapies" in general) was aptly satirized in a play popular in London at the end of the eighteenth century. Dr. Forceps rushes in to the hospital and asks Hellebore what the treatment for the day should be. Hellebore, sensibly enough, asks first "Why, what was done yesterday?"

FORCEPS: Sir, we bled the west ward and jalloped the north ["jalap" was a common purgative].
HELLEBORE: Did ye? Well then, bleed the north ward and jallop the west today.[43]

Earlier, in 1656, the poet-physician John Collop had argued for and against phlebotomy—another term for bleeding—in verse he hoped would be devastating. Arguing the affirmative, so to speak, Collop wrote: "The Courses Nature doth in Women take, / To open veins, shall we in men forsake? / Where Nature dictates, who will not submit?" Part of his negative take on the subject might well have given pause: "More merciful Turks thus blood do never spill, / Under pretense of help, nor do they kill."[44] Alas, neither verse, nor precept, nor common sense abolished the abuse for another two hundred years; only well into the nineteenth century did the careful statistical work appear that destroyed the rationale for bleeding.[45]

The whole issue of venesection was more complicated than it appears today. A generally accepted procedure that was virtually required by the old humoral theories, bleeding as a minimum provided doctors with something to do. Besides, many patients reported marked improvement in their symptoms after being bled. With this therapy so entrenched in the practice of the "experts," it would have been difficult to give it up altogether. Smith—noting the long convalescence needed in over-bled patients—advised caution; Sydenham (though he did not always have an entirely modern outlook on bleeding) had helped blaze the way, formulating many contra-indications to bleeding. Together, Sydenham, Wilson Philip, and finally Smith espoused attitudes toward bleeding that marked the beginning of its end as a cure-all.

Tradition has it that Smith campaigned fiercely against Cullen's antiphlogistic regimen and specifically taught that venesection was wrong. This he did not do. In some of his lectures, in fact, he explicitly advised bleeding and carefully taught correct techniques.[46] Furthermore, it is clear that he himself bled—or believed he should have—on occasion. Commenting on a patient who had died after a head injury, Smith observed that "perhaps if this person had been bled freely, fatal consequences would have been prevented."[47] In treating cases of catarrh, he went so far as to say that "[b]leeding is sometimes necessary when there is considerable excitement with local pain either in the head or breast," and that in these cases "[b]loodletting is very useful."[48] But note the "sometimes." Smith realized bleeding was not a procedure to be used for dogmatic reasons alone, as a matter of principle. "When there is an inflammatory disposition it has been highly useful but *as a general remedy it cannot be relied on* [emphasis added]."[49] In practice, he found fewer and fewer patients who needed to be bled, and he could be very blunt about the impropriety of bleeding. To treat a patient with a luxated arm, he said, antimony or tobacco should be given (instead of bleeding) to produce the necessary relaxation: "To bleed a patient to faintness because a shoulder is dislocated would be improper."[50]

This careful attention in Smith's teaching to the particulars of a case is also a clue to his practice. He damned venesection with faint praise. He knew and taught that treatment must be individualized. Diseases could and should be diagnosed and named, but it was the patient who must be treated. Theory was secondary. And therein lies the essential difference between Rush and Smith. To claim, as one historian has, that "Smith was a firm exponent of 'heroic medicine,' emphasizing bloodletting and the administration of large doses of emetics and cathartics to purge the body of waste material," and that Smith "was a follower of Benjamin Rush," is a most considerable misreading of Smith, who was famous already in his own time for his self-restraint.[51]

A Patient's Physician

Governing Nathan Smith's medical practice was his belief that "by diseased action, we are to understand an action begun and carried on in some part of the human system which is opposed to healthy action, and which tends either directly or indirectly to destroy life." He further held (and in his lectures proposed "to show by facts") that "the nature of diseased action depends principally upon 2 causes Viz. on the nature of the *exciting cause* and on the nature of the part affected."[52] Today this sounds so reasonable that the revolutionary nature of Smith's clear and simple understanding of what amounts to the difference between cause and effect is hard to fathom.

Though the record is of course incomplete, numerous stories have come down to us of Nathan Smith's successful treatment of satisfied patients, even if his explanations were not always as clear as he presumably thought. We have at least one story of a patient who was confused by the doctor's instructions and thus unable to carry them out. Smith's faithful friend Mills Olcott was the intermediary for a patient who had been seen by Smith. The "child's neck was rather better," he was told. "She had washed the Neck with Salt & Water [but] Had not persued Doctor Smith's Prescription as She could not understand perfectly how the Sponge was to be used & in what quantity."[53] Smith had probably prescribed burnt sponge to be taken orally, for its iodine content; assuming the patient had goiter, this would have been a sensible treatment. Rubbing the area with the sponge externally would do little good.

This rare case of Smith leaving confusion in his wake might be a sign of overwork—of which he complained on occasion, though usually only because it interfered with his collection of bills due. ("My business has been so very pressing this season," he wrote in one letter, and at another point, "I have been too busy this summer for my profit as I have been obliged to neglect collecting intirely."[54]) That he was busy was noted by others, too. In a letter that probably dates from late 1798 or early 1799, Nathan Noyes wrote to Lyman Spalding that "Doctor Smith was as usual very good and very busy."[55]

For the most part, however, busy or not, Smith was able to act (and to instruct others how to act) with a directness that left no one confused. A case in point is the dramatic story of how Smith treated William Jarvis, formerly United States Consul General to Spain. Jarvis, an active Federalist who had introduced Merino sheep to New England (giving local sheep breeders a boost), had retired to his farm in Vermont to enjoy the rewards of his successful import scheme:

Mr. Jarvis was very near losing his life. On awaking one night, he thought he heard some one in the house, and striking a light, without pausing to reflect, he went all over it without slippers or stockings. He took a violent cold, which resulted in quinsy [peritonsillar abscess], in so virulent a form as to defy the skill of his attendant physicians.[56] . . . Dr. Nathan Smith, of Hanover, was sent for. On his arrival he found the case so critical that he sat up with him. In the middle of the night the swelling in the throat had increased to such a degree that Mr. Jarvis was almost suffocated, and swooned.

Dr. Smith, with that presence of mind that characterizes great skill, instantly ordered a pitcher of cold water, and drawing the Consul by the shoulders over the side of the bed, dashed it violently into his face.

It occasioned a start, a struggle for breath, which broke the ulcer, and Mr. Jarvis was relieved. He often afterwards remarked that he owed his life to Dr. Smith, for whom he entertained the highest respect.[57]

Of course, we have no way of knowing how accurate or complete the above report was. Assuming it was both, one wonders why the skilled surgeon could not have lanced the abscess (something he recommended ten years later in his lectures on the treatment of quinsy) and spared Jarvis the dramatics. One wonders also whether he had tried to rupture the obstructing abscess manually, which has occasionally been done with success. Perhaps he was simply desperate to save his patient, and—not having any approved method of dealing with the problem—took drastic and immediate action, hoping the shock would work. He appears to have been lucky (as was Jarvis). Smith wrote about the case to Shattuck, saying matter-of-factly that he was "now in Weathersfield in the service of Mr. Jarvis, late consul at Lisbon who has been dangerously sick but is I think today out of danger."[58]

New methods of treatment interested Smith. What he did for the consul may have been part of his more general exploration of the possibilities of hydrotherapy, which he used to revolutionize the treatment of typhoid. In his essay on typhous fever, for example, he told in some detail the story of a case from 1798 ("the first year in which this fever occurred in my practice") where he experimented with external cold-water therapy. When twenty-four hours passed after the young man had undergone a warm-water treatment "without any symptoms of amendment," Smith

stripped him naked as he lay on a straw mattress, and poured [a] gallon of [cold] water over him from head to foot. He seemed to feel the shock, but did not speak. . . . No other internal remedies were administered. The next morning there was no alteration. The affusion of cold water was renewed as the day grew warm and the heat was kept down . . . . Before night, the patient recovered so as to speak . . . . From this period he became convalescent, and recovered without the use of any other remedy.[59]

Whatever one might think of pouring pitchers of cold water over ill patients (at least Smith had the young man moved to a dry bed after he was soaked), the treatment is striking for its simplicity.

Among Smith's contributions to medical practice was his careful examination of drugs prior to using them, which he taught his students to do, as well. To be sure, he recommended some drugs we now consider inadvisable, and many that have fallen into desuetude. But a careful analysis of his ledgers, year by year and drug by drug—for the five years before and the five years after his 1797 trip to Edinburgh and London—indicates that Smith made significant shifts in medical treatment.[60] There is no evidence that the changes were a result of the trip; rather, he simply prescribed what he found worked, not what was supposed to work.

The drugs Smith used in constant numbers in the two five-year periods would (with three exceptions) be acceptable today. They have all been used by modern physicians in similar doses for similar indications:

Paregoric, laudanum, and opium;
Castor oil, "cathartics," and Glauber's salts (sodium sulfate);
Corrosive sublimate (mercury bichloride), for skin disease;
Magnesium alba, for acidity;
Iron (in the form of flores martiales);
Quinine (in the form of Peruvian bark);
Gum arabic (a demulcent, i.e., a soothing—often oily—medicine or
   application);
Anise seeds (a carminative, i.e., something to reduce flatulence and
   assuage pain).

Out of favor today would be Nathan Smith's use of emetics (agents used to induce vomiting)—except as he sometimes used them in small doses, as simple expectorants; gum guaiac (a wood resin used to treat rheumatism); and Emplastrum epispasticum (blistering plaster), though some home-remedy enthusiasts still like mustard plasters.

The drugs Smith used increasingly after his return from Edinburgh are mostly acceptable today. The greater frequency with which they appear in his ledgers could be explained by the epidemics of typhoid, dysentery, and spotted fever that were rampant during the years around the turn of the century, for these were all drugs prescribed particularly for infectious diseases: Althea radix (marshmallow root, a demulcent); Balsam Copaiva, calomel, cantharides; Catechu, in diarrhea; cloves, in dentistry; Dover's Powders; Ipecac, iron, nitre, rhubarb, and sal soda (sodium carbonate). Digitalis (which he started using in 1800) seems to be the only new drug he learned to use while abroad.

Strikingly, the drugs Smith used in decreasing amounts were for the most part ones that have been discarded from today's pharmacopoeia (except in some instances by practitioners of alternative medicine): ammoniacum resin, cream of tartar, aloes, oil of sweet almonds, asafoetida, camphor, castor, cinnamon, columba, radix dcanthus (an anthelmintic—something to get rid of worms), various epispastics, myrrh, Elixir Proprietor of Paracelsus, sugar of lead (taken internally), and radix valerian (used as an antispasmodic). All of these Smith used in his first years; as he matured in practice, he discarded them.

Once again, student lecture notes provide the best evidence about Smith's practice—specifically, in this instance, about his conservative use of drugs. One drug that was commonly prescribed in his day was stramonium (made from the dried leaves and flowering tops of a plant colloquially called "thorn apple"). Smith told his students that although it had been given "with benefit in some cases," it was "difficult to point out the cases it which it would be useful and those in which it would not." Another student noted the same cautious attitude when Smith added the observation that the "immoderate use of [stramonium] may destroy vision."[61] Thus he implicitly taught his students not to use a drug until its efficacy and safety had been adequately substantiated. Another examination of Smith's materia medica shows that "Doctor Nathan Smith in his teaching was quite in accord with the accepted belief of his time"—but also "somewhat critical, and although a particular drug appeared to be of benefit in a single case, he was rather reluctant to infer that he had at hand a specific of uniform application."[62]

One example of how Smith used drugs in his practice comes from his lecture on acne (entitled "Eruptions of the Face of Young People"). He gave the following account: "I do not know whether the disease is local or not. I cured it in one case by a solution of *Arsenic*. It inflamed the skin considerably. The cuticle came off and the health was affected a short time. The affect of the skin was cured but I would not recommend a repetition of this practice." He then added two more encouraging accounts, one where "Fowlers solution" was applied and another where an ointment made by pounding the root of broad-leaved dock was used; the latter "at first produced inflammation," but in both cases the disease was cured.[63]

Like any truly competent practitioner, Smith recognized his limitations. He learned from his own mistakes, or tried to, and shared what he knew so that others would not repeat his errors. "I have had but two cases of tetanus and both terminated fatally," he acknowledged in a lecture, and then proceeded to detail what he had done and what the symptoms were.[64] If he was unfamiliar with a disease or condition, he did not pretend otherwise: "I never had much experience in the diseases produced by the bites of poisonous animals," he said; "I never saw a person under the influence of the bite of a Rattle Snake." The advice he then passed on was from a "physician who has seen many cases of this kind."[65]

In addition to lacking experience in some kinds of cases (and being aware of that deficiency), Smith could also be just plain wrong (and clearly unaware of it). In his lecture "Diseases affecting the Genital Organs of Women impairing their Functions," he delivered himself of the following profundities:

At the age of puberty there is a periodical discharge from the uterus resembling blood, but it differs from blood in as much as it wants some of the properties of blood. . . . When the menses flow in too great a quantity, either with or without pain, menstruation is not hemorrhage as the discharge *is not blood* [emphasis added].[66]

Not surprisingly, Smith also exhibited a few of the prejudices and confusions of his day with respect to tuberculosis, then known as "consumption." He began one set of lectures on the topic with the observation that to "the word consumption there is no definite meaning"[67]—which was true enough, but could well have left students uncertain what to make of the discussion that followed. Smith correctly pointed out that the "period of life at which it most commonly appears is from 15 to 30 years" (this had been known at least since the time of Hippocrates, who said the critical period was "between the ages of eighteen and thirty-five"[68]). Smith continued as follows: "[Consumption] is thought to be hereditary. It has as good a claim to this character as any other disease. It has been asserted by some that the disease is contagious. I have witnessed some facts which proved the opinion that it may be communicated to persons that have a predisposition to it."[69]

In other words, Smith's understanding of consumption was no better, but also no worse, than that of most of his contemporaries. As he ran through the various recommended treatments, he was—as usual—uncompromisingly blunt:

Many remedies have been proposed, but there is nothing that will prove successful in every case. . . . *Blood Root* has been beneficial, but when ulceration has taken place I never knew it successful. *Mercury* has been used with benefit. In one case I gave it . . . and it produced more effect on the mouth than I expected. During the salivation the patient was much relieved. When the salivation subsided the cough returned and the disease terminated fatally. . . . Formerly *Balsamics* were much given. It was supposed that they had a healing quality. This theory was fanciful. I never saw a case where I thought they were useful.[70]

Most striking, however, in all Smith's letters and student notes from his lectures is the repeated emphasis first on experience, and second on what makes the patient comfortable. Still talking about what to do in cases of consumption, Smith said:

Digitalis has been highly recommended by some physicians, but *experience has not justified their recommendations*, yet it ought not to be wholly disregarded. I have seen consumptive persons relieved by it. It should be used with caution and *if it disagrees with the patient lay it aside* [emphases added].[71]

He taught also that although it was appropriate for patients with enteritis (intestinal inflammation) to have their bowels evacuated, it should be done "by means of mild laxatives such as *senna*."[72] Smith was no disciple of heroic medicine; he was not interested in violent "purging and puking." As we saw in the excerpts from his essay on typhous fever, he repeatedly stressed the need to look for the gentler way to do things.

Smith's career was spent trying to apply the rapidly expanding knowledge of medicine to the treatment of patients, all the time watching closely the effect on individuals of whatever he did. His insistence on using what proved most efficacious for the patient bordered on the revolutionary. His genuine interest in seeing how human beings were affected by disease and how medicine could help them does much to explain his great

popularity; his shrewd guesses and careful follow-up show that his practice of medicine was quite modern compared to that of his more famous
contemporaries—the crusading Rush in Philadelphia, for example, or
Harvard's highly intellectual Waterhouse (who did not like seeing patients
anyway[73]). Both of those medical giants not only exasperated their colleagues, but propagated ideas that caused trouble for generations. Rush's
antiphlogistic regime in particular weakened the curative effectiveness of
his students. As one critic of Rush's insistence on his own system wrote in
the 1840s,

Now, one of the first and most inevitable effects of a belief in any *a priori* system
of medicine is an *utter disqualification of the mind for correct and trustworthy
observation*. No man with one of these hypothetical crotchets in his brain is to be
trusted. . . . He will always find what he expects to find; and he will always fail to
discover what he has concluded beforehand will not be present.[74]

Smith, in sharp contrast, rejected dogmatism in favor of close observation
and direct inquiry of the patient; in the process, he introduced many novel
medical and surgical treatments over the course of his career.

He also very much believed in treating patients as individuals. "Physicians have erred," he taught, "in attempting to generalize both diseases
and remedies."[75] And in his celebrated paper on necrosis (osteomyelitis),
he wrote that when a question arose over whether to operate, "the decision must be determined by contingent circumstances *like everything relating to our art* [emphasis added]."[76] He further advised listening to patients. With regard to diet for those with typhous fever, for instance, he indicated his belief that "if patients were left to select for themselves, without the interference of nurses and friends . . . they would generally decide
right."[77] Similarly, though "*[f]arinaceous food* is good for consumptive
patients," Smith insisted that meat ought not to be denied to those who
wished it. "When patients have craved it I have never prohibited its use
nor found it injurious when used in proper quantities."[78]

Well into the nineteenth century, it was fashionable for patients to dose
themselves,[79] but few doctors were prepared to acknowledge the legiti-
macy of their doing so. Smith was more willing than most physicians to
let patients make judgments for themselves and in this he anticipated by
more than a century the involvement of patients in their own care so prevalent today. Moreover, his attempt to treat the whole patient was suggestive of the current emphasis on patient-centered, "total care." He often
spoke of the importance of good nursing, or what he called "the general
management of the patient." Smith's description of how to "manage" the
care of a patient suffering from typhous fever could have been applied
with little or no modification to most other cases of serious illness. "If the
thing is practicable," he wrote, the patient

should be kept in a spacious room, the larger the better. . . . We should contrive to have a current of air pass over the bed by means of doors and windows.

. . . All the furniture should be removed, except such articles as are required for the patient's use. . . . The room should be kept as quiet as possible, since noise is injurious . . . . Cleanliness is absolutely essential to the patient's comfort. . . . [T]he bed and body linen should be changed every day . . . . The patient's body and limbs should be cleansed every day with a piece of sponge and warm water or soap and water.[80]

In other words: Do what you can to cure your patients, never forgetting to take advantage of the *vis medicatrix naturae*—and, above all else, keep your patients comfortable.

CHAPTER TEN

Nathan Smith's Surgical Practice

Devising New Techniques

Sat cito si sat bene.

[It is (done) fast enough,
if it is (done) well enough.]
— CATO [1]

THE PRACTICE OF internal medicine at the end of the eighteenth century was still very much governed by whatever system of medicine was dominant. Not so with surgery. This discipline was rigidly restricted in its advances by the lack of understanding of asepsis and anesthesia—ignorance that continued for nearly two more generations.[2] Wilderness accidents could be bizarre; surgical problems such as bladder stones, acute osteomyelitis in childhood, typhus-like brain abscesses, and carbuncle were demanding or insoluble. All of these were difficult, and even the most skilled surgeons treated them with varying degrees of success. The chronic diseases were even more puzzling, and surgery for them was less often attempted. Poorly understood pathology meant surgical treatment was as likely to introduce problems as it was to cure the condition.

A Varied Practice

A useful way to set the stage for examining the overall character of Nathan Smith's surgical practice is to review the description his Yale colleague Jonathan Knight gave of Smith's attributes as a surgeon. The following passage is notable for the sober and carefully chosen language Knight used in his assessment of Smith, and the details he included in his analysis.

For the duties of a practical surgeon, Dr. Smith was eminently qualified, and upon the manner in which he performed these duties, his reputation must, in a great measure, ultimately rest. To these, he brought a mind enterprising, but not rash; anxious, yet calm, in deliberation; bold, yet cautious, in operation. His first object was, to save his patients, if possible, from the necessity of an operation; and when this could be no longer avoided, to enter upon its performance, without reluctance or hesitation. In his operations, he was calm, collected and cautious.

He manifested no desire to gain the reputation of a rapid operator, a reputation, so ardently, and it is to be feared, so unfortunately sought for, by many surgeons of the present day. He who commences an important operation, with his eye upon the minute hand of a watch, starts in a race against time, in which the life of his patient is the stake, and often the forfeit. The true rule for the surgeon is, *sat, cito si sat bene*. Neither did he make any display, in the course of his operations, to gain the applause of bystanders. Hence there was no formidable array of instruments; no ostentatious preparation, so well calculated to excite the wonder of the ignorant, and to strike a dread into the mind of the patient. Every thing necessary was prepared, while all useless parade was avoided. When engaged in an operation, his whole mind was bent upon its proper performance. Every step was carefully examined, every occurrence narrowly watched; and if anything unusual appeared, he would ask the advice of those present, in whom he had confidence. In such cases, his promptness and decision, joined to what Chesselden[3] calls "a mind that was never ruffled nor disconcerted," were of singular utility. By the aid of these, he could look, with a steady eye, upon the varying features of the case, as they rose to his view, and adapt his measures, at once, to every emergency. By this cautious mode of proceeding, calculated to gain, not the applause of those who were present on a single occasion, but the enduring reputation of a judicious, skilful Surgeon, he performed with great success, the most important operations. That his success was great is fully attested by the facts, that of about thirty cases of Lithotomy, only three proved fatal; and that in the course of his practice, he lost no patient of hemorrhage, in consequence of an operation, either direct or secondary.[4]

Two particularly good examples of the way Smith's care focused on ensuring the comfort and welfare of his patients have come down to us, one from his lectures at Yale, the other from a letter to Mills Olcott. The first is a fine instance of Smith's preferring to "rather do too little than too much,"[5] as President William Allen of Bowdoin put it. No matter how damaged a hand, rather than amputate it entirely, Smith cautioned in a lecture that if "you can save one finger it will be best to save it. . . . A part of a hand would be of great use"[6]—sound advice indeed.

The second story vividly illustrates Smith's habit of staying with a patient even after there was little or nothing more he could do to cure. When Yale's President Timothy Dwight was dying of a painful cancer of the bladder, Smith never left his side; he performed many small and helpful acts of the sort that only a family doctor can. To Olcott he wrote in January of 1817, recounting the events as follows:

Dr. Dwight was better than he had been, but on the next morning he was suddenly attacked with a cold fit & shaking which continued sometime & when it went off he became comatous which continued through the day accompanied with fever &

quick pulse. When on the next day the comatous symptoms abated his mind became unsteady & occasionally wandering. He continued in this way till 3 O'clock on Saturday morning when he expired. I was with him nearly the whole time from Wednesday morning till he died when I closed his eye. It was truely melancholy to see so good and great a man leave the world in the midst of his usefullness & who but for the local complaint which distroyed his life had a constitution which bid fair to have sustained life to extreme old age. On the evening after Dr. Dwight's decease we obtained leave to examine the body & discovered that his disease was an inveterate cancer of the urinary bladder.[7]

Regrettably, although Smith listed operations in his ledgers and day books, we have no case histories apart from those he mentioned in his lectures and those few he mentioned in his *Essay on Typhous* and other publications, or the unpublished paper on cancer. Thus, to see what Smith's surgical practice entailed, we will continue to quote extensively from notes students took during the lectures in which Smith was engaged in teaching surgery. Once again, Worham L. Fitch's very extensive notes bring us close to pure Smith because of the way they report what Smith actually presented to his students. Accordingly, selections have been made from Fitch's notes with an emphasis on what Smith had to say in three main categories: ophthalmology, cancer, and orthopedics. We will begin by looking at the wide variety in his practice (including what his accounts for one year tell about its range) and then turn to observations on cases in general surgery and discussion of cases (from his correspondence), where possible.

The depth and scope of Smith's surgical practice becomes clear from analysis of his ledgers and day books, some of which are extant from both his years in Hanover and his New Haven period.[8] Accounts for the year 1800 (while Smith was at Dartmouth), for example, show the following major operations and charges:

Amputating a leg	$20.00
Operation [unspecified]	4.00
Lithotomy	4.00
Operation of trepanning	10.00
Extracting a tumor near an eye	5.00
Reducing a fractured clavicle	1.00
Operation [unspecified]	1.00
Reducing a fracture leg	3.00
Operation of trepanning	15.00
Extirpating a tumor on a hand	1.00
Operation of tapping	7.00
Amputating a thigh	25.00
Operation [unspecified] on a girl	1.00
Operation for hydrocele [a fluid-filled cyst, typically on the testicle or spermatic cord]	5.00
Extracting an eye	22.00

Operation for fistula in ano	5.00
Operation for hydrocele	5.00
Operation [unspecified]	11.00
Operation [unspecified]	1.00
Fixing on a truss	1.00
Reducing a luxated arm	2.50
Operation of castration	2.00
Extracting a pin from child's throat	.50
Reducing a luxated knee	8.00
Operation for a bubonocele [partial inguinal hernia]	12.00
Extirpating a breast	12.00
Operation for a harelip	6.00
Operation [unspecified]	20.00
Operation of trepanning	20.00
Dressing a ruptured artery	.25
Paracentesis [surgical puncture] of thorax	13.00
Reducing a fractured arm	1.00
Amputating a leg	30.00
Extirpating a tumor from a face	1.50
Extirpating a tumor on a side	1.00
Setting a dislocated arm	2.00
Operation for hydrocele	2.50
Operation for harelip	2.50
Operation [unspecified]	5.00
Operation [unspecified]	6.00
Operation for a hydrocele	10.00
Operation for a stone on a woman	20.00
Redressing a fractured leg	1.00
Extracting a wart	.25
Operation [unspecified] for a boy	2.00
Perforation [for osteomyelitis] of the bone for a boy	2.00

Smith's total charges for surgery for the year were $329.00; this amounted to just under 20 percent of what he charged that year for all practice, which amounted to $1,849.45.[9]

Quite possibly there were other cash calls that never got listed; records were important primarily where money was still owed. Bills were not apt to be paid very promptly—Smith knew plenty about that, from both sides of the ledger—making bills due a frequent (if incidental) topic of personal interest when one surgeon wrote to another. In a mid-August letter of 1820 to a medical colleague, Smith wrote:

I have had a very large share of operative surgery on my hands this summer. Since the first of May I have performed the following operations with many others of a less important nature, that is—three amputations, one trepanning case, one lithotomy, one tumor on the knee weighing four pounds and one on the thigh of nine pounds, and many smaller cases of cancer on the breast, twelve cases of couching, one case of inguinal aneurysm, for which I tied the external iliac artery. This was done twenty days since; I saw him Monday, the eighteenth day from the operation. Everything appeared favorable except that the ligature had not come away. The aneurysm tumor was chiefly gone and the edematous swelling of the thigh and leg had quite subsided and his symptoms were all favorable. I have also ligated a very large polypus in the vagina which has succeeded perfectly as all the others have. Alas if those tumor patients had all been such as some of your Boston nabobs I should not want for money at this time, but destruction of the doctor is the poverty of his patients.[10]

Smith worked against other handicaps besides those of slow or no payment. Some of these were of a sort that would thoroughly discourage most modern surgeons, if they could imagine them at all. Simply getting to his patients was often exhausting. In one of the most vivid accounts we have to illustrate the point, Smith's student Ezekiel Dodge Cushing wrote to his father in 1809, telling him what life was like for those making rounds with Dr. Smith. In that letter Cushing rattled on to his parents about how, even after several calls far from Hanover, the pace did not let up:

[Wednesday morning] all the way on horseback, next day we had two lectures, I went to bed early Wednesday night but all hands were called up at ten to go to see a boy that had broke his leg 12 miles off. I got home about 3 o'clock in the morning [Thursday]. Friday noon all hands were called to go with the Dr. to a boy that had fallen off a horse, upon his head the Dr. thought best to trepan him, which was accordingly done, he appeared entirely senseless but still was in great distress, and appeared to suffer as a person does in the night mare. The operation was unsuccessful and [he] died yesterday.[11]

Smith had no office in today's sense, not even in his home, and of course no hospital. Although he seems to have occasionally taken a patient in as a boarder for the duration of the illness,[12] most he treated in their own homes. Typically the patient resided miles away. For the first twenty-five years of Smith's practice the inadequate roads forced him to make all his calls on horseback; at times the trips were of forty or fifty miles or more. The serious nature of the illness at times required him to remain on hand ("I shall have to stay two or three days," he once wrote to Mills Olcott following an operation[13]). Unless he had brought along his students, which he sometimes did in considerable numbers, he would have to depend on unskilled aid during the operation—just as he himself had had his first taste of surgery as a farmer-teacher helping Josiah Goodhue perform an amputation in Chester, Vermont.

Good surgical instruments were also hard to obtain. More than once Smith wrote to friends and colleagues asking for assistance in finding what he needed or for advice on the latest invention; he was always on the lookout for anything that would make his work easier or the patient's recovery more comfortable. When Lyman Spalding was in Philadelphia (in 1810), for instance, Smith wrote him:

I wish you to procure me a Gorget for cutting for the stone according to the most improved plans such an one as Dr. Physic[k] will recommend. Tho, I have operated for the last four times with success, I suspect my Gorgets are not right. I have one according to Mr. Cline's plan & two according to Monro's—I wish also you would make diligent inquiry of Dr. Physic[k] respecting his mode of operating on the eyes & what kind of instrument he uses—& every thing else which will be interesting to me.[14]

These requests are significant, given that "cutting for the stone" and operating on eyes were two of the kinds of surgery for which Smith was already best known. Perhaps his success in these areas was directly connected to both his willingness to ask others for advice and his curiosity about the latest in equipment. Nor did this interest in having the newest and the best diminish as his reputation expanded further. Thirteen years later, from his outpost in Brunswick, Maine, he wrote to Shattuck in Boston:

Dr. Wells informs me that you have [Sir Astley] Cooper's newly invented instrument for extracting the stones through the urethra. We have a case in this village which I think is a proper one for such an instrument, and wish if you are willing that you would send it to me by the Captain of the vessel who will bring my chaise and I will immediately make use of it and send it safely to you. I have two objects in view, one to relieve the patient and the other to show it to Mr. Th. Eastman, a man of great ingenuity, whom [sic] I think having seen one can make another like it.[15]

Smith nowhere tells explicitly what he used to numb the pain of surgery (though he does on occasion mention that, following surgery, to "palliate the symptoms Opium is the best"[16]). We know he had misgivings about combining "strong brandy" with "large doses of laudanum and cantharides", but we also know that he bought—and sold, for that matter—great quantities of cider.[17] Whether this was simply or primarily for his own consumption, we cannot tell; cider was certainly drunk in quantities that seem startling today unless one is aware of the English tradition of "small cider" and "small beer" (well watered-down versions of those beverages).[18] If the cider Smith bought was "hard," he might have used some of it for pre-operative medication, though most New England farmers could of course supply their own; city dwellers of New Haven might have found cider in short supply.

Smith's success in operating without anesthesia was partly a result of his sympathetic response to patients, well illustrated by the story he is said to have told of a Mr. Stockwell. For some years the fellow had had a tumor in the side of his neck about the size of a goose egg; it changed its shape with moderate pressure. When it became too painful and inconvenient, Mr. Stockwell asked for surgical intervention if it would be of any use. Because the diagnosis was somewhat uncertain, and because Stockwell was apparently an extremely inquisitive man, a conversation enlivened most of the operation. A student wrote Smith's account of the episode in his lecture notebook:

I prepared for the operation and was assisted by Drs. Twitchell and Perkins.

After Mr. Stockwell was placed on the table and all things ready, the course and length of the incision determined, at the moment when the anxiety of the operator and assistants was at its worst he arose and said, "Dr. Smith is it best that I should submit to this operation? You see that it is a most critical time as it respects me." Answer, "Yes," "Dr. Twitchell is it your opinion also?" Yes. "Dr. Perkins is it yours?" Yes. "Are you all agreed?" All, "yes." "If you are disappointed in the appearance at any time let me know it." Through the stages of the operation he frequently inquired, "Are you deceived?" Answer, "no." "Are you all agreed?" Dr. Smith answered "The jury are agreed"; he says, "Very well I intend you should be jury but I mean to be Judge Advocate myself." He bore it without a complaint.[19]

Unfortunately, having apparently withstood the operation well, Stockwell died five weeks later.

Smith's sympathy for his patients emerges in another case, where he went out of his way to have the physician assisting him shield the young lad being operated on. "Hall," he said to him, "you know all about this boy's sufferings: at the moment we commence, bend over and across the bed to hide us from his sight, and do your best to comfort and sustain him."[20]

General Surgery

A further feature of Smith's skill was the speed with which he made decisions about how to proceed, even though he "manifested no desire to gain the reputation of a rapid operator" (as we learned from Jonathan Knight's remarks). His doctrine of limiting surgery to the least amount necessary helped keep his operations brief as well. More than most of his contemporaries, Smith also seems to have stressed cleanliness in general (recall his advice on hygiene in the essay on typhus); he frequently mentioned soap and water and thorough irrigation—still the best way short of aseptic technique to avoid one whole class of complications.

In addition, Smith exhibited a surprisingly modern reticence about changing dressings if the healing wound was clean: "After the wound is once dressed if it occasions no pain it will not be necessary to dress it again until it is entirely healed," he stressed.[21] Such measures as this, and his general attempts to keep patients comfortable, clean, rested, and free of pain, no doubt had much to do with his low morbidity and mortality rates.

Even more impressive is the frequent emphasis on what we speak of to-day as patient-centered care, already alluded to. Smith emphasized ways to make it possible for patients and their families to participate in their own recovery:

After a patient has learned [to pass a catheter] he will introduce it with more ease to himself than a surgeon can. Surgeons are apt to think that no body can do it but a practitioner, but an intelligent person may be taught so that he will do it better than nine tenths of the surgeons.[22]

In one case [of wound of the thorax] I drew off a pint of matter in this way [with a catheter] and instructed the family to introduce the cannula [small drain] and in the course of a week the patient was relieved.[23]

His consistent concern for a patient's comfort meant that, if there was a choice of treatments, he invariably recommended the one that was less painful for the patient: "Much has been said about this operation [treatment for fistula in ano] and many instruments used, and there has been a great degree of hemorrhage which has induced some to take a very cruel method to cure . . . ." Smith described two different methods, using instruments that would enable the surgeon to "cut all that is necessary and no more . . . . [It is] easier for the patient."[24]

Another standard procedure he objected to was pulling off the toenail to treat ingrown nails, which he said rarely succeeded ("when it grows again it will be inverted as much as before") and was "one of the most cruel operations in surgery." Instead, he advocated the following:

[S]crape the middle of the nail as thin as possible without coming to the quick. Cut off the end of the nail square and then with a probe insert lint between the flesh and the nail. . . . Then take a narrow strip of sticking plaster, put one end of it upon the flesh at the side of the affected nail and draw it obliquely around the toe so as to separate the flesh from the nail &c. The shoe should be made so as not to press on any part of the toe.[25]

Smith repeatedly gave his students practical advice on such general matters as the use of sutures, ligating arteries, and types of dressing, all of which provide insight into how he handled such things in his own practice. Advice on suturing varied, depending on the case: "Several kinds of Sutures are used. There has been a good deal of quibbling as to the kind . . . . It is better to have them waxed because they will slide better."[26] On the common interrupted suture, he said: "All the sutures should be passed that are necessary and then tied with the Surgeon's knot. It will remain firm enough by turning the thread two or three times over without tying the second knot. . . . They should never be kept in more than five days . . . ."[27] On ligating arteries, he had the following to say:

Some recommend silks, some linen and some leather . . . . All that is necessary is that it should be a small string, the smaller the better if of sufficient strength, and it should be drawn so tight as to destroy the vitality of the end of the artery . . . . It is said that leather will dissolve in the wound and that it will not be necessary to remove it. I have no doubt but this may be successful . . . . An artery should not be tied with a surgeon's knot, but with a common double knot.[28]

Bandaging, Smith believed, was a skill that deserved more attention than it sometimes received (in this, he was echoing Hippocrates[29]).

Sticking Plaster. There is more skill in applying this well than sutures . . . .
The Uniting Bandages may be used in some cases but if the sticking plaster is good it will hardly be necessary . . . . A certain degree of pressure disposes the wound to heal, but the bandage must press equally.[30]

Another favorite theme, as we have also already seen, was "simpler is better":

A man wounded his knee—he was covetous of his money and therefore got on to his horse and rode 2 miles to a physician who sewed it up as tight as a bug. In a few days it was found that a large quantity of blood had collected in it—and finally he lost the use of the joint. I believe it is better in all cases not [to] sew on a joint but to apply sticking plaster.
All the application necessary for a simple incised wound is *Simple Cerate* . . . . Time with these simple dressings is all that is necessary to affect a cure. . . .

A man whose father died of a stone in the bladder had symptoms of the same disease. I gave him *Soda* prepared with *Honey* in form of pills. In the course of 6 months every symptom of stone disappeared. The probability is that the stone was formed of uric acid. He continued the use of this remedy a long time after the symptoms of stone disappeared.[31]

"Operation for Stone in the Bladder" was a matter in which Smith had considerable experience:

Symptoms indicating the presence of stone in the bladder . . . are pain in the region of the bladder, pain in voiding urine—felt usually at the glans penis . . . . This pain takes place while the urine is flowing, but more particular as the last drops of urine are passed. . . . The patient has frequently to void his urine several times during the night. It is very common for the urine to be tinged with blood. Frequently there is pain in voiding feces . . . . Frequently the patient cannot ride in any kind of carriage. . . . The surest indication of the presence of stone is the evacuation of small ones with the urine. . . . A large stone is the most frequent cause of unfortunate operations. It is not the frequent introduction of the forceps that causes the death of the patient.
In one case I operated successfully where there were 40 stones in the bladder but they were small. The forceps were introduced a great number of times. . . . After the operation the bladder should be examined with the finger and after all the stones that can be found are removed, the bladder should be washed out with a syringe of warm water.[32]

Smith's discussions of gunshot wounds (which he described as a kind of puncture wound "accompanied with contusion") and injuries to the skull—"Where there is any foreign matter in the wound it should be removed if it can be done easily. . . . I believe such bodies should never be cut for unless their position can be ascertained"—were enlivened, as so much in his lectures was, by accounts of particular cases:

I know an instance where a ball was never found at all, but the limb was perfectly cured.[33]

A lady fell upon a log and injured her brain. At first she was sensible, but soon lost her sense, and stertorous breathing took place. I apprehended that blood was effused under the skull and performed the operation of trepanning and found the brain greatly compressed by a large quantity of blood. She did not recover.[34]

I have seen one case of compression followed by *Epileptic Fits* . . . this single case does not show that this slight compression which was not operated upon was the cause of Epilepsy.[35]

A boy was trepanned and at the second dressing the dura mater [the outermost membrane covering the brain] protruded and it appeared to be slipping out. I applied lint wet in a decoction of *White Oak Bark* and over this I applied pressure by means of a piece of pewter platter properly fitted to the skull. . . .
I believe we may lay it down as a general rule not to cut through the dura mater. When we have taken away what lies above it we have done all that we can do.[36]

A girl fractured her skull. . . . I was called in and found matter under the dressings of the wound and more than could come from the integuments. I cut down and found a fracture and matter pressing out through the crevice of the bone. I took out several little pieces of the bone and the matter was discharged and the girl recovered.[37]

Nathan Smith's criticism of colleagues usually consisted of little more than a passing mention that some other physician had previously been in attendance (and by implication had failed to do the job).[38] He could, however, be aroused, as remarks he made about distinguishing between "a tumour resembling the inguinal hernia" and a true hernia illustrate:

A man must be a great bungler not to be able to distinguish between these diseases. An enlarged testicle can generally be very readily distinguished from hernia. You can feel above the enlargement. An enlargement of the veins of the spermatic chord [sic] can be distinguished from hernia by several circumstances.[39]

Though he was for the most part remarkably sympathetic to the efforts of his colleagues, he did in one lecture say that the "lives of patients have been destroyed by the long perseverance and too violent force with the hands." Despite often having many students in tow, he knew that more hands were not necessarily better—at least not when it came to trying to repair a dislocated limb: "When too many physicians have been called, I have observed that the patient has generally died, in consequence of too many fruitless attempts at reduction."[40] Though he could lose patience, as we have seen, when someone appeared to have been "a great bungler," accounts of his having lost his temper are exceedingly rare. A colleague at Bowdoin said he saw Smith angry only once—over medical treatment he considered incompetent, rendered by one of his own graduates.[41]

Smith's own general skills ranged widely, as we have seen. He also developed extraordinary expertise in several areas, each of which encompasses several surgical specialties today. We will look at three of them.

Ophthalmology

Most notable in Smith's work in ophthalmology is what amounted to a one-man campaign against blindness carried out through aggressive surgical treatment of cataracts. While in Worcester, Massachusetts, during mid-March of 1811, Smith wrote a long letter to George Shattuck:

Today I have couched an eye for Governor [Levi] Lincoln and one for a little daughter of Judge [Nathaniel] Paine of this place. Both operations were attended with the most flattering prospects of success. In the governor's case the operation was exactly similar in all its circumstances to that I made on Mrs. Marston. The little girl's case was a very interesting one. She had lost one eye by a former operation. Her [remaining] eye was very unsteady, and the cataract membranous, but I contrived to fix the eye, and to perform the operation in about two minutes with the most heartfelt satisfaction to all present. . . . If these two cases succeed, as they promise, I shall be in danger of receiving more flattering and commendation than I can well bear.

Three days later he wrote again to Shattuck:

Since I wrote you last I have performed on an eye in Sutton. The case was a singular one, the cataract was as hard as a calculus. When touched with the needle it broke with an audible sound like that of glass which was heard by the bystanders, and a portion of it, about a third Part of it slipped through the pupil [here he provided a diagram] and popped into the anterior chamber.

He went on in some detail, observing that he thought the only harm likely to come of the extraordinary way the piece of the cataract remained below the pupil would be "the deformity, as it is white through the cornea." He also brought Shattuck up to date on the two earlier cases, cheerfully commenting: "Governor Lincoln and Miss Paine are both in a most hopeful and promising way. . . . I shall set out for Hanover tomorrow, covered with glory."

This was apparently an especially busy period for cataract operations.

A week later, Smith was once again writing to Shattuck on the same subject. He told how, having been delayed in Brattleboro, Vermont (waiting for the next stagecoach), on his way back to Hanover, he put the time to good use. After being "engaged to reduce a dislocated shoulder which had been dislocated nine weeks" (he succeeded in about half an hour), he was faced with a difficult decision:

Later on the same day a child was brought to me with cataracts in his eyes. The child was a beautiful and very sightly boy of three years old. The question, whether we should operate immediately and run the risk of failing in the operation from the restiveness of the child, or defer until the child was 10 or 12 years old. Considering how much the child must lose by being blind so many years and how very troublesome it would be for the parents, I determined to attempt an operation which was effected in the most safe and perfect manner, and I have no doubt of final success in the case.[42]

Then, two months later, he reported two more operations for cataracts, "both old men, one 72, the other 84 . . . . I have no doubt of the success of both cases. . . . All I expect in either case is the pleasure of doing good as they are both extremely poor."[43]

Despite the repeated expressions of confidence in his success, Smith did sometimes worry. "The first operation on Mr. Eliot's eye did not succeed to my liking," he once wrote to Mills Olcott; "I had to wait till the eye was recovered from that & yesterday I operated again very much to my satisfaction . . . ."[44] His students were, however, impressed at both the quantity and the quality of the couching operations Smith performed:

Doct. Smith has performed the operation of Couching five times within these Six weeks. They report to him from all parts of the Country, one person from the vicinity of Boston Came here Completely blind and had both Eyes operated upon about three weeks since, She can now see to read tolerably well by the assistance of Glasses.[45]

When it came to eyes, of course, cataract operations were not the only surgery Smith undertook, though he went into so much detail on different methods for couching that Fitch was able to fill several pages in his notebook with the discussion. In a later lecture, Smith also took up the subjects of "Dropsy of the Eye" (which he defined as the loss of vision as a result of "a collection of fluid within its coats"), the extirpation of cancerous eyes ("On the whole . . . a simple operation"), and operating on drooping eyelids (he described two methods but let students know which he thought preferable). Later yet, Smith dealt with tumors on the eyelids and (very briefly) with "Coagulated Substances on the Cornea."[46]

A further indication of Smith's reputation in ophthalmology appears in a notice on the back cover of a treatise, *On the Morbid Sensibility of the Eye . . .*, by John Stevenson ("Member of the Royal Society of Surgeons, etc."), which appeared in the United States in 1815. The publisher obviously thought it advantageous to broadcast the fact that Nathan Smith had deemed the book worthy; the company announcement and Smith's endorsement fill the space on the back cover of the little volume:

The publisher has been politely favored with the following recommendation of Stevenson on the Eye from Nathan Smith, M.D., Professor of the Theory and Practice of Surgery in Yale College.
Sir,

I have not only perused the treatise on the Morbid Sensibility of the Eye, by John Stevenson, but have had several opportunities of testing the correctness of his principles by applying them to practice. I am highly gratified with your proposals for reprinting the work, hoping by that means it may find its way to the Medical Gentlemen of this country by whom it is much wanted.[47]

Cancer

Smith in his lectures showed he had a grimly accurate understanding of many characteristics of cancer. Already in 1811 he began his lecture on cancer thus: "It is difficult to give any particular description of Cancer—it is a peculiar action in the system. What this kind of action is I do not pretend to tell—but when the system puts in this kind of morbid action, we have, as yet, found no remedies—and it generally ends in death."[48]

By the time he was lecturing to Worham Fitch's class at Yale, he was going into greater detail:

It is difficult to define cancer. There is considerable variety in its appearance. There are but few parts of the body [that are not] subject to it. It occurs in skin, bone, glands, cellular substance, and in many of the viscera. . . . It takes place in the rectum, urinary bladder, prostate gland, lips, glans penis, &c. which parts are particularly liable to it. Sometimes cancers almost immediately ulcerate, a scab at first appears and then when this is rubbed off an ulcer forms and spreads rapidly and extensively. . . .

A tumor in the breast will sometimes be accompanied with a tumor in the axilla; but sometimes the disease remains a long time before these take place. The breast is sometimes much enlarged. I performed the operation on a breast that weighed 9 lb. The wound soon healed after the operation. A few years after another tumor appeared which was removed and this also was healed.[49]

Smith proposed a quite modern definition of neoplasms: "A mere enlargement is not a disorganization of a part. I should define it to be a new substance or a part that has a new organization; or one that is different from what is natural. A clear idea of the different organizations of tumors cannot be given. It is not probably [sic] that any one man ever saw all the varieties."[50] As for operating on tumors, he had the following to say:

The size of a tumor is not a sufficient objection to an operation. If an artery should be wounded on the limbs it can be taken up and tied with safety. [Similarly, e]ven if the artery of the neck was wounded I believe I should not lose the patient. I could catch the artery with my thumb and finger and hold it till it could be tied.[51]

It was by no means his practice always to cut, however, and he learned from experience.

Where I have found several tumors in different parts of the body I have generally refused to operate . . . . I formerly operated in cases where I would not now. If the breast has contracted itself and the surface falls in I believe we ought never to operate. If white lines are to be discovered extending over the whole breast it is not best to operate because it will generally return again. It should be a rule never to operate unless you can operate so as to be sure you have cut off all the cancer.[52]

And of naevia materni (birth marks), he said:

They seem to be made up of a congeries of blood vessels . . . . Sometimes they grow or increase in size . . . . In such cases I have not attempted to cut them out . . . . Sometimes they have projected out into a considerable tumor. In such cases I have cut them out. When you do this you should cut on the outside of the tumor and not cut at all into it.

Once when I cut one out seated on the forehead I cut into it. It bled as much as a large artery and very much debilitated the child . . . . After extracting draw the parts together with plaster and dress it like any other wound.[53]

Probably in part because of his willingness to admit his errors to his students, as in the above instance, Smith's scorn was palpable for those who made claims beyond their knowledge or experience. In a later lecture, he said:

Where large scirrhus tumors are cured by *arsenic* the patient invariably dies. I challenge the whole world to bring an exception where the patient has not died within one or two years. The patient will live long enough to have it said the cancer is cured and for the quack to extend the fame of his remedy, and when the patient dies it will be attributed to some other disease.

The fact that *arsenic* mercury &c. have an effect on the system when applied to an ulcerated surface similar to the effect when taken internally is no evidence that I have cured the disease and the whole world ought to be advertised of it.[54]

In a letter to Lyman Spalding, Smith pursued the subject of the importance of not relying on "the famous Cancer Curers in Philadelphia & New York. We have lately had a melancholy proof of their power in this part of the country." He continued:

A Mr. Goodwin of Putney had a large tumor on his left side below the axilla which was of the cancerous kind. I extirpated the tumor & charged him & his physician to watch & if any new tumor arose to have it extirpated immediately   about six months after the operation a small tumor appeared in the site of the former. He came to see me on the subject after it was as large as a Walnut. I urged him to let me extirpate it as it was quite circumscribed. He promised to come & have it done soon but went to New York where something was done which caused the tumor to mortify, either by internal or external means   I do not know the particulars but, it left half a dozen behind worse than the first & in a short time so injured his health which was good when I saw him that he returned cancerated and in complete despair of a cure. I purpose to learn the particulars of the treatment & will then publish the Case for the benefit of the New York Cancer Curers.[55]

Smith included this case as the eleventh of the twenty-five he reported in his 1808 essay prepared for submission to the Boylston Prize contest (there the patient's name appears as "Goodnough").[56] But since he apparently never published that essay—and probably did not in the end submit it to the competition—no one other than Lyman Spalding (to whom he had written the letter) and George Shattuck (to whom he had sent a draft of the essay) ever benefited from this written exposure of the putative cancer curers against whom Smith railed.

"Cancer" makes a frequent appearance in Smith's account books. Judging from this and from the fact that he was able to select more than two dozen cancer cases that fit the criteria for the assigned Boylston essay topic, we can calculate that he probably saw as large a proportion of cases with cancer as a rural family practitioner would see today.[57]

Orthopedics

Smith had considerable experience with amputations of various limbs, and his pride in his record was justifiable. Both Jonathan Knight and Gilman Kimball—one of those Dartmouth students who had gotten into trouble over grave-robbing (he later became a distinguished physician in Lowell, Massachusetts)—mentioned that Smith never lost a patient to primary or secondary hemorrhage; Smith himself reported he had "never lost a patient from the operation [of amputation]. All that died, died in consequence of the wound they had received; or the disease with which they were previously affected; or a long time after the operation they have run into consumption."[58]

The indications for the major amputations Smith performed were for the most part acute trauma, infection, and arterial insufficiency with resulting gangrene. One such example he recounted as follows:

A miller's arm was caught by a rope across the fore arm near the elbow. The artery was not destroyed but the vein was. Mortification soon took place and the patient died. If you are convinced a limb will mortify you should operate immediately. It has been said that it is better to wait till suppuration takes place; but this I believe to be entirely improper.

If mortification takes place you cannot be at all certain that it will stop at the extent of the injury. It is of very great importance to decide right at first.[59]

In amputations below the knee, Smith stated that it is better to amputate as near the ankle as possible consistent with removing the disease. A long stump adequately covered with good soft tissue and skin would be preferable to the stump resulting from amputation at the conventional site for a below-the-knee amputation, likely to result in the amputee having to move around on his knees. He used as an illustration one patient with bilateral amputations, who had sufficiently long stumps to be able to walk on them.[60] (This is very reminiscent of Smith's urging that as much of a hand should be saved as possible, for the patient's sake.)

As we have seen in other instances, Smith was quite prepared to criticize his professional colleagues when he believed they had taken the wrong approach in therapy:

A young man had had a pain confined to a part of the [knee] joint which remained a long time and finally a protuberance of a small size appeared in the affected part. It was opened and the bone was rough. The attending surgeon thought this confined to the parts; and that only a piece of the bone was affected. He therefore attempted to produce exfoliation [a falling off of scales or layers of the bone]. I advised amputation but the surgeon still supposing the disease confined, applied the trephine and by a few turns of this he found the bone hollow. He removed as much of the affected part as he could, but the patient died in about 2 weeks.[61]

A Girl was attacked with a white swelling. The bone was at first supposed to be put out of its place by a bone setter and much force used to set it; afterwards blisters were applied, but they were productive of bad consequences. Any motion of the joint was painful I advised an apparatus to prevent the motion of the joint and it cured the disease without any other remedy. This could not cure where the bone was ulcerated or matter formed. [But t]his mode of treatment deserves consideration. I believe many more cases would be cured if the patient was confined. This ought to be tried before amputation if there is no certain evidence of matter being formed. . . . The patient had been under the care of Doct'r Sweet and he had attempted to set the bone. The patient was at the same time labouring with the Phthisis Pulmonalis. Therefore it was improper that amputation should be performed; but by confinement the disease of the limbs was much relieved before the consumption proved fatal.[62]

To treat curvature of the spine (probably tubercular spondylitis, i.e., inflammation of the vertebrae caused by tuberculosis), Smith's practice was as follows:

A woman had a curvature of the spine in consequence of an injury done to it. The curvature appeared a year after the accident . . . . Many remedies were employed that were of no benefit and at length a seton [probably intended to help drain the wound] was put in. This was too small and too low down, but it was evidently of benefit.

A year ago last spring when I saw her the lower limbs were perfectly insensible. I directed large issues to be formed on each side of the spine. She is now able to walk with crutches. The issues have been continued to the present time. The curvature is never removed after it has once taken place. . . . The curvature depends on a softening of the bodies of the vertebrae. Keep the patient in a horizontal position and prohibit exercise.[63]

Smith usually advised rest, as he did here, but obviously he was not altogether opposed to ambulation. While it was probably clear to him what was appropriate, it may have seemed to his students that he wanted to have it both ways. The master of clarity was not flawless.

Smith taught that when an orthopedist is faced with puncture wounds caused by open, or compound, fractures, "[n]o means should be taken to close the wound." He warned:

In all cases when matter forms under the fascia [i.e., when there is inflammation] the wound should be laid open. I have had some experience in cases of puncture and compound fractures.

A young lady had the tibia broken and the points of the bones extended through the external parts.

I laid open the wound and replaced the bone and the patient recovered as soon as though it had been a simple fracture.[64]

Smith cited cases of cancers of the breast that had metastasized to bone: "I have known of two cases where cancerous affection of the breast was attended with such a condition of the bones. I knew of no remedy."[65] He described how he dealt with exostoses (benign bony growths): "I once performed the operation on one arising from the fibula and inclined to the inner side of the leg. . . . The operation is simple and easily performed. Press the soft parts down on the tumor and from it as much as can be. Then cut down directly upon it and with Hey's saw cut off the projecting bone."[66]

Smith also reported in his lectures on how to deal with a variety of cases of dislocations—of the lower jaw, the humerus, elbow, wrist, thumb, knee, and ankle. "In almost every instance you can use the limb as a Lever with advantage and reduce it easier than by pulling directly," he pointed out. And later: "In dislocation of the shoulder you must not depend entirely on pulling. When the accident has frequently happened I can generally reduce a luxation without an assistant. Seat the patient low and use your knee as a fulcrum."[67]

The cases of fractured bones he discussed give ample evidence of his experience in this area. He frequently criticized standard practices:

It was supposed that if a bone was separated two weeks after it was first broken it would require as long a time to unite as it did when first fractured. This is not correct. . . .

All the necessity there is of setting a bone immediately after the fracture happens is it can be done with more ease before the parts are swelled and inflamed. . . .

By some practitioners, fractured bones have not been undressed till the bone was united, for fear of moving the bones and preventing their union. From such opinions patients have often suffered much. The limb has become swelled and the patient has suffered by confinement.

Many limbs have been lost by this treatment and when the dressings were taken off the limb has been found completely mortified. The application of force and pressure about a part to keep the bone in its place is very erroneous practice. No benefit can be produced by it.[68]

Once again on the principle of "less is more," Smith argued that for fractures of the humerus, "the only dressings necessary is [sic] a splint and roller"; the arm should be carried "in a sling." And as for fractures of the bones of the hands and fingers, he said it "is not necessary to apply splints. All that is necessary is to replace them as nearly as possible and apply a bandage. Sometimes it is convenient to bandage one finger to another."[69]

A fracture of the femur, however, Smith acknowledged as "the most difficult fracture to manage."[70] In addition to devoting considerable time in the lectures to a discussion of how to handle such injuries, Smith wrote two papers (published in 1825) on the subject.[71] (His son Ryno's claim notwithstanding, that "the apparatus which he invented . . . is altogether new, and has been adopted by some of the best surgeons in every part of our country as decidedly preferable to any in use,"[72] Nathan Smith's "new splint" was not one of the most favored among the numerous pieces of apparatus devised in the nineteenth century for coping with fractures of the body's longest, strongest bone.[73])

Another topic of considerable orthopedic interest to Smith was necrosis. Not only did he deal with the problem frequently—below, we will look at one of his more famous cases—but his essay, "Observations on the Pathology and Treatment of Necrosis,"[74] has had praise heaped upon it; various writers have called it valuable, a substantial contribution to the subject, and one of the classics in medical literature.[75] The disease, Smith insisted, could be found in "almost any part of the body,"[76] making an adequate discussion complex. When it comes to operating, he wrote, it is also true that "the cases which occur are so peculiar, and require such different methods, that nothing more than general directions can be given.— The object, however, in every case is the same; that is, to remove a piece of dead bone, which has become a foreign body as it relates to the living."[77]

Smith of course lectured on the surgical treatment of osteomyelitis, as well as having written on it. His discussion of necrosis opened with an observation directly relevant to the famous case already referred to: It "affects young persons altogether, at first generally those under 20 . . . . I never saw a person under 5 or 6 years of age affected . . . ."[78]

The technique Nathan Smith developed—"drilling, sawing, and removing dead bone in cases of osteomyelitis, thus preventing the unnecessary amputation of extremities"—was not standardized until more than

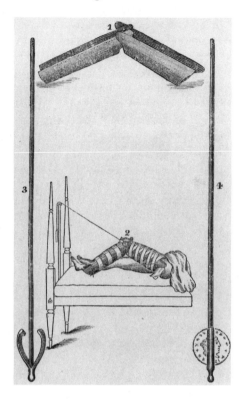

(1) Nathan Smith's leg splint; (2) the splint in use; (3) and (4) two views of Nathan Smith's instrument for removing coins from the esophagus. From N. R. Smith's Medical and Surgical Memoirs, *1831.* Courtesy of Yale University, Harvey Cushing/John Hay Whitney Medical Library.

one hundred years later. Thus when a young patient in Lebanon, New Hampshire, was suffering from osteomyelitis, probably in 1813, Nathan Smith was "the only physician in the United States at the time who had the vision, knowledge, and necessary surgical experience to deal success-fully" with the problem without amputating. Neither the young boy nor his mother wanted him to lose his leg.[79] The patient was Joseph Smith (no relative of Nathan's), none other than the future founder of the Church of Jesus Christ of Latter Day Saints.

The original accounts of the illness and the operation come from Joseph and his mother. Both give sufficient detail to make clear that the doctors in question were Nathan Smith and his medical school colleague (and, at the time, partner in practice) Cyrus Perkins, even though their names were not mentioned and no record of a fee that can with certainty be connected to this case appears in Smith's ledgers. The two separate descriptions of the surgery that circumvented the need for amputation both accord well with what is known about Nathan Smith's procedures (boring into the bone first on one side, then on the other, in order to be able to remove diseased portions of the bone). Thus, although we do not know positively that Smith himself performed the operation, we can be confident that he was the surgeon in charge.

Whether Nathan Smith can be credited with having saved Joseph Smith's life, certainly he saved the boy's leg. Who knows whether religious history might have turned out quite differently if Joseph Smith had been an amputee from early childhood?

An Innovative Surgeon Ahead of His Time

Nathan Smith performed more than the usual amount of elective surgery. Hence it is not surprising that he pioneered some procedures, and we do indeed find in his lectures, letters, and published articles (or in others' accounts) occasional references to or descriptions of operations that he was the first to perform. This excites the imagination: There is a certain glamour to the image of a surgeon bending over a patient to perform the first recorded operation of its kind, with resultant relief or cure for the grateful patient and progress for the medical profession as a whole. More important than performing radically new operations, however, is repeating an operation until all the ramifications of the one procedure are clear and the variations on the possible techniques have all been tried.

Smith repeated many operations with consistent success, and members of the medical profession frequently praised him for his surgical accomplishments. Gilman Kimball, for example, said Nathan Smith as a surgeon "was cautious and painstaking . . . . His ingenuity and manual adroitness are especially deserving of notice . . . ."[80] Another doctor, in describing Smith, stated simply that "[s]urgery was his masterpiece."[81]

Smith devised operations to remove ovarian tumors and to repair harelip and imperforate anus; he inserted a metal plate for traumatic skull defect and used the "Bigelow Maneuver" (before Bigelow) for reducing the dislocated hip; he performed many amputations. He became a veritable specialist at removing bladder stones. (Smith wrote Lyman Spalding on one occasion about a particularly dramatic case. His only recent bit of major surgery—"which proved very successful"—he reported, was "an operation for the Stone, or rarther stones, as there were 217 extracted."[82])

Smith's reputation rested more generally, however, on his repeated and splendid results in removal of cataracts, excision of a variety of cancers, repair of hernia, and drainage of osteomyelitis.

Of all Smith's surgical claims to fame, his treatment of osteomyelitis was among the most important. Not only did he perform a great many of these operations (Joseph Smith was one of numerous patients suffering from the condition), thereby enabling him to assist immensely in defining the pathophysiology of the condition; the operation as Smith performed it also brought out clearly the new and important surgical principle that prompt and wide drainage of suppurative processes is vitally important. He published a "clear and classical account" of the importance of the early removal of the sequestra a "year before [Benjamin] Brodie [1783–1862] performed the first operation on an abscessed tibia."[83] In that piece, he underscored the importance of drainage with characteristic bluntness: "The object of the surgeon . . . is to remove the sequestra." He ended with the following firm prognosis: "If the whole of the sequestra is removed, the cure will be perfect; but if any portion of it is left, it will keep up a discharge, somewhat in proportion to the quantity of dead bone left in the limb."[84] He thus contributed his share to the reduction of suffering and to the improvement of surgical principles for a later generation of surgeons.

A second basis for Smith's reputation as an innovative surgeon comes from the ovariotomy he performed on July 5, 1821[85]—the one thing those who know anything about Nathan Smith as a surgeon can be counted on to have heard about. Smith himself seems to have thought his operation was entirely original; in his very brief written account of the operation (it is the topic of one of the few case reports he wrote up),[86] he gives no hint that he knew of any other operation of the sort. And Smith's son, Ryno, referring to his father, wrote in the opening essay of his *Medical and Surgical Memoirs* that it "is believed that he was the first in this country to perform the bold operation of extirpating the ovarian tumour." In a note appended to the reprinted version of his father's account, however, Ryno went on to say, "I ought here to state, that the same operation has been performed in this country in several instances by Dr. McDowell, of Kentucky, and more recently by others. I am not confident that the first operation by Dr. McDowell was subsequent to that of my father."[87]

Surely Ryno was being disingenuous. There is no question that the Kentucky surgeon Ephraim McDowell (1771–1830) had performed the operation successfully as early as 1809. Because communication in those days was slow and difficult—Kentucky and New Hampshire were worlds apart, and McDowell did not publish an account of what he had done until 1817—it is possible that Smith really did know nothing of it.[88] Ryno's evasiveness is less excusable. Nonetheless, that Smith was apparently the *second* surgeon in this country to perform a successful ovariotomy does not detract from the significance of the operation. (McDowell's pioneering effort, incidentally, caused a much greater uproar; he was accused of "cutting people open and killing them."[89]) The tradition that has Smith bravely and successfully performing this bit of surgery without knowing that anyone else had attempted it is unnecessarily melodramatic in any case. Every operation is new to some extent.

McDowell was, however, merely the first in the United States. Robert Houstoun of the University of Glasgow had nearly a century earlier published an account of his successful operation for ovarian tumors. He ended on an instructive note: "The manifest Success of this Case, may be of use, and may shew, that we ought not to despair too soon, in Distempers that are seemingly most dangerous."[90] Since both Smith and McDowell had studied in Scotland, they could well have been (perhaps should have been) aware of Houstoun's paper.

If there was a special virtue to Smith's operation, apart from his having diagnosed the problem correctly, it was the fact that he used leather ligatures. Smith is also said to have "anticipated modern surgical technique by cutting the sutures short, dropping them back into the abdominal cavity, and completely closing the abdomen." But even five years after the operation, it is clear Smith had no strong feelings about the benefits of this kind of suturing material—though he knew it was said to be absorbable and though it may have occurred to him that healing would be faster if he tied the stump and allowed it to return to the abdomen.[91] For among the surgical techniques Nathan Smith helped establish or promote was the use of nonabsorbable ligatures. In tying off arteries, for example, he preferred a small waxed string with two ordinary knots (though in at least one instance he used "linen shoe-thread, made small and hard"[92]). The true novelty was his advice to "close the wound with a ligature and let the ligatures of the artery hang out of the wound."[93] Left to act as a kind of seton, ligatures—once they had accomplished their function— were loose and could be removed by gentle tugging.

Of particular interest is that Smith's case histories as they emerge from his lectures demonstrate both a modern approach to surgery and a high percentage of cures. Nor was this because he mentioned only his successes. He freely admitted his lack of knowledge ("We do not know what the state of the brain is in Apoplexy," and "How the seasons operate in producing the disease [dysentery] I am unable to say"), and he did not shrink from mentioning the death of a patient ("[A] family was poisoned. I gave *Calomel* as a cathartic and then *alum*. The man and wife recovered. The child died").[94] He acknowledged his mistakes, when he believed they taught valuable lessons to the students:

The last time I operated [for bladder stone] I cut the pedic artery. I directed an assistant to hold his finger upon the artery till I had removed the stone. By that time it had stopped bleeding and it was unnecessary to tie it. In another case I wounded the artery and took it up and tied it. This was done with as much ease as you would tie an artery upon the back of the hand. We have been very particularly cautioned as to cutting this artery but it is of little consequence.[95]

Patients knew Nathan Smith as a steady, skilled, and ingenious surgeon. He was probably among the first in the United States to perform staphylorrhaphy (surgical repair of a cleft palate),[96] the first to devise a good posterior splint for fractures of the thigh,[97] and the first in the United States to amputate at the knee joint.[98] If an instrument did not exist, Smith would invent it. He was the originator of both an extractor for foreign bodies in the esophagus[99] and a dilator of esophageal strictures.[100]

Always, he practiced by the principles he taught: For dislocations, discard pulleys and use the anatomic leverages of bone and ligament instead; for bullet wounds, limit probing, give up if you cannot find the foreign body accurately and quickly, and treat expectantly; for fractures, immobilize the limb in good position but allow for swelling; treat related lacerations, punctures, and bruises gently and thoroughly; for bleeding, carefully isolate the artery, cut it clean if it is jaggedly perforated, and try pressure alone before resorting to ligatures; for pus under pressure, particularly in acute osteomyelitis, cut widely and quickly.[101] Above all, he taught, do no more harm than necessary.

Indeed, Smith carried the principle of *primum non nocere* to its logical conclusion. Many times when called to operate, he found surgery unnecessary and prescribed supportive treatment only, with satisfactory results. Alexander Boyd once wrote from Hanover to William Boyd in Londonderry, New Hampshire: "I went to [Lisbon—some forty miles north of Hanover] with Doct. Smith and upwards of twenty of his students to see a limb taken off but when he got there he concluded that he could cure it without taking off the limb . . . ."[102] Such cases do not get listed among a surgeon's cures, but they are perhaps his greatest successes; they were especially rare in the days when most surgeons believed that once they had been called they had to do *something*.

There were other less dramatic cases where Smith exercised restraint. We find in Fitch's notes a number of remarks like these on hernias: "I never operated in cases of umbilical hernia. I never saw a case of this kind where an operation would be necessary,"[103] and in "cases of inguinal hernia it is always desirable to reduce it without an operation. The means are numerous . . . ."[104] Smith's skill and dexterity frequently allowed him to succeed by simple means; once, for example, he removed a uterine tumor by an uncomplicated vaginal procedure.[105]

"We now see," William H. Welch once said, "that he did more for the general advancement of medical and surgical practice than any of his predecessors or contemporaries in this country."[106] Small wonder that when Nathan Smith arrived in New Haven his surgery was promptly appreciated. Within a year he wrote to Mills Olcott in good humor: "The people in and about New Haven are very much elated with my mode of operating & are calling daily some wishing to have their legs & arms taken off and some to have that wished member remanded . . . ."[107] Even if Smith was joking a bit, Yale apparently struck him as a good place to be.

PART IV

AFTER DARTMOUTH

CHAPTER ELEVEN

A New Challenge

Woe unto thee, Dartmouth, for thy glory is departing—Dr. N. Smith has concluded to move to New Haven.   —HENRY BOND [1]

ON JULY 12, 1813, Nathan Smith offered his resignation to the Honorable President and Board of Trust of Dartmouth College, freeing him to join the faculty of the new medical institute being started
in New Haven.[2] He was re-appointed to teach courses at Dartmouth for
one term in 1816, but from 1813 on his attention was focused primarily
on events and institutions elsewhere.

Why did Smith leave Hanover, where he had fought so hard to build
his school? How could he bring himself to throw in his lot with an institution whose initial planning had been done without him? We must examine first the challenge unfolding at Yale, and then the disappointments
and frustrations at Dartmouth. Finally, we will look briefly at some features of Smith's years at Yale not already explored.

The Medical Institute of Yale College

Yale would no doubt have succeeded eventually in establishing a medical
school even if Nathan Smith had not answered the call to be part of its
first faculty. So great was his reputation as a medical educator, physician
and surgeon, however, that the would-be founders at Yale were utterly
convinced they needed him—and there is little doubt they were at least
partially right. Smith alone gave the new enterprise regional (even national) rather than merely local credibility; his presence did much to set
the new school on a firm foundation. Among the doctors involved in the
project at Yale from the beginning, only Nathan Smith had experience
running a formal institution of medical education. To this extent, then, he

is rightly counted as key among the founders of Yale Medical School, even though his relationship to its gestation and birth were unlike his connection with the medical school in Hanover. Nonetheless, it had been by no means a foregone conclusion that the great man could be wooed from Dartmouth.

Yale was established in 1701 (as the "Collegiate School of America") for the explicit purpose of preparing men for the Congregational ministry. In 1777, Ezra Stiles became president, and already in that year he had plans for creating a medical professorship, the first step toward adding a medical school and turning the college into a university.[3] Only after Timothy Dwight became president in 1795, however, did the plan begin to take shape.

Dwight, though not a physician, seems to have been the one who conceived the idea of a cooperative arrangement between the State Medical Society and Yale. This was in sharp contrast to the way medical schools were generally established in those days; cooperation in lieu of competition would, not surprisingly, prove beneficial to all.[4] In 1802, President Dwight took another important step by appointing Benjamin Silliman professor of chemistry and natural history in the college. Silliman was also not a physician, but he had taken courses in medicine at both Philadelphia and Edinburgh. The aim was never for him to practice or teach medicine, but rather simply to fit him for teaching the basic science courses as a member of the medical school faculty when it was created.

Characteristic of Dwight was the patient and thoughtful way he went to work setting up the new school. There were to be three important differences between Yale's Medical Institute and any previous medical school, quite apart from the unprecedented cooperation between the college and the profession alluded to above. First, the institute was to be created by the college as an integral part of the institution rather than to be attached to the college after being independently established by medical men. Second, each professor in the new school would be trained to teach a particular specialty. (Nathan Smith would turn out to be the sole exception by being appointed to teach more than one subject at a time; no doubt his general reputation as a physician and surgeon made it easy for others to assume he was capable of teaching whatever needed to be taught. But the blurred lines between the so-called specialties is evident from the way several members of the faculty played musical chairs over the next few years, moving from one academic assignment to another as colleagues moved away, retired, or died.)

Third, admission would be limited to students with a baccalaureate degree, or to those who were in college or demonstrably capable of college-level work. This last point may have been the most important. Though it was theoretically the aim of every medical school to enroll only college graduates, there had been little effort to enforce such a policy, anywhere. Thirty-one years earlier, the learned French physician Jean-François Coste, in a Latin discourse he presented when he received an honorary degree for "excellence in Medicine" from the University of Virginia, had advocated as much. Implicitly throwing down the gauntlet, he queried:

Why do those men assume indiscriminately that title of Doctor, whose lot it has never been to have even sipped from the surface of the streams of literature? Men to whom everything pertaining to the humane arts, to philosophy, to whatever is productive of the good & the wise is no less unknown than that knowledge which from its inherent nature is termed occult? Why do you greet as Doctors those who have never even saluted the threshold of a college?[5]

In fact, the very loose requirements for entrance to medical school and the casual licensing requirements of colonial days were not really corrected for another century. Yale, importantly, would be the first to come close to the standard Coste urged on American medical educators, and Smith—to his credit—seems to have concerned himself more and more with these matters at Yale. His own Harvard M.D. degree (awarded in 1811) was the result of that institution's decision to convert its M.B. degrees into M.D. degrees, apparently on the assumption that anyone who could earn a Bachelor of Medicine degree had an education equivalent to those who had earned a Bachelor of Arts degree. (Dartmouth in the same year converted each of its previously awarded M.B. degrees into M.D. degrees, and in 1812 started awarding the Doctor of Medicine degree to all its medical graduates; Smith had been given an honorary M.D. by Dartmouth in 1801.[6]) Smith's colleagues on the newly forming Yale medical faculty seemed to have a clear picture from the outset of what a doctor's degree should entail, and Smith came to approve heartily of the collegiate training the Institute required of its medical students.

Yale's new Medical Institute, then, was not the product of one man's dream, but the outcome of deliberate planning by several individuals endowed with foresight hoping to meet America's needs for physicians like those Coste had described. Between 1806 and 1813, a great deal of behind-the-scenes arguing and planning had gone on. A grant had to be sought from the Connecticut legislature; principles of cooperation notwithstanding, precisely how the responsibility for supervising instruction was to be apportioned between Yale and the Connecticut Medical Society needed to be worked out; and professors had to be chosen and assigned to specific chairs.[7] Already in 1806, the Reverend Dr. Nathan Strong and Professor Silliman had been appointed a committee by Yale's Board of Trustees to enquire about the feasibility of a medical professorship. Progress was slow, but perhaps no more so than was to be expected when such momentous undertakings were at issue. (Again, the contrast with the founding of Dartmouth's medical school at the impetus of a single man is sharp and instructive.) On September 11, 1810, the Board of Trustees recorded that "President Dwight and Professor Silliman were appointed a committee to unite with a committee from the medical society to lay before the General Assembly a report to apply for action on a new Medical School at Yale."[8] The next step came exactly a year later. On September 10, 1811, Lt. Governor John Cotton Smith joined Professor Silliman and the Reverend Strong on a new committee "to unite with the committee of the Medical Society" for carrying into execution the Medical Institute of Yale College.[9]

Among the first choices for a faculty position was Mason F. Cogswell (who, as we learned, was William Tully's first mentor), to be professor of surgery and anatomy; he, however, "had ever been loath to accept the professorship"[10]—not least because of "the ripening of the plans for helping his [deaf-mute] daughter Alice" in Hartford. Although he initially accepted the position offered on April 29, 1812, "[w]hen he heard that Dr. Nathan Smith of Hanover was available . . . he promptly retired in his favor."[11] Apparently no one had seriously expected him to accept (the offer was a gesture to show the esteem in which he was held). Jonathan Knight was another who was appointed early; he likewise accepted initially, only to resign fifteen months later. The resignation may have come from his not wanting to be a mere "Assistant" professor (to Cogswell or anyone else);[12] in the event, he was promptly re-appointed to a full professorship.[13]

The loss of Cogswell and the elevation of Knight meant the joint committee was obliged to rethink its strategy. Silliman himself was on the committee, and thus in an awkward position as a possible candidate for an appointment, yet he was the logical choice for professor of chemistry and pharmacy. Indeed, in all America the only chemist of comparable stature was Parker Cleaveland, who was fully engaged at Bowdoin College, in Maine. Further, President Dwight had clearly intended all along for his prize professor—to this day Silliman ranks as one of the most distinguished persons ever to have served on the Yale faculty—to help launch the medical school.

Another obvious choice was Eneas Munroe. No longer a young man, he was a revered member of the state Medical Society who would give an air of maturity to the faculty; his professorship of materia medica and botany was assured. Dr. Eli Ives would be assistant professor of materia medica and botany and would carry the bulk of the burden for teaching those subjects. (Ives, incidentally, would succeed to the chair of the theory and practice of physic on Smith's death, leaving the way open for William Tully to be appointed to Ives's old chair.)

Everyone was aware of the desirability of persuading Nathan Smith to take the surgical post. His national reputation would give the Institute a good start. William H. Welch, himself a great figure in medical history, would later say that when Nathan Smith went to New Haven from Hanover "he was already a star of the first magnitude in the medical firmament," and that he was "the most distinguished member of the first Medical Faculty of Yale."[14] The fifty or sixty students who were likely to follow Smith wherever he taught would also be an asset. (Most of the students' fees went directly to the individual professors rather than to the institution, but a sudden influx of students devoted to Smith would give the new school impressive enrollment figures to boast about in its first year.)

Some of the Connecticut doctors may have known that as early as 1808 Nathan Smith had been contemplating a move from Hanover. Certainly Jonathan Knight knew that Smith might look favorably on an opportunity to move to New Haven. Late in November 1810, one of Smith's Dartmouth students (Timothy J. Gridley, who would earn his M.D. there in 1812) had written to Knight, a college friend of his, as follows:

I was conversing with Dr. Smith, and during the course of the conversation I observed that a medical institution was contemplated at New Haven, and asked his opinion of the probability of its success. He answered that unquestionably in the course of a few years it would excel any medical school this side of Philadelphia. . . . I also expressed a wish that in case of a medical establishment at New Haven he could be one of the professors. He said if there was a vacancy, and the faculty of Yale College should request him to fill it, he would accept without the least hesitation, although by dissolving his relation to this college he might hazard considerable pecuniary loss.[15]

Smith almost certainly knew about this letter. He may even have been consciously allowing Gridley to test the waters for him, though it is curious if he thought he needed an intermediary. Gridley's letter goes on at such length and appears so carefully contrived to answer whatever questions a potential employer might raise that it seems likely Smith was involved in its composition and counted on Knight to pass it on. In any case, the letter gives us a picture of Smith at this stage of his career (whether it represents Gridley's independent view or Smith's self-assessment). Gridley continued thus:

One of [Smith's] reasons for removing from this place is the intolerable burden he has sustained for a number of years past, and which he feels unable to endure longer. He has lectured on Chemistry, Anatomy, Surgery, and the Theory and Practice of Physic, in addition to which he has constantly a very important and extensive run of practice. In case he was removed to Connecticut, he would probably undertake the anatomical and physical branches exclusively. It is, I presume, unnecessary to say anything respecting Dr. Smith's qualifications as a lecturer or operator. His reputation is extensive and well deserved. His lectures particularly on surgery are original and practical, the result of his own observation and experiences. He has made many and important improvements in operative surgery, and has discovered the origin as well as the cure of some diseases such as necrosis of the bone, . . . but his qualifications as a surgeon and Physician do not constitute the sum of his excellency. He is a man of general information, of an easy, familiar, but dignified deportment; communicative, agreeable in conversation, of equable temper, and of a charitable disposition. In short, wherever he is known he is admired and beloved. He has an extensive medical library, and a very reputable anatomical museum . . . . But the considerations of the greatest importance relative to Dr. Smith's admission to a professorship is that it would not only facilitate the acquisition of medical knowledge, but give the school an immediate and extensive reputation. . . . The Boston school [Harvard] would be deserted; even now the Boston students prefer a course under Dr. Smith . . . he would always command a large share of the students of New England as long as he chose to lecture.

What a pity we do not know more about the origin of this extraordinary document, a stunning letter of recommendation for a student to have written for his professor.

Smith clearly wanted his interest in Yale to be treated circumspectly. A few months earlier, he had written to Shattuck announcing his decision to leave Hanover, but he then added a postscript asking Shattuck to keep the information to himself:

I have at length determined to leave Hanover, but at present have not concluded on any certain place of future residence. The political parties are so very jealous of each other in this state, and so near a balance that I have nothing to expect from either as some ignorant person might be offended at any grant or assistance voted by the legislature to promote what they term "the cutting up of dead bodies."[16] No one will dare to advocate the measure, and I expect they will, if not deemed too unconstitutional, revoke the grant made for that purpose last year, and if that cannot be effected, they will enact laws which will inflict corporal punishment on any person who is concerned in digging or dissecting. If the thing should take this course, it will afford me a good pretext for leaving the College and State, a thing which will not be disagreeable to me. The proposal I made the state of giving land and the whole of my museum and apparatus was too much to give, but while engaged in promoting the school in this place, I felt willing to go all lengths in sacrificing on the Aesculapian altar, but the conduct of people and parties has cooled my ardor for laboring in my avocation in this place, and determined me to sell my talents in physic and surgery to the highest bidder. . . .

P.S. You will not at present mention publicly my intentions to remove from this place.[17]

Perhaps he was simply being shrewd, not wanting to seem too eager in case he was not wanted at Yale. He needn't have worried, really; from the outset, he was being considered, as Benjamin Silliman made explicit in a letter to Jonathan Knight late in 1812: "Ever since a medical school has been projected here Dr Smith's name has been much mentioned as a candidate for one of the places."[18]

Before Smith could be invited to go to Yale, however, the committee needed to ascertain where he stood religiously. Silliman, speaking with the confidence that came from knowing President Dwight's position well, continued his letter to Knight thus:

In the Opinion of many his claims were such that his reported infidelity[19] ought not debar him; but our Corporation & Pres[iden]t never countenanced the idea because they believed him an infidel & could not reconcile it with their duty to appoint any man of this description to a station in the College whatever might be his talents reputation & learning.

Nathan Smith was a good Episcopalian, at least by marriage (we noted earlier that he had apparently been an active layman at Trinity Church in Cornish). But Yale required all her faculty members to be Congregationalists, and much is made in accounts of the time of the resulting need for Smith to "achieve grace" before he would be acceptable to the Yale Corporation. He certainly would have understood the strength of the insistence on orthodoxy at Yale, after having taught for fifteen years in Eleazar Wheelock's College; he knew Eleazar had been forbidden to preach at Yale because of his Quaker leanings, even though his primary aim at Dartmouth was to train Congregational missionaries to serve the Indians.

Though the circumstances required Smith to trumpet his change of heart, it is not clear that his views on religion actually changed significantly. William Allen, in his obituary oration years later, said "Dr. Smith, until a later period of his life, did not seem to have adopted any established principles of religion" (though he had "purity of . . . moral character"). Allen also seemed to think that the death of a professor at Dartmouth in 1810, full of great religious "descantings," may have influenced Smith (he and others were, said Allen, "astonished").[20] Smith was in any case no one's fool; he was said to have announced his "state of grace" to his Dartmouth class of medical students with tears in his eyes.

Smith's professed discovery of his new "state" evidently did the trick. Silliman was sufficiently convinced to dispose of the troubling subject quite briskly later in that same long letter to Jonathan Knight:

We have it now on authority which cannot be questioned & with testimony which is satisfactory that Dr. Smith's sentiments on religious subjects have undergone an entire alteration. Those who know him best believe him too frank & high minded a man to allow them to credit the idea that he would be willing to practise duplicity to carry a point, and therefore the change is considered as real. He has fully renounced his infidelity in repeated conversations with intimate friends and to his class to whom he spoke in such terms of his past & present views as drew tears from speaker & hearers. . . . Dr Smith . . . is so frank as to say that he shall be happy to fill any place in the Institution for which he may be thought qualified.[21]

Silliman's letter went on to spell out in considerable detail how Smith's possibly joining the Yale faculty would affect Knight's position:

I have his letter before me & his remarks; "I have always considered New Haven as a place more favorably situated for a medical school than any other in New England, and, in my opinion at this time everything is propitious, and nothing is wanting but the united efforts of several persons suitably qualified to carry it into affect, & that a school may be shortly established that will very soon far exceed anything of the kind this side [of] Philadelphia." Although Dr. Smith's expectations may be over sanguine there can be no question that his reputation & exertions would go far towards realizing his views. You see then that Dr. Smith is willing to come & that we are on the whole disposed to invite him. His name is still in nomination & as the arrangements have never been definitely made by the corporation (except so far as you are concerned & Dr Coggswell) there is no impediment in the way of his appointment. You will not suppose that we are about to do anything that will militate with your claims or that we wish to do it. Dr Coggswell will decline accepting his appointment—he has never yet signified his acceptance—Dr Smith can be appointed in his room & as he will be on the spot the school will thus be filled & organized. It is not necessary now perhaps to determine precisely how the thing shall be ultimately arranged: the fact will be that the theory & practice—anatomy, surgery, & midwifery & materia medica & botany will lie among you Dr. Smith & Dr Ives & you can make such an apportionment of labour as shall be mutually satisfactory to you all. If these duties are all discharged no matter by whom of the three.— But for the sake of showing the practicability of this project—say that Dr Smith shall teach surgery & midwifery, [and] you anatomy (appropriately so called) & perhaps materia medica—Dr Ives theory & practice & as much botany as our circumstances admit of & I Chemistry & Pharmacy. Dr Smith's reputation in surgery & midwifery is unrivalled in New England—in this he could be of vast advantage to you both by Instruction & practice & by introducing you, while no young man can command public confidence immediately on these subjects. In the meantime you can be growing up to take his place by & by.

Anatomy is perhaps as good a department of medical instruction for a young professor to begin with as any because study and industry whether he has practice or not, will enable him to teach it. Dr. Coggswell Dr Dwight Dr Ives & myself all agree in opinion, that *Dr Smith, so far from standing in your way would be of great advantage to you in the ways mentioned above & also by causing the school at once to rise to a point which it would otherwise take years to attain.*—I have now with the advice of the President Dr Coggswell & Dr Ives stated this subject fully & frankly to you & we wish to know your sentiments as speedily as possible (allowing you however adequate time for reflections). No communication will be made from the College to Dr Smith till we hear first from you [emphasis added].[22]

This lengthy epistle, dealing as it does with a variety of topics, serves to remind us how complicated the matter before the committee at Yale was. Juggling expectations and egos with aspirations, reconciling religious concerns (a critical affair: Dwight, after all, was the author of a popular cautionary book called *The Triumph of Infidelity*; there could be no question about how serious an issue this was for him) with the desire to woo a famous professor from far away—all this took time and careful planning. No one in New Haven could know for sure what might motivate Nathan Smith to move, or what factors he would take into account.

Leaving Dartmouth

For Nathan Smith to extricate himself from Dartmouth and Hanover was no easy task. The Medical Building of which he was so proud had burdened him with heavy financial responsibilities. Furthermore, despite his efforts to keep requests for funding politically neutral, the cause of the medical school had become—perhaps inevitably—a "political affair" (as he had bemoaned in a letter to Shattuck[23]).

State politics were not the only political problems on Smith's horizon, as we also saw earlier. Internal institutional problems conspired to play into the hands of Smith's suitors in New Haven; going to Yale would give him a way out of what was becoming, increasingly, an uncomfortable situation—politically, educationally, and socially.

Furthermore, there were positive features about Yale that made it, by 1810, more and more appealing. Yale was in better financial shape than Dartmouth, and in Timothy Dwight it had a very strong president. The college itself would run the Medical Institute and provide professors in other departments, thus largely freeing the faculty from administrative responsibilities; Smith would be able to teach clinical subjects without the headaches that came with running the anatomy and chemistry departments.

Not that some of the concerns generally connected with teaching anatomy were not still on his mind. Even to teach surgery, he would need cadavers. New Haven being situated on Long Island Sound meant that "subjects" could be transported to the medical school from Boston or New York by water rather than overland; the dangers of anatomy riots would be sharply reduced. These are among the points in Gridley's communication to Knight that suggest Smith helped compose the letter:

The difficulty and danger of procuring subjects for dissection is another consideration which induces Dr. Smith to remove from this place. Without these, you may know, the study of anatomy is but trifling with time and expense, to say nothing of the danger to [which] the patient of the merely descriptive anatomist is subject in cases of difficult appreciation. . . . But the inhabitants within forty or fifty miles of this place are constantly on the watch, lest the silent repose of their departed friends be disturbed by the nocturnal visitations of medical students; . . . Boston is the nearest port from which subjects can be obtained without great hazard and difficulty. At New Haven the water communication with New York, and even with Philadelphia would completely obviate this difficulty, as subjects might be procured as frequently and as expeditiously as occasion might require.[24]

Connecticut had other attractive qualities for a medical man, not the least of which was that a goodly supply of distinguished physicians was in practice there. The prospect of a new medical school—which would mean the state's sons who wished to be doctors would no longer be entirely dependent on Massachusetts, New Hampshire, New York, and Pennsylvania to obtain formal medical training—could only add to New Haven's appeal.

In addition, the institutional contrasts between Dartmouth and Yale must also have seemed to be all in Yale's favor. The differences between Timothy Dwight and John Wheelock, already alluded to, were dramatic: the one a strong leader with a clearly articulated vision for the future of his institution, the other an embattled administrator who had probably always been in over his head and who now faced the greatest threat possible not only to his position but to the future of the young institution itself.[25] Smith's personal sympathy for Wheelock made it increasingly difficult to remain neutral in the controversy between the Board of Trust and Wheelock. Furthermore, Smith's partnership with Cyrus Perkins had its awkward features, given the overt nature of Perkins's commitment to the university side in the debate over Dartmouth's institutional governance, which we also saw earlier. And when it came to colleagues, neither Cyrus Perkins nor anyone else Dartmouth would hire in the next few years was in the same class as Yale's distinguished Benjamin Silliman.

Smith may also have begun to realize how overextended he was financially. He had started using the new Coös bank in Haverhill, New Hampshire—Mills Olcott was one of the trustees—in 1806, when Olcott deposited $88.02 there for him. In 1808, he borrowed $600.00 from the bank.[26] Later, having been sued by the bank, he was forced to pay $622.04 and $25.55 in costs when the Superior Court of Grafton County issued a judgment against him because of his failure to repay the loan on time.[27] When Lyman Spalding turned to him for financial help (Spalding should have known better), Smith wrote back in July of 1809 as follows:

My affairs are at the present very much embarrassed on account of some purchases of land which I made two years since, and the money which I have been obliged to expend for the Medical Establishment has reduced my finances very low. It will be impossible for me to help you from the money granted for a Medical Building . . . [as] that money is granted for an express purpose, and put into the hands of the committee for the purpose, so that it cannot be touched by me.[28]

In general, the value of Smith's land was going down. The extent of his financial difficulties throughout the period before he left Dartmouth is evident from an extraordinary note that Mills Olcott penned in October of 1813, as Smith was preparing to go to Yale:

Whereas Dr. Nathan Smith is indebted to Pres. Wheelock in a sum of about three thousand Dollars & some interest, & is indebted on account of the Sheriffs liabilities in consequence of the neglect of his Deputy Jedediah Baldwin (for E Baldwins neglect the sᵈ Smith being bound to the Sheriff); in a sum of Eleven Hundred seventy eight 41/Dollars for neglect with six different debts & for sᵈ last sum 1,000 Smith has this day given his notes to me and is also indebted to Samuel Poole in the sum of about Six Hundred Dollars — And whereas sᵈ· Smith has lodged sundry notes & accounts with me to collect & also given me an order on Wm. H. Woodward, Esqr. for the avails of what demands if his s^{d.} Smiths are in his E. Woodwards hands for collection, & from the avails of those & such other demands as s^d Smith shall hereafter deliver s^d Olcott he wishes to discharge the above described debts of s^d Smith—And whereas s^d Smith wishes to provide for the payment of his above described debts from such as and shall be in my hands, I have agreed with him to take the risk of making any advances upon myself for such sums as shall have to be paid sooner than collection can be made from s^d Smiths debts—& if I have occasion to hire money for that purpose upon any premium or extra interest, I am to bear that loss myself, & also to free s^d Smith for all expense which he may be put to in consequence of any suits—& although at my own expense I may procure any delay I wish with s^d debts, I am still to indemnify s^d Smith from all cost or expense, & for all I advance before collection, I am to receive interest to be reimbursed—It is understood that Dr Smith has mortgaged his farm to the Pres. for security of his debt & I am to settle s^d debt within a legal period of redeeming land recovered in mortgage if the Pres. should sue the same.[29]

These were large sums in 1813. Quite apart from the questions this document raises about why Olcott was willing to undertake a task that must at times have appeared hopeless if not thankless, it turns out that Smith's mortgaging his farm to President Wheelock was not enough. Smith remained in financial difficulties, deep enough to seem insoluble at times. On December 29, 1814—a year after he had moved to Yale—he succeeded in getting Yale to offer him $3,000 in exchange for his release to the university of all his Hanover land near Ebenezer Woodward's property. This amounted to a mortgage loan from Yale College to Smith,[30] and it must have given him some further relief (though, as we shall see, this was by no means the end of financial problems for Nathan Smith or his family).

Quite possibly, anatomy department troubles—real or imagined, past or potential—were the critical factor in Nathan Smith's decision to resign from Dartmouth and move to Yale. And whether it was with misgivings or sadness that he left Hanover, we cannot tell. But by July 12, 1813, the overtures from Yale were too much to resist. On that date, Smith wrote the following letter of resignation:

This may certify to the Honble president & Board of Trust of Dartmouth College that I do hereby propose to resign my office of professor in said College at the next annual meeting of the Honble Board of Trust & therefore wish them to appoint if they think proper some other person to the office I now hold in the College—[31]

The New Haven Years

In November 1813, Nathan Smith commenced his surgical course in the new medical institution at Yale with about forty pupils.[32] Right away, he was busy—and in trouble:

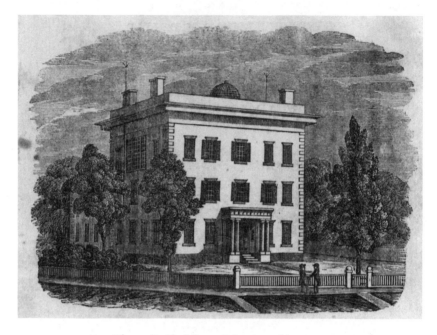

The medical building at Yale, pictured in 1839.
Courtesy of Yale University, Harvey Cushing/John Hay Whitney Medical Library.

Immediately on coming into New Haven I fell into such a run of business that it being very dark, one evening, I run my leg against a plank with such violence I have it a pretty severe contusion not so bad, however, as to confine me at once, but in a few days, after, I was suddenly attacked with violent pains accompanied with fever which has confined me flat on my back till today, & now I barely set up to write. I think however that the difficulty is chiefly over & that I shall soon be sailing again as brisk as ever . . . . The people here seem to speak me favor & give me a little money . . . . [R]especting our school it is very much as I expected the numbers who attend are not large but very respectable. I perceive there will be much for me to do if I continue here.[33]

A few weeks later he wrote to Olcott again, in a similar vein: "I intended to have come to Hanover this vacation, but at present I happen to be so much engaged in business that I can not without too great a sacrifice. I have lately performed several important operations which will require my attendance for a time."[34]

Smith had not completely cut his ties with Hanover: His family, all his property, his debts and his assets—including much of the scattered acreage his land speculation had brought him—all were still there. At least on some issues, however, he found it easy to decide in favor of Yale; he apparently had no qualms about taking with him some of the teaching materials he had accumulated originally for use at Dartmouth. He wrote to Silliman in March 1813:

[R]especting the Anatomical Museum and Library, I wrote [Cogswell] that I would furnish something toward a museum and that I had between five and six hundred vols. of books, chiefly medical, which should contribute to build up the intended Institution at New Haven.[35]

The question of ownership of these objects was settled in Smith's mind. He seems to have believed he had earned title to the museum specimens by fighting the battle of Alexander Ramsay (he had, it will be recalled, paid Ramsay's salary himself) and by dealing with local problems of finding subjects. He had spent a considerable amount of money on his library—some of it for nought, as his medical students often borrowed and failed to return (or stole) books paid for with his own money. As he complained in a letter to Shattuck,

Since you left this place, I have suffered a prodigious loss of books. On getting my library together since the close of last years course of lectures, we find that 22 no's of the *Medical and Physical Journal, Medical Museum and Medical Repository* are missing with about 20 volumes of other books. Have since brought my library into my own house and suffered no one to take a book without my knowledge.[36]

Smith frequently commented on adding books to his library, but it is rarely possible to tell whether he meant personal books—as when he mentioned (in another letter to Shattuck, several years later) adding fifty-two volumes "to my library of historical works"—or books purchased for the medical school library.[37] No one seems to have questioned his purchases, even when they were made with funds granted by the New Hampshire legislature (despite the fact that books were not specifically referred to in the legislative agreement).

Smith remained in Hanover during the summer of 1813. His family was still there, and his finances were in a precarious condition. Correspondence with Mills Olcott shows he maintained an ongoing interest in and concern with affairs in Hanover; severing ties was not easy. More upsetting than his financial situation, however, was the terrible meningitis epidemic that was increasing in severity, as the March letter to Silliman just quoted made clear:

[W]e were visited by a very fatal epidemic and instances of sickness and mortality became so frequent that I was afraid to leave my family in such perilous times; and my fears were not groundless,—four of my children have lately been visited by sickness.[38]

In 1816, Smith returned to Hanover when the Yale trustees allowed him to be re-appointed to teach at Dartmouth. But, as we have seen, Smith found the return to Hanover less congenial than he had expected, what with the ongoing political controversies in the College. Except for that one-term reprise in Hanover when Dartmouth rehired him, Smith was from 1813 until the end of his career identified as a professor at Yale.

The understanding with Yale after the fall term of 1816 was that Smith would thenceforth lecture there exclusively. (In 1821, however, the trustees relented and once again voted to allow Smith to lecture elsewhere; see chapters 12 and 13 for the stories at Bowdoin and the University of Vermont, respectively. Perhaps by that time they were more confident that their man would stay.) On April 22, 1817, the Board of Trustees voted for "hardship" an annual increase of four hundred dollars to Nathan Smith above the salary of the other professors to raise his income from the institution, for the year, to no more than $1,000. Only then, in a letter to the Board quoted in the Minutes of the Corporation, did Nathan Smith accept the offer and promise to move his family promptly to New Haven.[39] The pattern established when he moved to Hanover (without his family, at first) was repeated.

The tug between the two institutions continued, however. Yale, in increasing Smith's salary and refusing him permission to continue at Dartmouth, was firmly putting down its institutional foot. Dartmouth, on the other hand, would have liked to hold onto Smith. Wheelock had been replaced as president of the College by the Rev. Francis Brown, but the rift between those who wanted to preserve Dartmouth College and those who envisioned a Dartmouth University had not yet been settled. (Nor would it be, until the Dartmouth College Case had gone all the way to the United States Supreme Court. Daniel Webster's emotional plea to the Court in March of 1819 on behalf of the "small College" had carried the day; Dartmouth was not to become a university. The case was of national importance because the Court's decision made explicit that the state could not use its financial assistance to the College to override the property rights accorded it—by charter—as a private institution.[40]) President Brown had written to Smith in August 1817, saying he had hoped Smith "would find it consistent with your interest and your feelings to remain connected with us during the remainder of your useful life"—but he admitted that "a cloud still hangs over the College."[41]

One suspects Brown was not surprised, however much he may have been disappointed, to receive Smith's reply a week later, in which he resigned from Dartmouth for a second time: "[U]nder existing circumstances I think but to resign my office as professor in Dartmouth College. . . . I beg leave through you to request the Honorable Board of Trust for Dartmouth College to consider my office as vacant."[42]

Smith went on to say he had "several reasons for taking this resolution," but he may have been somewhat disingenuous when he insisted that the chief reason was the tangled web of controversy between the State and the College. This was, to be sure, a serious enough concern; as Smith indicated, he had been appointed by the Board of Trust for the *College*—whose authority the legislature had attempted to strike down. Until that matter was settled, it was legitimate for anyone to hesitate to teach under the auspices of the College, though Brown himself never wavered in carrying out his functions as president. What makes Smith's remarks seem less than forthright is his letter to Silliman the previous November.

The correspondence between Smith and Olcott gives ample evidence that even after he was settled at Yale, Nathan Smith was unable to separate himself wholly from Dartmouth business. "Since I left Hanover the affairs of Dartmouth College & University as well as the church difficulties have pressed considerably on my mind . . . ."[43] And in another letter to Mills Olcott he indicated that he was prepared to cooperate with Dartmouth folk: "I rec'd a letter from President Brown some time since in which he expressed a wish to hire my house & land the same as last year. I am willing he should have it & if in a letter to me you will give me a form of the lease I will execute one and send to him."[44]

Smith's interest in Dartmouth and her problems finally began to wane. In early 1822, he wrote to Mills Olcott in a rather different mood. "I perceive you have at length found a President for Dartmouth. . . . I do not know much about Colleges & take much less interest in them than I did. I do not think it can make such a mighty difference in the world as to who learn boys hic, hac [sic], hoc."[45]

By 1817, at the age of fifty-five, Smith was well settled into his life in New Haven. For the first time in his career, teaching was the focus of his professional activities. At Dartmouth his students had shared actively in the work of his practice, which loomed large in the way Nathan Smith spent his days. In New Haven his practice became secondary, and students were less likely to go with him on calls—though his reports of cases continued to serve as important examples for points he wanted to make in his lectures. The larger faculty at Yale and the resulting expanded curriculum allowed for more detail in each individual course. This is turn required a greater emphasis on pedagogy as such. Further, Smith's enthusiasm for academic instruction over and above what could be learned from a preceptorship gave a renewed urgency to his interest in formal medical education.

Though one imagines he must have felt overworked on occasion, Smith undertook to teach at two other medical schools for a brief period during his tenure at Yale; this is perhaps not altogether surprising, given his success as a teacher. But the tour de force could not last. Being pulled in three directions simultaneously was undeniably a strain. (Other professors of medicine would at times follow Smith's pattern of teaching concurrently at more than one institution, but rarely was anyone on three faculties at once.) We learn much about Smith's commitment to education and the esteem in which he was held from the fact that he was sought out by other institutions and apparently felt a responsibility to respond to such calls. Nathan Smith truly came into his own as a medical educator during his years at Yale.

He was busy in New Haven, and for the most part he was content. In the late spring of 1818, he confided to Olcott: "I have had rarther a busy winter in giving lectures examining & practice & tho not so profitable as I could have wished. The prospect however brightens a little at present."[46]

His mood shifted, perhaps not surprisingly, as local circumstances altered. A year later, as the struggle over legitimizing anatomy continued, he sputtered in a letter to Olcott: "I wish I had nothing to trouble me more than the cry of Joab about the dead. The souvereign Male the Legislature of Connecticut have a bill before thim [sic] which if it passes will put an end to our school in this place & will absolve me from my obligation to them, like the Christian of old if they persecute me in one city I shall flee to another."[47]

A month after that, he was still in a less-than-sanguine mood. Irked at some unspecified difficulty, he wrote to his old student Ezekiel Dodge Cushing: "Entre Nous I am not well satisfied with my situation and contemplate a removal but do not know yet whether it will be towards the North or South. Medical Science will never flourish in Connecticut; the soil is too dry."[48] But a few years later, he was writing rather more cheerfully once again. In mid-August of 1824, Smith recorded for George Shattuck his very real pleasure at how things were going in New Haven at that point in his career: "I have just located myself in the medical house which is fitted up in good style and makes a very commodious house for my family."[49] And in another sign of satisfaction with the situation at Yale, another three years after that, Smith wrote again to Shattuck to report proudly, "Our school [at Yale] flourishes . . . a class of 90 . . . better than any class previous."[50]

As mentioned earlier, much of what we know about Smith's Yale years can be inferred from the lecture notes taken by one or another of his students there. The record is, of course, frustratingly incomplete. How consistently Smith continued to inspire his students even after he was so much in demand that he was frequently absent from New Haven we do not know. That he was a very busy man we can tell from letters like one he wrote to Olcott explaining a change of plans. He had not gone to Hanover on that particular occasion, he said, because "our lectures had commenced at this place [Yale] before I left Burlington."[51] In other words, he was already behind schedule when the term started. Thus it would hardly have been surprising if his teaching had suffered as a consequence, but we have only rare documented criticisms of him as a teacher (leaving aside William Tully's distress over Smith's colloquial speech and too-casual manner). Earlier in 1823, Datus Williams wrote to Mason F. Cogswell reviewing his experience as a medical student at Yale:

[T]he Lectures of Professors Ives and Silliman have been all that one could wish Dr Knight's have been good but you have probably been informed that they were interrupted for 3 or 4 weeks in Dec. owing to some disturbance in N. York . . . .— & Dr Smith Lects. I will leave for you to draw your own conclusions . . . he spends I should guess about ten or eleven weeks with us . . . & has sought better quarters . . . I think if his chair was well filled . . . a better set of professors could not be found in the U. States.[52]

We do not know how many students reacted this way, but Smith was probably aware that his lectures did not meet the highest standards. On at least one occasion (five years before that, in 1818), he acknowledged as much in a letter to Spalding: "I have been very closely engaged in delivering my lectures on which I have been more full & particular than heretofore."[53] Williams's complaint came late in Smith's career; it is possible that—like many professors as they move toward retirement—Smith was no longer paying such scrupulous attention to his lectures. (Smith had passed his sixtieth birthday half a year before Williams wrote to Cogswell.) But that may not have been the whole story. Another student, Henry Ingersoll, had a good deal earlier (1811) jotted down in his notebook that "Doct. Smith by delivering his lectures extemporaneously is less methodical [than whom, is not specified] together with occasional repetition."[54]

Despite his busy life and the intense pace he typically kept up, Smith's health was remarkably good. One exception he noted in early March of 1825: "I have had a pretty hard winters work but have done very well till the last week when I was overtaken by the prevailing epidemic and though it has not stopped the career of my business it has made me pretty uncomfortable . . . ."[55]

That year was a signal one for Smith in a nonmedical way. In January of 1825, a committee of medical students in the Class of 1826 at Yale engaged Samuel F. B. Morse to paint Smith's portrait for $100; thanks to their initiative, we have a fine picture of what Nathan Smith the mature physician, respected surgeon, and distinguished professor looked like in his prime.[56] He continued to be busy and involved. When a group of Connecticut's medical men succeeded in their effort to establish a state hospital the next year, Smith was very much a part of the endeavor; his name came first in the list of incorporators.[57]

No one could have guessed that Nathan Smith would live less than three more years; when he died on January 26, 1829, he had turned sixty-six only a few months earlier. As Jonathan Knight said in his obituary oration, "Such as he has been for many years past, so useful, so honored and so beloved, we fondly hoped he might continue to be, for many succeeding years."[58] It was not to be. Nonetheless, it is probably fair to say—as one writer has—that the "first two decades of the Yale Medical School were dominated by him" (even though that period extends past Smith's death), and that it was "at Yale that Smith made his greatest contributions to surgery, as a teacher, practitioner, and politician."[59] One of Knight's summarizing comments underscores the point:

To this place [Yale] have resorted for many years past, from seventy to ninety young men; and it is no injustice to Dr. Smith's associates [of whom, of course, Knight was one] to say, that a principal object has been to learn from his wisdom and experience, the practical parts of their profession. Here, the sick and unfortunate, from every part of the country, have collected, to receive the benefit of his skill. In addition to his practice in the immediate vicinity, he has been called to visit, professionally, every county, and almost every town in this state, as well as many more distant places in the neighboring states.[60]

What he said about the "neighboring states" is certainly true. During his years in New Haven, Yale's professor of surgery became also a surgeon to all New England.

CHAPTER TWELVE

A Growing Reputation

[M]any are physicians by repute, very few are such in reality. He who is going truly to acquire an understanding of medicine must enjoy natural ability . . . . Moreover, he must apply diligence for a long period, in order that learning, becoming second nature, may reap a fine and abundant harvest.

— HIPPOCRATES [1]

The Medical School of Maine

BOWDOIN COLLEGE in Brunswick, Maine, was chartered in 1794 with a grant by James Bowdoin (1726–1790) of Boston and opened in 1802. Three years later, Parker Cleaveland (1780–1858) joined the faculty. A 1795 graduate of Harvard, he had concentrated his studies under Aaron Dexter. He added uncommon luster to the new school; he was as famous in chemistry and pharmacy as Benjamin Silliman at Yale, and the support his courses would give for a true medical department may well have been a factor in attracting Nathan Smith to Bowdoin. In any case, by 1821 events in Brunswick proved Maine had indeed been ripe for a medical school.[2]

Why Smith should have been interested in starting yet another medical school is unclear. One Bowdoin College historian has pointed out that two acts of the state legislature in 1821 were involved before the Medical School of Maine could come into being. The first was to increase the size of the college's board of trustees, making it "constitutionally eligible" for aid from the state; the second was to establish the medical school "in connection with the college, with an annual grant of $1,000 during the pleasure of the Legislature" (which turned out to be until 1834). We are told that nothing would have come of the project that "originated with President [William] Allen," unless he had "fortunately secured the services of the eminent Dr. Nathan Smith, of the Medical Department of Yale College, to inaugurate the enterprise."[3] A second chronicler of the college's

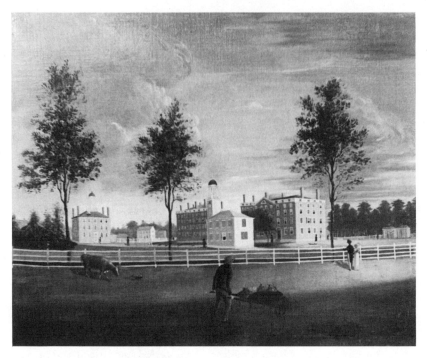

The medical building (far left) at Bowdoin, pictured in ca. 1822. Oil on canvas, by John G. Brown. Bowdoin College Museum of Art, Brunswick, Maine; gift of Mr. Harold L. Berry. Used by permission.

history echoed this, saying that as soon as Allen accepted the presidency he proposed to Nathan Smith that medical instruction should begin in Maine.[4] And yet another historian explicitly claimed that Bowdoin's success with the Maine legislature was "in no small part due to the fact that Nathan Smith had been previously consulted on the subject of being its head."[5]

One aspect of the proposal that might have appealed to Smith is that traveling to and from Maine would give Smith opportunities and excuses for long side trips to Hanover as well—at the time the idea was first broached, Sally had not yet moved to New Haven; he loved riding horseback in any case. Journeys of this sort also enabled him to make rounds, so to speak. He could usually travel in easy stages because he had former students and patients and friends in so many towns. In his correspondence Smith often mentioned or asked after people he had treated in a wide range of places. In addition, he was beginning to be called upon to consult or to operate in many places far from both New Haven and Hanover. Because his treatments were generally successful, it is easy to imagine that, for Smith, travels through New England were less an ordeal than a kind of triumphal progress, the exertions more likely to serve as medicinal tonic than to bring on exhaustion. Being known far and wide as an expert surgeon must have pleased him. (Recall the satisfaction with which he reported to Mills Olcott the praise he received in Massachusetts when his cataract couching cured former Governor Lincoln and the young Miss Paine.)

Besides, we know that Smith was restless, and for all his general contentment in New Haven, the unaccustomed and perhaps unexpected conservatism of Connecticut may have made him itch to get away at times. One wonders what Professor Silliman and President Dwight and others at Yale would have said or done if they had been privy—as they surely were not—to Smith's honest assessment of his Connecticut colleagues as expressed in a letter to Shattuck in 1818, five years after he had professed his new-found state of grace:

The people in this state [Connecticut] . . . are lower in point of knowledge and morals than they are in Mass. or N.H. or Vermont. I do not know what to attribute it to except it be a puritanic spirit of religion which I am convinced never warmed the heart of man with love towards his Creator or his fellow mortal. It is like the curst wind that blights everything that it touched being in itself the most illiberal kind of paganism. These remarks you must not expose out of your own family.[6]

(This, from the self-same Nathan Smith who had written to Mason F. Cogswell thus: "Respecting Dr. Dwight's former objections to me, I freely acknowledge that they were well founded and such as a wise and good man would always consider as all important. My earnest prayer now is to live to undo all the evil I have done by expressing my doubts as to the truth of Divine Revelation . . . ."[7])

Maine, on the other hand, only recently separated from Massachusetts, still had an air of independence about it that Smith probably found refreshing. At the end of 1819, he noted in a letter to Mills Olcott his pleasure at what was happening in Maine:

President Allen [the same son-in-law of John Wheelock who had been briefly president of Dartmouth University] is appointed president of Bowdin [sic] College which I am very much rejoiced to learn, as I think him well qualified for that office . . . . I think that the new State of Maine will retain something of the spirit of Old Massachusetts & will not suffer so important an Institution to languish for want of money.[8]

Smith seems here to be hinting that he thought he would be able, if called upon, to repeat his New Hampshire feat of getting a grant for the school from the state legislature. His optimism about state finances in Maine was in sharp contrast to his running complaints about his personal finances.

In another letter to Olcott just three weeks later, he was sputtering as usual about money problems: "The want of money in this region seems rather to increase and is so general that I find it next to impossible to collect the smallest debt. I however continue to charge the divils as usual . . . ."[9]

Quite apart from the support Smith anticipated in what he assumed would be an independently minded legislature, he was drawn to Maine by his philosophy of medical education. Rooted deep in his early experiences in Cornish was the firm belief that each state should have a medical school of its own, since it "does more toward ameliorating conditions of mankind than any other institution."[10] The key to why he would have supported so enthusiastically the founding of a medical school in Maine lies, perhaps, in this sentiment.

Bowdoin was not, however, without its money concerns. Several years before undertaking to establish a medical school, the trustees at Bowdoin had decided (in 1816) to try to persuade the state legislature to permit raising funds through a lottery. This is reminiscent of Nathan Smith's 1791 petition to the New Hampshire Legislature for a "Lottery in the value of £100, the proceeds to be devoted to purchasing a medical library for the instruction of medical students and practitioners . . . ,"[11] an effort that failed. (Nehemiah Cleaveland—a younger cousin of Parker Cleaveland and once a student of Smith's at Bowdoin—declaimed from a lofty seat on his moralistic high horse when he wrote his history of Bowdoin College: "This extravagant and iniquitous way of raising money was, at that period, often resorted to by literary and even by benevolent institutions."[12])

By 1820, however, the situation had improved. The Medical School of Maine was established on June 27 of that year, and the first series of lectures was given in the spring of 1821. The faculty comprised Nathan Smith, Parker Cleaveland, and John Doane Wells.[13] In early January of that year, Smith had announced to George Cheyne Shattuck his decision to go to Brunswick: "I have engaged to go to Bowdoin College and to deliver a course of lectures which will continue about ten weeks, for which I am to have $600." As usual, however, the challenge of finding the "subjects" necessary for teaching anatomy and surgery effectively was much on his mind, and—also as usual—he undertook to draw his young friend into the project:

President Allen has written me saying that there is a young physician in Boston by the name of Arnold who has had considerable experience in dissecting, and wishes me to consult him about going on with me, and to ascertain what compensation would satisfy him. It is not possible that his services will be wanted more than five or six weeks. Will thank you to feel of him on the subject, if you think he would be a suitable person, and learn his terms if he is inclined to go with me.

I have one more favor to ask of you, and that is to see if you can find some young man in Boston who would agree to furnish us with two or three subjects.

They could be sent to Portland and by Water. The college expects to pay the expenses and will be willing to give a reasonable compensation. Perhaps some young man who wants cash might be willing to furnish two or three. They will not be wanted until sometime in March.[14]

Getting Yale to release Smith for a teaching course was no small matter. That the effort might fail caused the Bowdoin trustees from the start to be ready to replace Smith at a moment's notice; it must have been an anxious time for them. Much though they wanted Smith, they also did not want to be left without an instructor. At the same meeting where it was voted that members of the senior class would be permitted "to attend the course of lectures on Anatomy and Surgery [to be given by Smith] by paying $10 for a ticket of admission, and that all who are minors must also obtain the permissions of their parents or guardians," Professor John Abbot was also authorized to proceed "to Boston to make enquiries for Dr. Smith." Should he ascertain that Dr. Smith would be unable to give the medical lectures at the college for the present season, he was to offer a sum of $550 to Dr. Nathan Noyes "to give 2 courses of lectures viz. on Anatomy and Surgery and on the Theory and Practice of Physic."[15]

Fortunately Smith was able to get away, though to do so entailed—by his own admission—squeezing things a bit at Yale. (Recall Datus Williams's letter of complaint to Cogswell.) Some weeks before that cautious action by the Bowdoin trustees, Smith wrote to Shattuck:

We have a good class of medical students in this institution [Yale], about sixty very reputable young men. I have pushed on my course of lectures with a view to my engagement at Bowdin. I am through the Theory and Practice and have advanced some ways in Surgery. I shall go to Brunswick by the way of Boston and will then see you. This will be the forepart of next month. I have performed many surgical operations the last year, and some of great importance. My success was very great as respects curing, and if my patients had been of the right sort [financially] my business would have been very good, but, alas . . . .[16]

Shortly after arriving in Brunswick to begin teaching, Smith wrote to Mills Olcott with satisfaction, "Our business in the College goes on very well. We have 30 students all good men & true." With money ever on his mind (at least, in correspondence with Olcott) he added, "That means those who pay well."[17] The happy prospect of income helps explain Smith's contentment at Bowdoin; another factor emerges comes from a letter he wrote just a couple of days later to Harvey Bissell of Suffield, Connecticut. Apropos his belief that President Allen was "very happily situated [at Bowdoin] much more so than he could have been at Dartmouth," Smith asserted that "Bowdoin College is not inlisted in any party either religious or political."[18] A year later, he wrote to Olcott cheerfully, "There is but one sentiment in the state regarding Bowdoin College and that is to built [sic] it up by every possible means."[19] To the extent this was true, it must have been a relief to Smith after the politics of Hanover and the religious fervor of New Haven, both of which had left him disenchanted.

The young John Doane Wells, hired to help Smith as an assistant dissector, had graduated from Harvard College in 1817 and received his Doctor of Medicine degree there in 1820.[20] His early career nicely exemplifies the kinds of connections between Smith and his students, and among Smith's students who later became colleagues: Wells had apprenticed in Boston with none other than George Shattuck. Then at Bowdoin, under Smith's watchful eye, he gained additional experience. A memorial tribute to Wells tells us:

In the course of the winter, the Professor [Smith] found it convenient frequently to call upon his assistant to take his place in the lecture room. This, Dr. Wells did with so much ability and so much to the satisfaction of all who heard him, that, in the following May, the Faculty at Brunswick appointed him Professor of Anatomy and Surgery, Dr. Smith having determined to resign as soon as [some]one could be found to fill his place.[21]

In fact Smith did not abandon Bowdoin that abruptly, as we shall see. But the role he played in bringing Wells along as a medical educator in his own mold is clear. In addition to assisting Smith (and having the opportunity to fill in for him), Wells imitated Smith in going abroad better to prepare himself for his teaching. In 1823 he was appointed physician to the Boston Dispensary for three years, and in 1826 he was unanimously elected professor of anatomy and physiology in the Berkshire Medical Institution. With Smith—juggling assignments at Yale and Bowdoin—as a role model, Wells doubtless saw no problem in accepting that appointment while continuing at Bowdoin; the lectures, after all, came at different seasons of the year. He was regarded—again in the words of the memorial tribute published shortly after his death at thirty-one (he obviously did not have Smith's stamina)—as the "pride, the ornament and the support, of the Brunswick Medical School."[22]

Not surprisingly, Smith found his assistant both well trained and a good teacher. He did not hesitate to praise Wells, clearly more concerned about the future of the school than about the possibility that Wells might usurp his position at Bowdoin: "Dr. Wells gives a very good course on Anatomy and is popular with the class. I think the school is now established,"[23] he wrote to Shattuck in April of 1823.

After his first session at Bowdoin, Smith was back teaching at Yale in the autumn of 1821. "I found a large class of medical students assembled at New Haven & have been able to keep up my usual number [of] lectures each week & to do a goodeal of profitable business," he wrote to Olcott that November. "Besides the operation today which amounts to 100.00 dollars I have operations enough engaged to come to another hundred, so that though I have been absent a long time [I] have not lost any business in this place."[24] He seems to be trying to justify his widespread travels to his business agent.

Who would hold exactly what title among those teaching at Bowdoin emerges somewhat confusingly from the record of votes taken by the trustees. On May 21, 1821—in other words, at the end of Smith's first term at Bowdoin—there is a record that, "Dr. Smith having resigned the Lectureship of anatomy," those present voted to choose a replacement: "On examination of the ballots it appears that Dr. John D. Wells of Boston is unanimously chosen." Yet on February 13, 1822 (and thus in time for the following spring's term), the record shows that it was "[v]oted in consequence of the absence of the [Professor of] Anatomy and Physiology [Wells] to proceed to the choice of a Lecturer . . . . On examination of the ballots it appears that Nathan Smith is unanimously chosen."[25] This latter vote, re-appointing Nathan Smith, was a response to Wells having gone to Europe.[26] Making Smith "lecturer" rather than "professor" may have been a way of appeasing Yale; it is quite possible that the officers of the University in New Haven wished their professor to hold that title only at Yale if he was going to teach elsewhere concurrently.

In any case, in the spring of 1822, Smith again taught at Bowdoin. After the term ended, he traveled farther than even he was accustomed to doing. Having been asked by a Mr. Bates—a wealthy inhabitant of Eastport, Maine—to make the trip of three hundred miles and charge what he would for the visit, he set off "Down East." He recounted the adventure for Parker Cleaveland in a long letter, after he had returned to Connecticut:

As you recollect I left Brunswick on monday about 11 o.c. & proceeded to Gardner where I staid there till 9 o.c. the next day, from thence went to Hallowell, called on Mr. [Charles] Vaughn, [an overseer of Bowdoin] & Dr. Allen [?] & reached Vasselborough that night. The next day [Wednesday] couched two eyes & lodged at Dixmont from thence reached Bangor by 11. o.c. [Thursday] A.M. The next day was there delayed till the next day [Friday] 9 o.c. A.M. on account of a patient who could not swallow. From Bangor I proceeded to Machias without interruption, engaged some business on my return. Set out on monday morning from Machias to Eastport in a boat. Reached Eastport the same day in the evening.
Found Mr. Bates' case to be a paralysis of the lower extremities; he is gaining a little from the use of Nux-Vomica [a bitter tonic and central-nervous-system stimulant]. I have seen many other patients. Last Wednesday I went to Deer Island to operate on a young man for a stone in the bladder. The operation was performed & a stone weight about 8 ounces extracted. I say about eight ounces because the stone being broken into fragments & very much comminuted could not all be collected. The patient we consider is out of danger. The people have all agreed that Mr. Bates shall be charged 500. dollars. I shall probably set out for home on thursday next & be about a week on my way. . . . I am the tempest tossed & much enduring man.[27]

Smith returned to Bowdoin several times; he lectured on the theory and practice of physic, as well as on both surgery and anatomy. His association with Bowdoin lasted five years.[28] Obviously pleased with his accomplishments there, he boasted to Mills Olcott in the early spring of 1823: "The medical school in this place [Brunswick] is pretty well anchored. We have the best anatomical museum and the best library to be found in New England and a fine class of students, I think in point of learning & talent the best I have seen together."[29] This was not the only time Smith announced that the best medical students he had ever met were at Bowdoin. In a letter written two months later, he made much the same claim: "We have a class of 51 medical students [at Bowdoin] among whom there is not an idler or a dissipated character. Upon the whole I have never seen so fine a class of medical students together."[30] Perhaps the group in the spring term of 1823 really was an extraordinary set of would-be physicians. In any case Smith seems to have believed, at least in the midst of his experience with those particular Bowdoin students, that Maine boys would make unusually good doctors.

Though the names of Smith's students from those years do not today leap off the page as figures famous for their accomplishments, still Smith would have had reason, looking back, to be pleased. Two thirds or more of the medical graduates in 1823 and 1824 served small New England towns (many of them in Maine) as physicians; several later taught at medical schools elsewhere. Malthus Ward, whom we met as a student at Dartmouth years earlier, became professor of natural history at the University of Georgia; John Bell became professor of anatomy and physiology at the University of Vermont; a striking number went on to become members of the state legislature in Maine or New Hampshire. One such, Ezra Carter, also served a term as president of the New Hampshire Medical Society.[31]

In addition to the kind of praise Smith typically gave the Medical School of Maine in letters, he performed many services for Bowdoin; one, oddly enough, seems to have been inspecting a possible new fire engine for the college (perhaps as a matter of public health and safety). A great fire on March 4, 1822, had gutted Maine Hall, a dormitory built in 1808. Although the conflagration did not affect the medical school as such, it alerted the college authorities to the risk of fire. The prompt and effective public campaign to raise money to repair the damage impressed Smith, perhaps a factor in his willingness to help assess the merits of purchasing a particular fire engine:

I have visited the Society [of Shakers] at Canterbury [New Hampshire] and saw an Engine for extinguishing fire which I thought a very good one. Was informed that it would throw the water 70 feet farther than the best engine at Concord which cost over 400 dollars. This engine was made by the Shakers and they informed me that they could make another on the same plan & size for 300 Dollars. If the College should conclude to get an Engine, I think it would be best to engage the Shakes to make it. . . . [Y]ou may depend on its being faithfully made in every part of it.[32]

Perhaps it is not surprising that Yale eventually grew impatient with its perambulating professor of medicine. Less than two years after having explicitly voted Nathan Smith permission to lecture elsewhere (in September 1823—the same meeting at which the Yale trustees formally defined the laws and rules of the Medical Institute), the corporation insisted that he focus more of his attention on Yale. Smith formally resigned from Bowdoin, this time for good. How genuine his regret was, we do not know. In July 1825, Smith wrote to Bowdoin's President Allen as follows: "Since my return to New-Haven I find my fellow professors & and the good people generally so much opposed to my going abroad to lecture any more, that I have concluded to give up my connection with Bowdoin College. . . . I shall always cherish the recollection of the pleasant days."[33]

Nearly a year later, correspondence with Cleaveland shows Smith had by no means stopped being concerned about a wide range of issues connected with the medical school in Brunswick. One matter of some urgency was finding someone to replace Smith himself on the faculty:

Respecting a Professor of Theory and Practice [of Medicine] I have not been able to find one with which I am satisfied and who would be likely to accept the appointment. . . .

There is a Dr. Harry Bond of Philadelphia who was educated at Hanover while I was there [A.B. 1813, M.D. 1817] and afterwards practiced in Concord, N.H. from whence he went to Philadelphia where he has given private lectures I believe in Anatomy. Dr. Bond was a very excellent schollar and did himself great credit in his examinations and from a letter I once received from him on his hearing I was [considering] going to Brunswick I thought he would have then liked an appointment in Bowdoin College but how he is now situated I do not know. If he could be obtained, I should think he would do better for you than Mussey & Mussey would do better than Childs.[34]

Smith also advised in the same letter on administrative matters, the most important being the pitfalls in the usual manner of medical school financing:

It is generally better for all concerned to have the notes [students typically paid in promissory notes rather than cash] settled in a reasonable time. Besides, if you grant too much indulgence it becomes a kind of law and when you depart from it will give more offense than it would if you had begun right at first. This was exemplified last fall at the medical school at Castleton, Vt.

They had formerly, to get great numbers, taken notes without interest or indorsers, payable in four years. Then last fall they demanded pay down or notes indorsed and the class [lost] 20 [who] left and their professors were obliged to comply with their former terms or have no class.

The Vermont Medical Academy in Castleton, where Smith's former student Theodore Woodward[35] was registrar and taught surgery, had had even more financial trouble than Dartmouth; Smith was eager that Bowdoin should avoid the folly of accepting unsecured notes for tuition. This concern may have had to do with his characteristic worry about the effect of any new undertaking on his own finances. He tried to make clear to Cleaveland that he could not go on teaching at Bowdoin if doing so would require him to make further monetary sacrifices.

Whatever was going to be done about finances, however, Smith ended his letter to Parker Cleaveland on a note of general solicitude and personal friendliness, with a promise to do anything he could to help.[36]

Back to Yale

One Bowdoin College historian wrote that "Dr. Smith's connection with the school was severed in 1825, when his duties in New Haven had become such as to forbid his absence."[37] Certainly evidence can be found that Smith had no desire to alienate those in charge at Yale. Already in the early days, when he went back to Hanover to be with his family after teaching one term at Yale, he had written to Silliman—both to apprise him of the continuing financial difficulties he labored under and to assure him he would not renege on his commitment to Yale, regardless of what those at Dartmouth who wanted him back should offer:

I can simply imagine how the report came, that I should not remove my family to New Haven. The people in this place have indicated that idea [and] have taken all honest means to prevent it. . . . I found they were taking measures to effect that object by liberal offers of a pecuniary nature but I have not changed my plans. I have to[o] much regard for my honor to retrograde in a business which I have begun with so much success. I will not however conceal from you my real situation. I have not personal property sufficient to pay all my debts here & remove to N. Haven.[38]

Mortgaging his property helped on the economic front, and in the end Yale was very good to Smith in a number of ways. No doubt that fact, as much as the press of "duties," played a part in his decision to cease dividing his energies between Bowdoin and Yale. There may have been other reasons, as well. We know he continued to be plagued by financial problems despite all Yale had done; if the extra teaching at Bowdoin was not proving to be economically advantageous, that would likely also have influenced him. In the spring of 1826, after severing his formal ties with Bowdoin, Smith wrote Shattuck a letter that indicates his earnings there were relatively modest and that he was months overdue in being paid:

In my letter to you last winter respecting my dues at Bowdoin College I made a mistake of $200, which leaves me but $400 due there, and from a letter I received from Mr. Cleaveland some time since I fear there will be more delay about paying that than I had expected. I have written to [him] stating that I should expect the notes to be put in suit immediately or that the Board approve the debt and pay me the money. The notes are given to the faculty of the college. What they will do about it I do not know. Be that as it may I can pay the money to you if necessary about or not long after the time proposed.[39]

In any case, two months after Smith had written to Allen announcing his intent "to give up my connection with Bowdoin," at a meeting of the Faculty of Medicine of Bowdoin College in September 1825, it was "[v]oted that Nathan Noyes be appointed Lecturer on the Theory and Practice of Physic in the Medical School of Maine in the place of Nathan Smith M.D. who resigned."[40] Noyes declined, however, and Henry H. Childs was appointed in his stead. Childs, it will be recalled, was one of those recommended to Cleaveland by Smith initially, albeit as his third choice.

Later, his second choice—Reuben D. Mussey, Smith's protégé who had succeeded him at Dartmouth—followed in his footsteps at Bowdoin, too. In October of 1830, Mussey wrote to Parker Cleaveland from Hanover to "accept the appointment of Lecturer on Anatomy & Surgery for the next course in your Institution." He went on, raising several questions, among them a perennial one that would have been familiar to Smith (though the presumption with which Mussey ends his communication makes him seem more optimistic than Smith had usually been): "How many subjects have you usually had at each course & are they already provided? If not, I shall presume that you will be able to have them in readiness in season . . . ."[41] In this manner Nathan Smith's influence on the Medical School of Maine continued, even after his departure from Bowdoin and his death.

Smith had no grounds for misgivings about Bowdoin, either during his official association with the institution or later. As we have seen, he himself more than once acknowledged that the school was well established. Moreover, with Parker Cleaveland and John Wells on the faculty, there was reason to be confident about the institution's future. (In fact, the school continued to serve Maine for more than a century, until 1936—not a bad run for a small country medical school.)

Yale's refusal to permit Smith to continue at Bowdoin, which he re-iterated in a letter to Parker Cleaveland in late August 1826,[42] had indirect advantages for Smith. In a letter to Shattuck earlier that year, he admitted that business was looking up in New Haven, probably at least in part as a consequence of his not hurrying away to Brunswick. "Since I made my determination not to go abroad any more to give lectures my business in this city has increased and is increasing. I have had a good deal of surgery this winter, a part of which was [performed] before the class."[43]

Smith's departure from Bowdoin did nothing to diminish anyone's sense of his importance. Just how considerable that was understood to be is clear from the resolution drawn up at the time of Smith's death by a committee that consisted of Wells and Cleaveland:

> Whereas the Medical School of Maine from its Commencement in 1821 for 5 successive years enjoyed the instructions and profited by the force of the late Pro. Smith who was highly distinguished in this profession and who by years of arduous exertion and by possession of rich stores of experience had peculiarly qualified for the duties of Medical Instructor and whereas it has pleased Divine Providence to remove this individual from life, the Medical Faculty of this College in justice to the offices they hold as well as to their own feelings would pay the tribute of high respect for his character and grateful recollections for his professional services; therefore:
>
> Resolved that the Faculty deeply sympathize with the Profession in the loss of a public benefactor whose reputation as a lecturer, a skillful surgeon, and a successful physician, distinguished by accuracy of opinion, clearness of judgment, and benevolence of feeling are universally acknowledged and that they will ever cherish the memory of one who has contributed so much to the improvement of Medical education and the advancement of Medical science.[44]

Thus did another New England state retrospectively acknowledge its debt to Nathan Smith.

During the early 1820s Maine had not, however, been alone in luring Smith from Connecticut. Before Yale finally restricted his teaching to New Haven, he had also been persuaded to take his teaching skills to Vermont.

CHAPTER THIRTEEN

Surgeon to New England

❧

The very high reputation universally accorded to Dr. Smith at that period, not only in New Hampshire but throughout New England—perhaps a reputation never before so generally awarded to any member of the profession in this part of our Country—had inspired me with a respect;—almost with awe—for one so distinguished.   —A. T. LOWE [1]

To JUDGE FROM the insistence of the Yale trustees that Smith resign his position at Bowdoin, there was perhaps some anxiety that the public would be confused about Smith's academic loyalties. For students, this was less of a problem; they often followed a professor from one institution to another. A case in point, indicating that Nathan Smith's reputation could draw students from all across New England, is Edward H. Leffingwell.

We know Leffingwell was a student of Smith's at Yale; after earning his A.B. degree there in 1822, he went on to earn a Yale M.D. two years later. Furthermore, the ticket issued to him by Nathan Smith and admitting him to the "Lectures on the Theory & Practice of Physic Surgery & Midwifery" at Yale, in 1823, can still be seen today.[2] Then there is a letter Smith wrote to Edward's father, William Leffingwell, Esq., from Brunswick in May of 1823, touting the benefits of the medical instruction being offered at Bowdoin at the time.[3] For all we know this is what tipped the scales in favor of Edward's spending time at Bowdoin as well; in any case, his name appears in the official Bowdoin records as a nongraduate in the class of 1825.[4] Another ticket admitted the same young man to Smith's lectures "commencing September 10th, 1823 at the University of Vermont,"[5] where Smith was also teaching at the time even while he continued as a member of the Yale faculty. Although Leffingwell's name does not appear on the rolls at Burlington, given that he was sufficiently eager (ambitious?) to attend Smith's lectures at Bowdoin after he had already earned his M.D. at

University of Vermont.

LECTURES

ON

Theory and Practice of Physic and Surgery,

BY

NATHAN SMITH, M. D.

ADMIT *Mr. Edward H. Leffingwell*

TO THE COURSE COMMENCING *10th September, 1823.*

Burlington, *Nathan Smith*

Edward H. Leffingwell's admission ticket, University of Vermont, 1823. Courtesy of Yale University, Harvey Cushing/John Hay Whitney Medical Library.

Yale, he may indeed have followed his mentor to Burlington as well. Of course there are other explanations for the UVM ticket; Smith may have been so busy as to be periodically confused about which students were planning to follow him where. In any case, Leffingwell was clearly among those who attended Smith's lectures in at least two medical schools.

This was by no means unique or even particularly unusual. With the short course terms, it was fairly common for professors to lecture at more than one institution. Most students were required to attend a minimum of two courses of lectures before they could earn their degrees, and following their own professor to his next assignment meant finishing sooner (and was no doubt easier because the very lectures would already have been heard). Even when students were not required to take a second course, many professors recommended that they do so. Lyman Spalding, in his inaugural address as the first president of the College of Physicians and Surgeons in Fairfield, New York, had made a point of saying that students should not limit themselves to a single course: "[N]o man, without having attended several courses of lectures, thinks his medical education complete."[6]

Educational Advisor

Meanwhile, Smith's growing reputation turned him into a perambulating pedagogue throughout New England. Maine was not the only state beyond New Hampshire and Connecticut in which Nathan Smith's assistance in improving medical education seemed desirable. In Burlington,

Vermont, plans for yet another medical school had been brewing for some time. Nathan Smith's advice was sought.

Vermont, to be sure, had had a small medical school: the Vermont Academy of Medicine, in Castleton. This was the institution with which Jo Gallup and Theodore Woodward, among others, were associated, as mentioned earlier. But efforts had been underway for some time to start a medical school in Burlington, where the University of Vermont (UVM) and the State Agricultural College had been established in 1791. The driving force behind the effort was Dr. John Pomeroy.[7]

Already in 1804, Pomeroy had been elected to serve as the whole faculty of a medical department or medical school, such as it was. He seems to have been actively engaged in teaching a number of apprentices who gathered in Burlington to study under him, just as Smith's apprentices had gone with him to Hanover when he first gave lectures there; thus there were parallels between the origins of the medical schools at Vermont and at Dartmouth.

From 1814 on, increasing efforts were made by the Vermont trustees to strengthen the teaching of medicine at their university; Pomeroy was not in fact holding forth on the UVM campus itself, and to that extent it was difficult to claim the university had a medical department (let alone a medical school). Pomeroy apparently met and exchanged professional opinions with Smith as part of the process of trying to organize matters in Burlington.[8] But regardless of whether Pomeroy was interested primarily in the benefits he knew would accrue from having a man of Nathan Smith's reputation associated with the school, or whether he simply made the very practical calculation that Nathan Smith was the most experienced man around, the two men clearly shared the view that attaching a medical school to an academic institution was good strategy. They seem also to have agreed about the importance of establishing such a school with an eye to training physicians who would serve the surrounding rural area.[9]

Significant differences existed between the school in Hanover and the one in Burlington, however. For starters, Pomeroy could lean on Smith for advice, as he apparently did. Secondly, although the idea for a school and the first students in Burlington were Pomeroy's, unless one counts the years before the school in Burlington was fully organized, he himself was never the sole member of the medical faculty. In 1804, for example, Pomeroy was appointed lecturer in anatomy and "chirurgy" (surgery), and in 1809 professor of physic and surgery. Indeed, at various times he held chairs of physiology, anatomy, and surgery—but the "faculty appointments which Pomeroy held were all without remuneration as far as the students and the University were concerned." Thus although Pomeroy was certainly "among the founders of the medical school at Burlington," he was, in those early years, teaching in the university rather than in anything formally designated as a medical school or a medical department. Furthermore, others (John LeConte Cazier, Jairus Kennan, and Pomeroy's own son) were soon also part of the informal medical faculty, another way in which the Burlington story was rather different from that in Hanover.[10]

But on March 21, 1821 (just when the Maine Medical School was taking shape in Brunswick) the University of Vermont trustees took a crucial vote, that "a Com^tee of two be appointed to confer with the Medical Gentlemen in Town, on the subject of delivering Lectures in the College." On the following day, the committee duly reported, and the appointments were made. John Pomeroy was to be a member of the "Prudential Committee," and the new school's professors were named as follows: William Paddock for theory and practice and for materia medica, Arthur L. Porter for chemistry and pharmacopoeia, and Nathan Ryno Smith—the son, not (as one might have expected) Nathan Smith the father—for anatomy and physiology.[11] Ryno had begun to practice medicine in Burlington, where he had settled;[12] thus appointing the young man to the faculty made more sense than trying to persuade his father to accept yet another professorship. This proved a very satisfactory arrangement (and one we can imagine would give a proud father considerable pleasure).

Nathan Smith was not, however, left entirely out of the picture. Appointed "Lecturer" (just as he had been at Bowdoin, and perhaps for similar reasons), he lectured at the University of Vermont on several different occasions from 1822 to 1825.[13] Letters make clear that he spent a fair amount of time in Burlington, and that at least part of the family was with him during some of those periods. In September 1822, for instance, Smith referred to his wife and son in a letter written to Mills Olcott from Burlington: "Mrs. Smith and Morven will leave for Hanover some time this week"; in mid-July of 1824, Smith wrote to Olcott from New Haven, indicating he had just returned from Burlington—but not by way of Hanover, as he usually did, because of "Mrs. Smith's illness."[14]

Once the University of Vermont not only had a medical school but could boast of having the Smiths, père et fils, on the faculty, Pomeroy had reason to consider his efforts a success. Though the initial appointments do not include Pomeroy among the faculty members, by 1822–23 he seems to have held the chair of surgery in the new school, and he surely has to count as a principal figure among the founders. Nathan Smith did not work alone to bring formal medical education to Burlington, and his relation to the university there was neither so extensive nor so clearly defined as his affiliation with Bowdoin had been. But he played an undeniably important role, not least in helping to put the medical school on a secure footing.[15] One writer, while insisting it is not clear why anyone would claim that Smith "founded with the aid of his son the medical school at the University of Vermont" and that "we are not willing to accept either Smith as the founder of our medical college," nonetheless gives Nathan Smith his due. "It would appear," we are told,

that the elder Smith's influence and enormous prestige were back of the school from an early date and certainly played a great role in the final decision to organize the school. His presence on the campus certainly coincided with the period of greatest prosperity of the enterprise.[16]

From the outset, Smith was well satisfied. Early on, he wrote to Olcott from Burlington: "Our Medical School flourishes well—so far we have a class of 24 all good and true men which is a greater number than any other medical school in the United States has commenced with." The proprietary tone extended to praise of at least one of his colleagues as well: "Dr. [Arthur L.] Porter succeeds well in his lectures and gives great satisfaction to those who attend . . . ."[17]

Smith was also pleased with the physical arrangements. Even his recent enthusiasm for the rapidity with which Bowdoin rebuilt after its fire[18] did not overshadow his pleasure at what he found at UVM: "Burlington has one advantage over the others & that is good rooms & accommodations for medical purposes . . . . [The] College too will soon be in funds sufficient to aid the school."[19] This concern with the physical arrangements was typical; from the time before building the New Medical House at Hanover, Smith was always interested in the accommodations he might arrange for his school and his family. Two years later, in 1824, he was exulting to Mills Olcott, with characteristic dry humor, about the new situation at Yale:

I am going into the medical house in a fortnight which is fitting up in a splendid manner. The lecture rooms are cut off from the rest of the house so that the students do not come in contact or in sight of the part which is occupied by the family. The appearance of the house is quite splindid & unites as many conveniences for a family as any house in the city. I have the use free from rent during my professorship, on the condition that I keep off ghosts, witches and such imaginary beings all of which I have covenanted to do being considered here as the master of magicians.[20]

Apart from lecturing at the institution, Nathan Smith contributed to UVM indirectly. Having his name associated with it added to its stature. Furthermore, in addition to having supported Pomeroy's idea of affiliating with the university, Smith helped secure a grant from the Vermont legislature. Early in 1823, he wrote to Mills Olcott, enlisting his aid for the forthcoming struggle with the Vermont legislature:

We are making every adept to build up the College & Medical School at Burlington & so far the prospect is quite flattering. But there is one thing must be effected
& that is the patronage of the state & we wish to engage you in the case and must
request you to write a speech for us to make before the legislature next autumn. I
shall see you before that time & we must plan the attack so as to enter the weak-
est side. I have a long string of reasons why the medical school of the state should
be located at Burlington in preference to any other place. You know I have been
rather successful with Legislatures & therefore shall not be easily discouraged.[21]

Smith was not being immodest; he had indeed by this time become an
old hand at persuading officials on the state level that they should support
local medical education. He was quite conscious of his past successes, as
well as of the burden he was assuming once again. Two months later, in
March of 1823, he wrote to Olcott again in this vein:

The next thing which I wish to effect is to place the medical school at Burlington
on as good a foundation as [Bowdoin] is. To do this the Legislature of Vermont
must be pressed into service. You know I have seen a little service of this sort &
am not quite a novice in the management of petitions to the Honble members of
the court, though a year ago I did not think of engaging again in a campaign of
that sort. But you know it is not in many to direct his own steps. However irk-
some this kind of service may be where we are obliged to come in on our marrow
bones before the Honble Legislature it is not quite so bad as to stand candidate for
Governor which I shall always decline.[22]

Despite what would seem to many like an unmanageably busy life, filled
among other things with responsibilities for three medical schools in three
different states, Smith had not lost his sense of humor. Most of the time he
was drawn in too many directions to give the guidance and support to his
colleagues that he might have desired; the distractions were often personal or financial. The previous autumn (October 1822) he had written
Olcott from Burlington in some frustration, saying "I am so scattered that
13 moons must pass and worse before I can collect all the fragments [of
real estate] at Hanover . . . ."[23]

A letter from Nathan Smith to George Shattuck in early 1823 indicated
that Smith thought he was through establishing medical schools: "I think
the four schools which I have been concerned in bringing forward will in
addition [to Harvard] be as much as New England will bear and I think
these will not be too many. Any State should have one medical [school]
and no more."[24]

Toward the end of 1824, Smith wrote Shattuck soberly, "I have agreed
to go to Burlington for six weeks which will be the last time probably that
I shall leave New Haven for the purpose of lecturing in any other place."[25]
With that, Smith's direct participation in the UVM medical school ended.
As we have seen, however, he was involved in Burlington during a period
of critical importance to the school.[26]

We do not know how much attention Smith paid to the institutions in Burlington and Brunswick between 1825, when his official affiliations ended, and his death in 1829. Both schools would go through trying times in the next generation, struggling with many changes in medical education. But the Medical School of Maine closed only after a century of training doctors, and UVM still has its medical school today, as do Dartmouth and Yale. These successes warrant calling Smith one of the all-time great founders of institutions for medical education.

Expert Witness

Much of Smith's current reputation rests on his far-flung efforts to improve medical education; in his day he was known for other kinds of expertise as well. As revealing of Smith's character and talents as anything was his success in medico-legal work. He was called in for the defense in at least one murder case, and he helped resolve a difficult battle over the supposed malpractice of two Maine physicians.

The medico-legal case we know Smith was involved in occurred during his early years at Dartmouth, when he alone constituted its medical faculty. His reputation was enhanced when he attacked local physicians for arousing the countryside with their pseudo-scientific investigation of a case of sudden death in Alstead, New Hampshire (nearly sixty miles from Hanover, but only three miles from Walpole, where Smith's mother then lived).[27]

The dead man's friends asked Smith to look into the cause of death. His careful and precise analysis simply exploded the case, the bare facts of which are as follows: In September 1806, Benjamin Fay of Alstead died and was buried. When rumors arose that Fay had been poisoned by his step-mother,[28] Mrs. Margery Fay, she was arrested, and Fay's body was exhumed for examination. Most of the physicians on hand were convinced that Mr. Fay had been poisoned, and they quickly found evidence —so they said—to support their assumptions: The body was found swollen; the pit of the stomach was "mortified"; and the contents of the stomach, which tarnished a knife blade when boiled, revealed a metal all resembling arsenic.[29] Thus the charges against Mrs. Fay, which had begun in gossip, were significantly strengthened by the judgment of the local physicians. Mrs. Fay was bound over for trial.

Smith, unconvinced by the findings of the local physicians, investigated—and promptly wrote a defense for Mrs. Fay. He pointed out that for people truly acquainted with the effects of arsenic, nothing more than a recital of their opinions was required to expose the "ignorance and folly of the physicians." But "as the assertions of medical men frequently obtain more credence than comported with the good of society," he wished to make a few observations of his own:

That Mr. B. Fay died by poison seems to have been inferred from the suddenness of his death, tho' there was not one circumstance which could induce that belief . . . . He died in an apoplectic state without any evacuations . . . convulsions, pain or distress, being perfectly insensible from the moment he was discovered to be indisposed, till he expired. Compare this with the effects of arsenic . . . which are, as stated by the best authorities, nausea, vomiting, purging, hickuping, violent pains in the stomach, convulsions, twitching of the tendons, increased flow of saliva, . . . asphyxia, syncope and death . . . . That a body, eleven days after it was committed to the earth, should swell and turn a livid color, should surprise none but learned physicians all other persons knowing it to be the course of nature.—But as to the substance found on the pit of the stomach . . . we should have called on the learned gentlemen to shew how it could have found its way through the integuments of the body, and, like a night-mare, have couched itself upon the pit of the stomach; but the substance being produced in open court was found . . . to be a small scab, the most trifling thing in the world.—The next object of their invetigation was the contents of the stomach . . . . They first heated a quantity of it boiling hot, and then put several polished metals into it, which being tarnished, they inferred it contained arsenic. [I]t should be noticed that the contents of the stomach were principally apples, bread and milk. Every one knows that the acid of apples will tarnish metals.—The last experiment . . . was a kind of firey ordeal. They took a quart of the contents of the stomach . . . and subjected it to a red hot heat for the space of three hours. The result . . . was a metallic substance in the bottom of the vessel; but [if it had been arsenic, which is of a volatile nature] it would have been dissipated, with that degree of heat, in less than one fourth part of the time. Thus from causes so slight, being magnified by the ignorance, I had almost said fatuity, of some of the learned faculty, and the credulity of others, the whole country was alarmed with the report of a most horrid murder . . . . But when [the report was] examined by the touch-stone of legal evidence, vanished like a scroll[?], leaving not the least shadow of reason to believe, or even suspect, that the man died by poison. This case will shew how careful judges and persons ought to be, when life and character are at stake, in giving credit to the reports and testimony of gentlemen of the faculty, at least in matters of opinion depending on their professional knowledge.[30]

This direct attack on the competence of the local medical men appeared in the newspaper for all to read, with Smith's name appended. In a letter to Lyman Spalding a week later, Smith explained the circumstances surrounding the publication of his statement:

Perhaps you may if you [still] take one of the Walpole Papers [Spalding had practiced there earlier] observe a publication respecting the death of Benj. Fay, of Alstead, who was supposed to be poisoned. The piece signed by my name I wrote at the request of the friends of the deceased, but did not put my name to it, but sent it to them to do as they pleased as to publishing it. They, either ignorantly or willfully, mistook my intention as respects signing my name and put it to the piece.
You will perceive that some of the learned Faculty are pretty severely lashed.

What effect it will have or how they will behave toward me, I do not know, nor do I much care, being confident that they merited the whole of what they have received, and more also, as you will see by the history of their conduct.[31]

We can only guess that Smith may not have been altogether averse to having his views—including his unbridled contempt for incompetent medical men—made public.[32]

A second murder case in which Smith is said to have been involved occurred years later, in 1823. It had several similar features: enraged citizens, doubtful guilt, and the defense of a man who—if not as guiltless as Mrs. Fay—at least had not committed premeditated murder. The scene was Samuel Coombs's blacksmith's shop, in Portland, Maine. When a customer, Patrick Cole, complained about service rendered by Coombs, "A high dispute soon arose with violent and irritating language [and the two men] agreed to fight," according to the newspaper account. Each of the adversaries grabbed the other's collar with the left hand and struck blows with the right; in the end, Coombs lay dead. "The testimony of the surgeon, who examined the body, was, that the death was caused by strangulation"—again according to the news report. No indication is given that Smith was the surgeon in question, nor—although he was teaching at the time at Bowdoin and might have been called in as an expert witness—has any evidence been found that he testified at the trial. The only reason for thinking Smith participated in the case is a letter he wrote to George Shattuck from Brunswick saying that he was going to Portland, where he expected to be "detained . . . the whole week, as a witness in a case of a late murder."[33]

Despite testimony from defense counsel that Coombs might inadvertently have tightened his own cravat, Cole was found guilty and was sentenced to "three month solitary confinement and four years hard labor."[34]

A year earlier another Maine case began in which we know for certain Nathan Smith was called to give expert testimony; this was a considerably more complicated case of much greater medical importance.[35] Interest was high and widespread for several reasons. In addition to complex and unusual issues, there was the spectacle of the Harvard faculty pitted against the Bowdoin medical faculty (in the person of Smith) and the splenetic rodomontade of the plaintiff, Charles Lowell, who traveled about the countryside limping pitifully and swearing vigorously at "those doctors."

The time was June of 1822; the place was Washington County, Maine. Lowell, from Lubec, Maine, had fallen from his horse—a common enough source of injury. But in this case, the horse landed on top of the rider in such a fashion as to dislocate his hip. Or so he thought. The local doctor, John Faxon, had been called, and he had asked the help of a nearby surgeon, Dr. Micajah Hawkes. Neither had ever reduced a dislocated hip; a measure of their inexperience was that, when they had done their work, they asked whether the bystanders thought the reduction complete.

Two weeks after the accident and contrary to medical advice, Lowell got out of bed and walked 150 rods or more. He soon found that the hip was lame, painful, and getting worse. He went to Boston, where he told a story that enlisted the sympathies of John Collins Warren at the new Massachusetts General Hospital. Warren thought the hip in poor shape and used pulleys and all the arts of tobacco and antimony (presumably as muscle relaxants or antispasmodics) to weaken the hip into submission, but without effect.[36] In June 1822, Lowell sued Faxon and Hawkes, and the trial court awarded him damages amounting to $1,962.[37]

The defendants appealed; in response the plaintiff brought in Nathan Smith as his expert witness. Once Smith had examined Lowell, however —stripping him, measuring him, and watching him walk (witnesses to the examination later testified it was "done thoroughly and deliberately"[38]), he decided to support the defense. For Smith had concluded that a fracture was involved, not a dislocation, and that the doctors had done as well as they could have (it is unclear why he thought they were not remiss for their failure to diagnose the fracture).

Rivalries between the hometowns of the major players in the case— Eastport and Lubec—did not help matters. The opinionated jury in the second trial (September 1822) was unable to agree and was accordingly discharged. Newspaper accounts aroused popular interest; the case gained in notoriety. A third trial before Justice Nathan Weston nearly two years later was a more rational affair all around. An impartial jury (no residents of either Eastport or Lubec were selected this time) and first-rate attorneys helped. Nathan Smith testified, for the defense, in part as follows:

I examined Charles Lowell. . . . My examination was lengthy and critical, and my opinion then was, that the thigh bone was not out of joint; and I have not altered my opinion since. From the nature of the injury as described to me by said Lowell, it could hardly be possible that the hip should be dislocated. A fall on the hip, with the weight of a horse upon it, would be likely to break the bones of the pelvis, and might drive the head of the bone through the bottom of the socket, but could not dislocate the joint; and, in my opinion, if there is any derangement of the bones, it is a fracture, and not a dislocation. In that case, it would not have been in the power of [the defendants] or any other medical man to have rendered the said Lowell any effectual assistance, more than to have administered remedies to keep down inflammation; they could not have altered the situation of the bones.
    . . . I do not think that the mechanical powers, such as the wheel and axles, or the pullies, are necessary to reduce a dislocated hip, or any other dislocation. They have sometimes been used with effect, but they have oftener been injurious; and what can be effected with them, can be effected without them.[39]

The third trial ended when the jury acquitted Faxon and sat deliberating about Hawkes; the Chief Justice suggested that the parties settle. Lowell agreed to end the case in non-suit, and the defendants were assessed no costs.[40] But then began the battle of broadsides. In January 1825, Lowell published a pamphlet attacking Faxon and Hawkes, Nathan Smith, Judge Nathan Weston, and—for good measure—Sir Astley Cooper, personal physician to the King of England. In the autumn, friends of Judge Weston answered Lowell, and in the process criticized Warren. He, in turn, could not let it go; incensed by what he considered a personal attack in the pamphlet (he had been "accused of 'ignorance of anatomy and surgery,'" among other things),[41] in 1826 Warren published an extensive dissertation on hip dislocations. He appended documents from the trial (having removed names), including Nathan Smith's deposition. The resulting *Letter to the Hon. Isaac Parker* ran to 142 pages. Though it is an able discussion, Warren also sounds very much on the defensive in places (fittingly, perhaps, given that his side had lost).[42]

In a way, however, Warren did have the last word. When Lowell died in 1858, an autopsy was done by Dr. Henry K. Oliver of Boston at Warren's request at Massachusetts General Hospital. (Lowell had demanded this as his right, seeing it as his chance for postmortem vindication.) Oliver, perhaps out of loyalty to Warren, reported that he found an unreduced dislocation with the ligamentum teres (femoris)—the ligament at the head of the femur—intact, and that the injury "was just what Dr. Warren always believed it to be, a simple dislocation."[43] Oliver sent Lowell's whole pelvis to the Warren Museum.

Yet that was not quite the end of the story, either. In 1959, the then-curator of the Warren Museum, Dr. Paul Yakovlev, located the pelvis and allowed X-rays to be taken. The hip was displayed at a meeting of the Trustees of the Boston Medical Library during a talk on Nathan Smith, and orthopedic specialists in the audience examined the hip carefully. Thanks in part to the hip joint having been tremendously overcast with new bone, opinions were still divided. The fact that Dr. Oliver had found the ligamentum teres intact (even though the head of the femur was far out of its socket), combined with the latter-day X-ray picture that shows fracture, forces the conclusion that a displaced fracture of the acetabulum accompanied the dislocation of the femur.[44] To this extent, then, Smith was right: There was a fracture, and the case was so complicated that Faxon and Hawkes had done the best they could have been expected to. Smith was apparently wrong, however, in saying there was no dislocation.

The trial aroused many passions. Perhaps Maine people would have been disinclined to agree with a doctor from Boston regardless of the circumstances. But particularly when the Boston man's word was up against that of their new professor of medicine at Bowdoin College, there was nothing to discuss. Smith in any case probably had a way with a jury (if he could persuade state legislatures, why not trial juries?); when he said the result was as good as any man could rightly expect, most laymen would be likely to agree with him.[45] To top it off, the defense attorney had ended his summation by insisting Smith could not be doubted, alluding to "a recent trial in Maine in which this surgeon was eulogized as the brightest light in the medical firmament of today."[46]

When Warren's pamphlet was published, its unmistakable attack on Smith's testimony roused Nathan Ryno Smith—ever loyal to his father— to insert the following brief comment on Warren's work in his *Philadelphia Monthly Journal of Medicine and Surgery*:

> The subject of this volume is one of no little interest to us, and will, we think, if freely and candidly discussed, lead to the exposition of certain erroneous principles in surgery, better substantiated by authority than by fact and inference. We have the subject under consideration, and only request that our brethren will suspend their opinions till the discussion is completed.[47]

Oddly, Ryno seems not to have been alert to the ambiguity of what he wrote or to the difficulty in figuring out whom he supported. That "erroneous principles in surgery" had been "substantiated by authority" was presumably meant to refer to the way Warren tried to make his case; his position at Harvard could be said to give him "authority" in the eyes of many. Determining things "by fact and inference" sounds like what Ryno would have wanted to attribute to his father. Yet Warren, in his published discussion, had made a snide remark about it not being necessary "to point out the incorrectness of the deponent's inference from the supposed fact."[48] Relying on "fact and inference" could cut both ways.

Smith, for his part, had written to George Shattuck in early January 1826 asking him to send on by mail "a report of the trial" (a reference in all likelihood to Warren's book, which had been published the previous year) inadvertently left in Boston, because "[s]ome of our fraternity here [in New Haven] having seen some sparring about the case wish to see the report. . . ." He went on—whether disingenuously or not, we cannot tell—"For myself, I care very little about it or what the newspaper folks say about it."[49]

Of other medico-legal cases in New England in which Smith might have played a role we have no record. Quite likely there were some; we have at the very least the reference (quoted earlier) to a "recent trial"—which may of course have been something other than the dueling case. We do know Smith complied when he was asked to prepare a "careful affidavit" concerning a malpractice suit in Austinburgh, Ohio, in 1827, involving Dr. Orestes Hawley. A patient had fallen in such a way that his knee had been damaged and the ankle badly dislocated. Though the ankle seemed to have been set perfectly, Dr. Hawley amputated. The patient, when he had time to think about it, decided he had been subjected to unnecessary surgery and sued.

Smith explained that dislocation at the ankle never occurred without the fracture of one or more of the bones of the leg, and that in his practice, even when he had achieved a perfect reduction, he was often forced to amputate later because of infection—always a terrible danger in a compound fracture.[50] Without knowing the judicial outcome of this case, we cannot be sure, but it seems probable that Smith's deposition—which left little doubt that the problem was one more likely to have required major surgery than not—was dispositive. This was, after all, expert testimony from New England's best and most famous surgeon, "the brightest star in the medical firmament" of the day.

Medical Consultant

Smith's advice was sought not only in medico-legal cases; he was often called in as a consultant, attending physician, or surgeon in charge. One such instance was the case in Norwich, Vermont, where he performed his famous ovariotomy, when he no longer lived across the Connecticut River in Hanover, but had to ride up from New Haven.

"Dr. Smith's life during his sixth decade [especially] was incredibly full," we are told. "He visited and operated on patients over the length and breadth of New England. . . . [H]e performed operations wherever he found himself."[51] A handful of examples not cited before will suffice to illustrate the point: An 1812 letter from a Brattleboro physician, Willard Arms, inquired on behalf of "Esq. Stockwell" when Smith would again be in town (easily seventy miles from Hanover) to follow up on his patient.[52] Correspondence a few years later between Smith in New Haven and Mason F. Cogswell in Hartford concerned Smith's advice on what to do about "Mr. Hart's" hydrocele.[53] Also that year, Dr. Thomas Chadbourne of Concord, New Hampshire, sought Smith's help in persuading the New Hampshire Medical Society not to support one Dr. J. D. Kittredge in the promotion of his "Vegetable Rheumatic Ointment" (which Chadbourne referred to as "Quack Medicine").[54] This request for help is all the more interesting given that Smith had by mid-1815 largely severed his ties with New Hampshire and thus with the New Hampshire Medical Society (of which he had been president in 1811). But Chadbourne knew his man; more than once in lectures, Smith railed against "irregulars" who promoted themselves as competent "bone setters" and were called when "regular surgeons" were what was needed.[55]

As was the custom at the time, largely because of the expense and difficulty of travel, physicians were often consulted in writing. In 1817, after he was settled in New Haven, Smith received a letter from the Hall family of Charlestown, New Hampshire: "My Brothers mental malady continues and I think grows more alarming. We are fearful that next Fall and Winter will find him considerably worse. What would you advise in the case? It is now impossible to pursuade or control him.—Your advice will have great weight with us."[56] One rather hopes Smith had been involved in "Brother" Hall's case earlier; the letter provided little enough basis for a professional assessment. (But then, there often was not much to go on—and in any case, more than one physician might be consulted. In 1828, when Daniel Webster's wife became ill, he wrote to both Nathan Smith and Philip Syng Physick in Philadelphia seeking help.[57])

Though Lyman Spalding may not have been directly seeking advice when he expounded his theories on goiter to Smith in 1819, his observations elicited a long commentary from the senior physician.[58] When another physician's patients consulted Smith, he had the courtesy to let the primary care physician know: In late 1826 he wrote to Dr. Fuller of Columbia, Connecticut, "Your patient Mr. A. Bailey has consulted me respecting his eye . . . a prolapsus of the iris."[59]

Scattered through the literature of early New England towns are numerous anecdotes about Smith, which, though undocumented, add substance to the claim that he was indeed a physician for all of New England. One comes from Sutton, Massachusetts, and tells how "the noted surgeon, Dr. Nathan Smith" was called to relieve "Lame David" Dudley (who may have been a relative of Smith's on his wife's side), of the "breach and stoppage" he experienced after eating "Vermont plums, stones and all." If accurate, it adds to the picture of Smith as a doctor with ingenuity as well as commonsense. Smith

got out the stones and relieved him, but could not heal the ruptured intestine, so his excremental discharges always afterward passed out of the aperture made by the doctor. By wearing a belt and a cloth over the aperture he was made quite comfortable, and able to work some for several years; he died at last from drowning.[60]

Another local history gives us a story of Smith accompanying Dr. Daniel Adams (a former student) on a call in Keene, New Hampshire; the patient, the Rev. Mr. Sprague, is said to have greeted Smith with "I am happy to see you, sir; I have often heard of you as an eminent surgeon."[61] Smith was undeniably both well known and respected.

PART V

THE SMITH LEGACY

CHAPTER FOURTEEN

A Man of Many Parts

❦

[F]ull of honors, if not of means—He was an extraordinary man.
— JOSEPH PERRY [1]

O F NECESSITY, the story of a person's life can be told only in part. Particularly when so many years have passed, the picture that emerges is frustratingly incomplete. We can infer only so much about Nathan Smith's sense of humor or kindheartedness, for example, from his letters or the handful of contemporary accounts of his life. What was it like to be his friend or acquaintance, or a member of his family? We can be impressed, but learn little—one has to be cautious about taking eulogistic remarks literally—from claims made in obituary notices, like the one that Smith "was the favorite of a wider circle of personal acquaintances and friends than any other man probably ever enjoyed in New England."[2]

More tellingly specific is a hint that lies buried in a letter Roswell Shurtleff, professor of divinity at Dartmouth, wrote to George Shattuck in 1810. The topic was whether Shattuck could be persuaded to join his good friend Nathan Smith on the slowly expanding medical faculty at Dartmouth. "Will you consent to be professor here? . . . Dr. Smith, as Prof. [Ebenezer] A[dams] informed you, wishes for it. But we apprehend that Col. [Rufus] Graves would be glad to Lecture, & possibly Dr. Smith with his usual accommodation will consent while conversing with Graves. Prof. A and myself think this will not do . . . ."[3]

What emerges is Smith, a man who has generally seemed quite capable of getting his own way, being characterized by a colleague as likely to back down simply to accommodate someone of lesser ability. Perhaps he was not so driven as we might have thought. Shurtleff's "usual accommodation" makes Smith sound habitually inclined to compromise to keep the peace. Of course other interpretations are possible, but Shurtleff's comment reminds us that we do not know the man Smith fully.

We have only scattered and incomplete glimpses into the impression Smith made on people. One of the most valuable is a posthumous remark by Nehemiah Cleaveland, who—while a student at Bowdoin College— had "joined [Smith's] class, attended the lectures, [been] present at most of his operations in the neighborhood, and [seen] much of him in society." In his history of Bowdoin, Cleaveland said about Smith (in his early sixties and at the height of his fame):

Dr. Smith was a large man, a little clumsy, and of a somewhat shambling gait. [He had an] expressive and genial countenance . . . . Those to whom Dr. Smith had been known only by fame might be disappointed in their first impressions. He was rather slow of movement and of speech, and in his manners often there was an air of indifference. There was no show of learning, no attempt at brilliancy, no assumption of dignity or superiority. The admiration which was felt for his ability and wisdom—a feeling shared by all who knew him—could be accounted for only by his possession of those attributes.[4]

In an attempt to understand this man of "expressive and genial countenance" more completely, we must look at some aspects of his life and career so far touched on only tangentially. Important though the roles of medical-school founder, professor, and practicing physician and surgeon were, there was much more to the man.

Medical Author

By 1804 Nathan Smith had been in practice nearly two decades and had been a medical professor for seven years. He wrote to a fellow physician that he was contemplating writing up "the history of some of the most important cases which have occurred to me in practice such especially as tend to illustrate particular principles in Physiology . . . ."[5] Unfortunately, no notes for such a paper seem to have survived.

In a letter to Shattuck in early 1823, Smith wrote, "I shall also . . . finish a book on Surgery which will contain about two hundred pages, which I shall publish in the course of the present year."[6] Distractions abounded, however, and more than four years later, he still had not finished the book. Late in 1827, he wrote Shattuck again on the subject: "Respecting my Surgery, I have written a considerable part of it, and expect to get through it the next summer. I should have probably accomplished it before but have been obliged to write some for my son's Journal and several essays to deliver before medical meetings, etc. . . ."[7] (The journal in question was the *Philadelphia Monthly Journal of Medicine and Surgery*, which Ryno founded in 1827, and which lasted only one year before merging with another journal.) Evidence has not been found that this planned text on surgery was ever completed, let alone published, though Smith was apparently sufficiently confident about finishing it to allow a prospectus to be published.[8]

Nathan Smith did finish some writing, however, and more than one of his publications stood the test of time remarkably well. The most famous is his *Practical Essay on Typhous Fever* of 1824, the importance of which was recognized immediately. A review appeared, almost as soon as the book was published, in *The Medical Review and Analectic Journal* (also in Philadelphia). The reviewer was John Eberle, M.D., one of the journal's editors; he observed that the essay had been written by "one of our most enlightened and experienced physicians." It was, he continued, "a plain, sensible, and instructive exposition of the author's views and experience concerning the nature and treatment of typhous fever—a disease respecting which, medical opinion is as yet exceedingly unsettled, and, in many respects, unsatisfactory."[9] Eberle was not afraid to criticize some of what Smith had to say. "With regard to the value of medical treatment in typhus, Dr. Smith holds sentiments which we cannot advocate in their full extent," he wrote; and on the issue of whether the disease could be controlled or interrupted "the weight of authority is, we think, decidedly against him."[10] For the most part, though, Eberle was enthusiastic. He quoted one passage at length, because Smith's "observations . . . appear to us so rational and interesting," and he praised the author's account of the symptoms of typhous fever as "methodical and clear, and evidently drawn from much close observation."[11]

Not everyone was so favorably impressed. Dr. Thomas Miner of Middletown, Connecticut, a Yale graduate, annotated his copy of the *Typhous* essay with mostly malicious marginalia, which serve above all to expose him as a reactionary practitioner who disparaged any therapies that did not accord with his.[12] A more public criticism appeared in an anonymous review in the *New York Medical & Physical Journal*. Negative from the first page, it was a devastating attack; time, however, proved Smith (and Eberle) more correct than this anonymous critic.[13]

Smith's son Ryno had joined John Eberle and George McClellan as an editor of their journal; Nathan's own name was later added to the masthead. Whether the senior Smith was expected to serve as a working editor or was included simply to reflect his promise to make frequent contributions to the journal is not clear. Both his "Observations on Fractures of the Femur, with an account of a new splint" and his "Account of a New Instrument for the extraction of coins and other foreign substances from the esophagus" appeared in early issues of this journal (in 1825),[14] along with an editorial note by Eberle following the first of these:

We are confident, that our readers will be highly gratified with the above account of professor Smith's apparatus for fractured thigh. We regard it as the most valuable paper, on the subject of fractures, which we have for a long time seen . . . .

This distinguished and original practitioner, from an almost unequalled experience in the practice of surgery, has accumulated a fund of original observations, which have not yet been communicated to the public but through his lectures. We are happy to announce that, hereafter, probably every number of our journal will be enriched with something from his pen.[15]

Three additional essays were published in subsequent issues: "Observations on Fractures of the Leg, with an account of a new support" (1825), "On amputation at the knee-joint" (also 1825), and "Suture of the Palate" (1826).[16]

Another notable contribution to medical science published by Nathan Smith is his "Observations on the Pathology and Treatment of Necrosis" (1827); it was published in both the *American Medical Review & Journal*, of which Ryno was one of the editors, and in Ryno's own *Philadelphia Monthly Journal*.[17] Ryno then reprinted this and the typhous fever essay in his *Medical and Surgical Memoirs* of 1831 (with no indication that they had been previously published), along with a small number of his father's other papers. Earlier, Nathan himself had published (in the form of a letter to John Coakley Lettsom) "Observations on the Position of Patients in the Operation for Lithotomy" (1805) in the *Memoirs of the Medical Society of London*. A second piece by Smith, on the medicinal properties of bloodroot, also appeared in London; written in 1807, it was included in the first issue of a new version of the Society's journal in 1810.[18]

The single largest publishing endeavor Smith engaged in was one in which he served as editor rather than author: He prepared the second American edition (published in Hartford, Connecticut, in 1816) of the multi-volume *Treatise on Febrile Diseases* by Alexander Philips Wilson Philip[19] (originally published in England in 1799).

A. P. Wilson Philip's work was a massive treatise (the American edition, printed in two volumes, totals more than eight hundred pages), which thoroughly covered the subject of fevers as then understood. Wilson Philip described each disease and discussed its treatment in scholarly fashion; text and notes alike made reference to, discussed, cited, or quoted dozens of authors both modern and ancient, European and American. The task Smith set himself as editor frankly pales next to the work done by the author, notwithstanding comments made by A. T. Lowe, a former student. Smith's "additions to this work were highly valued by the physicians of his time, for their strong sense and close, logical reasoning," Lowe said. Furthermore, the work on Wilson Philip illustrated "Dr. Smith's industry, as well as his ability. Occasionally in our long rides, when we were kept from home for a night Dr. Smith would retire to his room and write a chapter or a few pages . . . ."[20]

Most of the numerous notes that appear in the Smith-edited version are in fact Wilson Philip's own, however. The point of an American edition of an English or European book was to cope as briskly as possible with the unusual manifestations of disease assumed to be present in the New World. Hence, "New World" editors added to (rather than revised) "Old World" classics and published them as if they were new texts. (Ryno alluded to this custom in a prefatory remark to his father's essay on "Typhous Fever" as it appeared in the Memoirs: "[T]he author treats of Typhus as it presented itself to him, and not as he had studied it in books. His sketch is from nature . . . . The climate and soil of New England are peculiar, and we look for corresponding modifications of the disease."[21])

A meticulous comparison of the third London edition of Wilson Philip's work and the second American edition derived from it yields no evidence of changes in the text itself, and only brief commentary in a few appended notes. Volume 1, in addition to the introductory essay on nosological classification (already mentioned in chapter 9), has only four notes of varying length by Smith and one appendix (not listed in the table of contents) from his hand; Volume 2 has five notes, an essay on dysentery, and an appendix on the modus operandi of morbid poisons. Smith did not even bother to give page numbers for the cross references he made in two different places to other notes of his own. Moreover, his additions are hardly a model of scholarly rigor. The most dramatic example of his casual style comes late in the second volume, when he cited an experiment by "Dr. [Reuben] Mussey, a pupil of mine, and since that time a young gentleman from Albany whose name I do not recall . . . ." Earlier, in what he called "Dr. Smith's Note on Dysentery," he acknowledged he was quoting extensively from Moseley—though he did not bother to give either Moseley's first name (Benjamin) or the title of the essay in question (*Observations on the Dysentery of the West-Indies*)—and he made additions and bridged paragraphs (and played so fast and loose with quotation marks) as to make it impossible to determine how much is Smith and how much is Moseley.[22] On the other hand, in a letter to Lyman Spalding shortly after the book came out, Smith sounded like every other author who cares deeply about a book he has worked on. He wrote, with annoyance:

Last spring a year ago I wrote some notes on Wilson [Philip] on febrile disease. If you should happen to look into it you will observe many blunders by the printer. The cause was, that Mr. Cook never sent me a proof sheet nor a book but printed and distributed the Books while I was waiting for a proof sheet.[23]

Printer's errors and casual scholarship apart, the additions to Wilson Philip's text nonetheless do have value, not least in the evidence they give of Smith's reliance on experience and practice rather than theory—which, as we have seen, was so central to his style both as a physician and as a

professor of medicine. At the end of the section "Of the Causes of Inter-
mitting Fevers," Smith added a half-page note that relied explicitly on his
"twenty-eight years of practice on the banks of the Connecticut River."[24]
When he appended a short note to the section "Of Scarlet Fever," he likewise commented on his own experience, this time during the winter of
1813 in Vermont and New Hampshire.[25] The appendix he added to the
first volume—"Dr. Smith's Treatise on Dropsy"—was offered, he said,
for the sake of those who had not read Lachlan MacLean's book on hydrothorax; though "not copied" from MacLean, Smith said, his essay
"contains nearly the same principles . . . with the addition of some remedies which from my own experience I have found efficacious in dropsy."[26]

In Volume 2, Smith used case reports from his practice to qualify what
Wilson Philip said; although he sometimes took issue or criticized mildly
("The causes of haemorrhage here assigned are not very satisfactory"[27]),
he occasionally affirmed, too ("Respecting epidemic catarrh, the efficient
cause is still wrapped up in mystery . . . . The author has justly observed . . ."[28]). Smith emerged in purest form in his note on spotted fever,
a popular topic because it was such a common malady at the time: "We
should always suspect, when an overdose of medicine is given without
producing its appropriate effect, that the medicine is not adapted to the
case, and that something else should be done . . . rather than to repeat the
same remedy."[29]

In the end, perhaps the greatest importance of Smith's work on Wilson
Philip is that it helped establish Smith as an expert on fevers. From his Harvard "Dissertation on the causes and effects of spasm in fevers" in 1790
to his classic paper on typhous fever twenty-five years later, he was consistently interested in the subject. Together, these works show an unusually clear understanding—as Osler's later remark (quoted in chapter 9) reminds us—of a subject whose significance in early nineteenth-century
medicine can hardly be exaggerated.

One could wish that Smith had managed to find time to write more, or
at least more extensive works, in published form. The practical details
generally found in his lectures, judging from his students' notes, showed
up elsewhere in the care with which he expressed himself when he was especially concerned about getting some medical matter exactly right. In a
long letter to Shattuck, Smith discussed a "dissertation on Cancer" he
was in the process of writing. There he exhibited the kind of attention to
detail that would probably have made the finished product as valuable as
his other best work:

I fear I have not in my observations on cancer and scirrhus been so particular in
some parts of it as I should have been respecting the definition of the word "scirrhus." If that word means only a diseased gland I am incorrect, or rather the defi-

Title page of Nathan Smith's unpublished "Dissertation on scirrhous & Cancerous affections," 1808. Courtesy of Beinecke
Rare Book and Manuscript Library, Yale University.

nition is defective, for from the cases I have related it appears that a scirrhus tumor often arises in a part of the body where there are no glands of any kind . . . .
Another point perhaps I have not sufficiently insisted on, that is, that when cancer begins in any particular part of the body and if it produces its likeness in another part of the body it is in a similar part, viz; if it begins in a bone it will next appear in some other part of the cellular substance, etc. . . .

I fear too that I have not explained myself sufficiently on the question respecting cancer being a general or local disease. I think, however, it will appear that I consider it often as a general disease.[30]

Apparently he had intended to submit the essay to the annual competition for the Boylston Prize given in Boston. Certainly one of the assigned topics that year looks as if it could have been the inspiration for what he wrote: A gold medal (worth $33.00) was to be given for the best essay on each of three questions, one of which was "On the Diagnostics of Scirrhous and Cancerous Tumors with the comparative advantages of extirpation by the knife and by caustic." He seems not to have turned in the essay, however, perhaps because he was still working on it as the deadline for submission approached.[31] He had sent Shattuck a copy of the paper, with comments attached about places where he thought Shattuck might help polish it, adding, "You are perfectly at liberty to make what alterations you please in this hasty performance . . . ."[32] In the end, however, by his own admission, he had sought Shattuck's help too late:

If you have time to make any alterations in what I have written . . . I wish you to do it, but I fear you had it too late and that the thing will be found too imperfect to make anything of it this year; if so let it lay over, we can do something with it hereafter.[33]

We do not have copies (published or even in manuscript) of everything Smith wrote. He is said to have given talks on more than one occasion before the New Hampshire Medical Society, and the topics attributed to him —"Pathology and Physiology of Arteries," "Spontaneous Stopping of Hemorrhage in Wounded Arteries," "Spontaneous Hemorrhage," and "An Artificial Joint in the Thigh Bone Cured by an Operation"[34]—are all plausible subjects, given his interests. Unfortunately, none of these papers seems to have survived. Smith also once wrote to Lyman Spalding expressing a desire to speak on quackery before the New Hampshire Medical Society,[35] but we do not have a copy of that talk, either. Regardless, despite his success as a lecturer before students—testified to both by his great repute as a teacher and by the clarity of his students' notes—Smith did not think of himself as much of a public speaker. Concerned that the public was to be admitted to a meeting of the Medical Society before which he was supposed to pronounce an "oration, as you are pleased to call it," he wrote Lyman Spalding:

You know what my former habits have been viz. to deliver my sentiments in as plain and simple a style as possible and, as this method has raised me to honor, and my pupils to a rank at least equal to any medical man's pupils in New England, I should not like to depart from my former practice and especially, as what I have to say to the Society will be wholly confined to the theory and treatment of one or two diseases which can only interest medical men, I should think it highly improper to deliver my sentiments before a public audience. You will therefore advertize that the discourse (for I should not like to call it an oration, lest from the name I should be inclined to try to play the orator) will be delivered before the Society, in their Hall.[36]

If the high style required for orating was not to Smith's liking, it may be that the polished prose required for publishing was something for which he simply had too little time. Nevertheless, the result is a surprisingly long publication list, ranging from very short notes or reports of single cases to a few carefully worked-out articles, addressing a wide variety of medical and surgical issues of the day. (See Bibliography of Works by Nathan Smith, pages 337–39.)

Man of Business

Frequent references have been made to Nathan Smith's financial difficulties. Some of his problems were characteristic of the economy in which he lived: Cash in the young United States was scarce, and it often consisted of state scrip that was liable to unpredictable discounts in Boston;[37] furthermore, there were no banks in the North Country until about 1805. Although letters were carried by stage satisfactorily, enclosing money was generally deemed imprudent.

A very common practice was to pay by promissory note any debts not paid in kind. This could work well, but bills were often paid by someone else's note; thus transactions that began in straightforward fashion could turn into a very complicated affair especially when, as frequently happened, notes were passed more than once or were simply lost. Smith himself often admitted in correspondence to Olcott that he had misplaced a note or was unaware of its amount; on occasion he even signed legal papers testifying to problems of this sort.[38]

Smith's ledger books are in places nearly illegible today, and not only because the ink is fading. Various categories of charges and payments are mixed together; some entries are undated, and even the dated ones are not always in chronological order. Furthermore, many financial transactions were written on scraps of paper; the folders full of notes, receipts, and memos in the Dartmouth College Archives are evidence enough for that. In a letter to Shattuck, he once wrote: "I wish you to call on Mrs. Derby, and say to her I do not recollect whether I took the money which I deposited with her or not. If she gave it to me it is safe in my sock at Leominster. . . ."[39]

We cannot infer from any of this that Smith was unusually careless, however, or that he was incompetent when it came to finances. His method of keeping accounts was standard enough, if far from perfect. But bookkeeping could be exceedingly complicated under the circumstances of the day; getting paid was likely to involve prolonged and idiosyncratic financial arrangements. Early in August 1801, for example, Sylvester Day, a medical student acting as agent for Nathan Smith, signed a receipt given to Sherman Minott for three certificates totalling $48.78. One was for $21.41, bearing interest at six percent; another was for $10.71 "deferred stock"; and the third was for $16.66, bearing interest at three percent.[40] Legal action might well be required before such dealings could be straightened out. Thus the Keene, New Hampshire, Court of Common Pleas shows Nathan Smith on the docket on numerous occasions for several different suits in 1795–97,[41] for instance, and letters from Smith to Olcott frequently refer to payments and charges connected with court appearances that the lawyer or his deputy made on Smith's behalf.[42]

On the other hand, financial matters could be handled perfectly smoothly. When Hezekiah Ensworth was ready to pay Nathan Smith the $8.25 due him for medication and house calls between June 11 and July 13, 1816 (seven visits, at intervals of one to three days), the money was apparently simply sent to Smith's daughter Gratia Eliza, in New Haven—no questions asked. No explanation appears on the receipt.[43]

Ongoing concerns about shaky finances may have been among the reasons Smith was slow to make a permanent move to New Haven. After one course at Yale he returned to Hanover, as we have seen. He wrote Silliman from there in August 1814, of his continuing problems:

Now I want to mortgage the whole [of his real property, worth—he said—"about eight thousand dollars"] for four thousand dollars which would enable me to remove without any sacrifice & relieve me from all embaresment so that I should be able to devote all my labors both of body and mind to my professional business in New Haven. The property which I would give in security is the house and land where I live & two other farms with wild land in this state & in Vermont. The house & land where I live I think will sell within a year for the four thousand dollars & the other if necessary could be sold at some price so as to meet a payment in a reasonable time.[44]

Time would demonstrate that money matters for Smith were neither much worse nor particularly better in New Haven than they had been in Hanover (just as we saw, in chapter 12, that the additional teaching at Bowdoin had not noticeably improved his financial situation). In October 1815, he wrote a letter to Olcott that probably had a kernel of honest apprehension behind the jokingly avaricious remark he appended: "I concluded to stay [in New Haven] till our school was organized & the lectures advanced a little before I returned home [to Hanover] fearing that if

I was absent at the beginning I should not get my share of the money . . .
which promised to be considerable."[45]

One particularly complicated bit of business from Smith's New Haven
days can stand for the hundreds of transactions that took place over the
years between him and others. The following letter to Olcott from late
1817 shows both that financial dealings continued to concern Smith and
that he still relied, long after he left Hanover, on the services of the faithful Mills Olcott:

Last summer I bought a horse of a man in Corinth [Vt.] whose name I have forgotten, the note is out the first of January next. I wish to have him paid the note
was 90 dollars & I gave him an order on Capt Lovell who died soon after which
was to be indorsed on the note which would reduce the note to 78 dollars   Now
I wish to have Dr. Kimball pay the note of Dr. Burnham of Brookfield their sons
are with me & they will be owing me to that amount I have written thim on the
subject I have written to them both fearing that one or the other of them might not
have the money on hand, now I wish you to write to some one whom you may
know in Corinth to call on the widdow of Capt. Lovell who will know the man of
whom I purchased the horse & then let him know how I have provided to pay him
& also to let you know his name. ——

I wrote you some time since informing that as I was obliged to meet the payment of Mr. Pools note of 5000. dollars it would prevent my sending back as
much money as I intended to pay my debts in N. Hampshire I wish therefore if it
is possible that you would transmit to Dr. Torry of Windsor one hundred Dollars
to pay over to Judge Kingsbury of Claremont as he will want it about this time[46]
and also if you could discharge the mortgage which Willm Woodward has it
would oblige him.

I shall be able to forward you some money in the course of the winter I have
not yet rec'd any thing but the 500. dollar premium for removing my family which
is taken up in paying Pools note the other 750. dollars I have not rec'd & it will
not be convenient for them to pay it immediately & I feel some delicacy in pressing them for every cent as soon as I get into town — [47]

Late in Smith's life, he was as dependent on Olcott as ever. "Will you
be kind enough to drop me a line informing [me] respecting the money
due to me about the Norwich farm and when the next payment will probably be made, as I have forgotten the particulars," he wrote somewhat
plaintively in a letter from late 1828—only two months prior to his death,
as it turned out. Occasionally, as is true of that same letter, he also paid
testimony to the close bond that had grown up between their families:
"My family are all well," he went on, "and send much love to you and
yours."[48]

Smith's financial difficulties did not turn him into a miser; far from it.
He often forgave bills his patients could not pay without hardship, and
his philosophy about money was expressed somewhat roguishly in a letter to Olcott in May 1818: "You thot if I had money it would do me no
good because I should spent [sic] it. Now I always thought that spending

money was all the fun of it as it does no good while we keep it."[49] His sense of humor remained intact.

He did not, however, learn his lessons. Nathan Smith managed again and again to get himself into financial difficulty. To a great extent, this was a result of the way that he engaged in land speculation throughout his adult life, buying and selling property (frequently at a loss) wherever and whenever he could. If his father really was a surveyor, as tradition has it, perhaps Smith's interest in land began there. In any case, a precedent for making frequent real estate transactions was evident in what happened to the family property in Chester, Vermont. The land that Nathan's mother, Elizabeth Smith, inherited when her husband died, she deeded over to her son John when she remarried in October of 1779. Six years later, the north half of the one-hundred-acre parcel was deeded by John to Nathan. Two years after that, there is another deed of property, this time to John from Nathan. A few months later, John and his wife Olive (Gilkey) Smith in turn deeded the Smith land to Thomas Charles Chandler, thus finally moving it out of the family.[50]

Land transfers were not the only business matters within the family, incidentally; there is evidence that Nathan Smith borrowed money from his relatives, as well as from friends. Among the extant scraps of paper showing receipts for amounts both large and small, due and paid, are slips indicating Smith had financial dealings with both Jonathan and Dudley Chase, for example. And in 1803, Hall and Chase names appear along with Nathan Smith's on an "action of Ejectment in favour of Doct.ʳ Nathan Smith against Aaron Batchellor."[51]

Nathan Smith's land deals combine to make up the most unpleasant chapter in his life. He was a failure, to put it bluntly, probably as a farmer and definitely—completely and cataclysmically—as an investor in real estate. Certainly Smith never made any profit in either of these endeavors. Every indication is that he ruined his fortunes by trying to be a gentleman farmer and engaging in land speculation. Any question about whether he ever achieved solvency—never mind security—can be answered by analyzing the correspondence between Olcott and one or another of the Smiths after Nathan died, and of the Court of Probate records in New Haven. Nothing shocking or ignominious is to be found, only much that is sad.[52]

During Smith's childhood, fortunes had been made and lost in land speculation along the Connecticut River, particularly in Vermont, and that may have affected (not to say infected) him. Chester, Vermont, was one of the towns created by Governor John Wentworth of New Hampshire expressly for land development and speculation. The history of early Vermont turns on the varied fortunes of the New Hampshire and New York speculators who tried to make money from the Royal Grants. Among the most successful of the speculators was Jonathan Chase, another possible influence on Smith in his propensity for acquiring real estate. Before Smith moved to Hanover, he inherited large tracts of land in Cornish and elsewhere from his father-in-law, as we learned earlier.[53] He wanted a farm in Hanover. He bought a good one, with fine orchards. He had ten pleasant acres (in what became College Park) for grazing his horses. In Norwich he had what he intended as a model farm, but which was notoriously unprofitable; one tenant after another served above all to demonstrate that tenant farming was not working. Still he bought property.

Smith purchased a house in Hanover in early 1805, where his family lived until they moved to Yale in 1815. He enlarged his holdings with numerous subsequent purchases. He bought several parcels of land in Hanover in 1806 and 1807, for example, from several members of the Woodward family: William, Bezaleel, Mary, and James.[54] By the time he moved to New Haven, he owned a good portion of Hanover.

When Smith left Hanover and was no longer able to supervise his affairs in person, he felt forced to sell, even though no one was particularly eager to buy (thanks in part to the unsettled social situation in town, caused by the controversy that culminated in the Dartmouth College Case). Early in September of 1815 he wrote to Olcott:

I intended to have talked with the president on the subject [of selling the farm] before I left Hanover, but the great battle between him & the Trustees put it out of my power to speak to him [on] minor matters. I thought probably he might be willing to purchase the farm & to pay me in a note against the Trustees providing I would sell it immediately all which I should be willing to do—provided he would give me in that way 6000 dollars for the farm—or if he would advance the money 5000.[55]

In early March of 1822, Smith still had not sold his house or land in Hanover, and he offered his "estate" to Professor Ebenezer Adams for "six thousand dollars down in Boston money or silver money." He then added, wryly, affecting a humorous frame of mind in unpleasant circumstances: "If I cannot sell it for that I will punish Hanover by living on it myself."[56]

One reason Smith kept buying more land was that patients sometimes paid big surgical bills by offering to turn property over to him. But the bills were typically equivalent to only a small part of the value of the land; to acquire the land (and thus payment at all), Smith had to lay out money of his own. And so he did. In addition to his land in and around Hanover, he had property thirty miles south in Springfield, New Hampshire, and off to the west in Orange, Vermont, as well as his holdings from Jonathan Chase's estate. The taxes were appreciable. Worse was the need to keep track of it all, which he did not always succeed in doing. In March of

1821, he confided to Olcott, "I have been informed that my land in Orange, N.H. has been sold for taxes . . . ."[57]

The land in Hanover would have been a good investment if he had held it long enough. But that is often the case, and Smith seems to have been less able than most to retain property. In fact most of Smith's trouble with banks and creditors can be traced to his real estate deals, rather than to the building of the Medical School or to poor fee collection. Even Olcott, his very experienced lawyer—a successful entrepreneur on his own behalf, "a man of remarkable sagacity and enterprise in business affairs"[58] —seems to have been unable to turn Smith's dealings into a profitable venture.

Family Matters

The picture we have of Smith family life is like an old painting in need of restoration. Some portions are blurred or faded beyond recognition, a few are caked with the grime of two hundred years. Fortunately, a few areas of this canvas are still in good repair. In Nathan we see a man of many talents whose life was full of professional activity, a man with a great deal on his mind—but also one who through it all does not seem to have wavered in his concern for his family. A touching letter written home to Sally in March of 1814, during the trying period when the family was still split between Hanover and New Haven, gives sharp expression to his mood and this side of his character:

My Dearly and Well-beloved:
    I fear my absence has been severely felt by you and the children. For my own part I have had a dreary winter of it; you may rest assured that I will never leave you and the dear children so long a time during my lifetime. I think I shall be able to get home by the middle of April.
    . . . Do kiss all the children for me and tell them that papa will come home and never leave them again.[59]

Though we are told Sally was "bright and gifted,"[60] we do not actually know much about her. Born and raised in Cornish, New Hampshire, Sarah Chase married Nathan Smith—as we saw earlier—after his first wife, her half-sister Elizabeth, died. She seems to have been a woman with an independent streak, who led a life largely separate from her husband's and generally uninfluenced in its everyday details by the fact that she was a doctor's wife. Left at home with a young child, and pregnant with the second when her husband set off for Scotland and England, must have cherished a farewell letter that gave evidence of his concern both for her and for his little son.[61] A letter he wrote home from Edinburgh in early February of 1797 is full of similar expressions of homesickness and ended thus: "I am, my dear Sally, yours with the fondest love and conjugal affection till Death, which God grant may be at a late day. Adieu, my dear, for a little."[62]

Unfortunately, no letters from Sally to Nathan appear to have survived. Was she content to be left behind under the watchful eyes of her parents? How early did she have hints of what a terrible businessman her husband was—of his constant inclination to buy land he could ill afford and his too-generous nature? How soon did she begin to understand that his restless desire to educate a new generation of physicians would have him leaving home repeatedly to found new medical departments in four New England states? How symbolic is it that, after Hanover, the move to Yale was the only one she made with her husband? (Sally did, however, occasionally accompany Nathan on his professional travels, as we know. He wrote to Parker Cleaveland at Bowdoin from New Haven, late in August 1822: "I find my family all well, I shall take Mrs. Smith & little Sarah [the youngest child, who had just turned three] with me to Burlington. From thence I shall return home the last week in Oct.r"[63])

Sally Smith's situation was not unusual for her time; it was normal then for a woman to live in the background of her husband's prominent career. Accounts of the life led by other nineteenth-century doctors typically leave out all but the barest mention of the wife.[64] In Sally's case, at least there are occasional signs that she did not sit wholly in the shadows. The deed conveying to the State of New Hampshire land for the new "brick and stone" Medical House in Hanover, for example, was signed by both Nathan Smith and "Sally his wife." They "personally appeared and severally acknowledged" the deed.[65]

The move from Hanover to New Haven was in some ways more complicated for Nathan than the move from Cornish to Hanover had been, even though he was being asked to help organize a medical department at Yale, instead of taking the initiative as he had at Dartmouth. The chief problem, as we have seen, was religion. This has to have been a concern for Sally as well; she was the one with the Episcopalian background. Perhaps because of that, the Smiths maintained full membership in their old Cornish church, and they never signed the Covenant for the Congregational Church (organized in 1805) in Hanover, even though the entire Mills Olcott family, as well as most of the others in the College community, did. In 1811, Smith bought from Jedediah Baldwin the No. 1 pew, presumably for family use, but that was his only known association with the Hanover church.[66]

This helped make Smith look like an "infidel" to the strict Congregationalists at Yale. How much this mattered to Sally we cannot tell, any more than we know what she made of her husband's achieving a new "state of grace" or whether she shared it with him. Our only knowledge of her attitude toward religion is that we are told she "was a pious woman and read her bible through in course as often as she could. When she died her book-mark was at one of the Psalms."[67] (It was also said, long after she had died—at the funeral of one of her sons—that Sally Smith "did not make a public profession of religion until after the death of her husband when she united with the North Congregational Church in New Haven."[68])

Further independence is shown by Sally's being even slower to move to New Haven than she had been to settle in Hanover. In the summer of 1814, Malleville Allen wrote to her husband—the Rev. William Allen, Dartmouth's acting president at that point—that Smith's "family are opposed to going, Mrs. S. says *she won't go* and when I see them started I shall believe it and not till then."[69]

In January of 1816 Smith wrote to Olcott for help:

I feel very anxious about my family & have heard that Plumley [a student boarder[70] and hired hand] has not been kind & attentive   I wish you would call on Mrs. Smith & if any thing is wanting to make her comfortable during this cold & stormy season. If you will lend her the necessary cash I will remunerate you if I live as I trust I shall.[71]

After a delay of four years, Sally finally consented to the move, and Smith went to get her. Whether it took Sally that long—watching from a distance—to become convinced that her husband would be happy on the Yale faculty, or whether she simply had personal reasons for hesitating, we will probably never learn. (Perhaps in the end the $500 incentive Yale paid Smith for moving his family was persuasive.[72]) We do know there were times when Sally was not well (bearing ten children might have had something to do with it). On more than one occasion Smith expressed concern about her health. In a letter to Mills Olcott written after Sally and the children had finally moved to New Haven, Smith commented that "Mrs. Smith has been quite sick since we arrived here but is recovering."[73] Another letter (written several years later) with a similar theme was worded more strongly: "I did not return by Hanover as I intended on account of information from home of Mrs Smith's sickness. I . . . found her alarmingly out of health. She is now much better & I think her health will be restored . . . ."[74]

For the most part, Sally could see more of her husband in New Haven, especially in the later years when he had reduced his teaching responsibilities in other places. But her life was never completely easy. In addition to her natural concerns for her own children, she still had to deal with student boarders; a vexatious example was Olcott's son Charles, who worried the Smiths with his drinking.[75]

Letter to Mills Olcott from Nathan Smith, expressing concern over the health of his wife, Sally. Courtesy of Dartmouth College Library.

Like Father, Like Son

Nathan and Sally Smith were the parents of ten children. With the exception of the death at sixteen of their eldest daughter, Sarah (Sally) Malvina, they seem to have been spared the sorrows and pains of childhood mortality so common for parents in those days (and experienced by Nathan's own father each of the four times his first wife had a child). To be sure, young Sally's death was an important exception; her death, we are told, was "the first break in the home circle and came as a crushing sorrow, never to be entirely outlived."[76]

We have surprisingly little documentation on Nathan Smith's relationship with or concern for his children. He did occasionally write about aspects of their education, a subject in which he took a particular interest. During the period when the boys were still quite young, for example, in a letter that fairly bursts with fatherly pride, Smith wrote to Shattuck expressing his pleasure (he sounds frankly amazed) over Ryno's success at school. Professor Shurtleff had been on hand when Ryno was being examined in arithmetic and volunteered the remark that it was the "best ex-

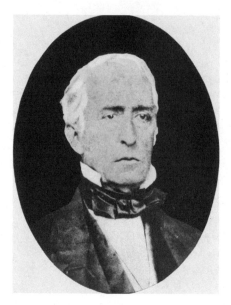

David Solon Chase Hall Smith, 1795–1859.
From Emily A. Smith's *Life & Letters of Nathan
Smith* (Yale University Press, 1914). Yale University,
Harvey Cushing/John Hay Whitney Medical Library.

amination on the principles of arithmetic he ever witnessed in any person
of his age." Smith went on to say, "I have great reason also to be satisfied
with the progress Solon made during my absence & the little girls have
exceeded my most sanguine hopes in their improvements."[77]

Fifteen years later the fatherly concern over the same two sons (both
physicians by that time) is evident in another letter to Shattuck:

I want three hundred dollars to enable my son [Solon] at Sutton to pay for a house
and land which he has purchased, and if you will lend that sum to him, and me,
with our joint security I will see it forthcoming to you in the month of June next.
. . . I believe N[athan] R[yno] is getting on very well at Philadelphia. They have
110 students who pay $15 each which is much better than I expected.[78]

Much later, in a rare indication that he was worried about his offspring's
future—or was it his old real-estate concerns surfacing?—he wrote to Olcott asking him to keep an eye on the house in Hanover (still not sold!),
which he had rented out. He seemed less interested in the rent money than
in making sure the premises would be protected "against the depreda-
tions of medical students etc. . . . The main object is to keep the place in
repare [sic] till some of my children want it to hire out . . . ."[79]

From the somewhat fragmentary evidence that remains to us, there is no reason to think the parents concerned themselves less with the girls than with the boys. The times being what they were, however, the information we have about the six daughters is much thinner than it is about the four sons, all of whom became physicians.

The first son, David Solon Chase Hall Smith, was born in Cornish on June 27, 1795. Like several of his siblings to follow, he was generally called by his second name, Solon.[80] Although he was more interested in botany than anything else, he received his M.D. from Yale in 1816.

In addition to being the eldest, Solon was also the first to marry. On July 26, 1820, he married Lucy Hall, from Sutton, Massachusetts, where he had settled down to practice the previous year. The town already had three physicians, but Solon's "thorough training and the prestige of his father's name" gave him a boost, and he is said to have soon become "one of the most popular physicians in that part of the country."[81] The proud father once wrote to Shattuck, "I believe Solon is getting into considerable repute at Sutton."[82]

Solon was, in fact, much like his father in being a skilled diagnostician.[83] Another trait he shared with his father was generosity, coupled with sincere concern for those worse off than he. A telling anecdote appears in the Sutton history:

Like his father he . . . never became rich; indeed at one time he was quite poor, deeply in debt, and his creditors attached his horse, so that he had no way to visit patients, and he became discouraged. One day a man came for him to go to Thompson [Thomaston?], Ct., but he told him that he could not go, for he had no horse; the man told him that he would take him up there in his own carriage and bring him back. 'Well,' said the doctor, 'if you will do that I will go'; so he went. When he reached home the man asked him what was to pay. 'Oh, nothing,' said the doctor, 'you have had trouble enough to get me there already.' 'But I am going to pay you for all that.' He gave him a ten dollar bill and left. The next day a man came for him to go and see a poor family in the south part of the town. He said, 'If they are poor I'll go, for I am poor myself.' When he reached there he found they were poor indeed, and he said starvation was all that ailed them; so he took out his ten dollar bill and gave it to the poor woman to buy wholesome food for her sick children. It was all the money he had. He thought their rich neighbors could doctor that family as well as he could.[84]

Of all the sons of Nathan Smith, the one who most closely followed his career was his namesake, Nathan Ryno Smith, born May 21, 1797. Ryno received his M.D. degree from Yale in 1823. He was in at least two important ways more like his father than any of his brothers were: He taught in several medical schools (primarily anatomy and surgery) and was involved in establishing more than one.

Ryno was practicing medicine in Burlington, Vermont (as we saw earlier), when steps were being taken to found a medical school at the University of Vermont. Appointed the first professor of anatomy and physiology there, he was on the faculty with his father. After only two years at UVM, however, Ryno went to Philadelphia to study at the University of Pennsylvania. In 1827 he became professor of anatomy at the new Jefferson Medical College.[85] Both an editor (of the *American Medical Review*[86]) and a writer, Ryno soon published a *Physiological Essay on Digestion*. In 1827, as we also saw earlier, he founded and edited a journal of his own.

Two years after his father's death, Ryno published what purported to be his father's *Medical and Surgical Memoirs*. The book contained more of his own papers than of his father's; Ryno seems to have taken advantage of the opportunity that presented itself to him by fleshing out the volume with his own work.[87] This bespoke no lack of respect or affection, however; the tender concern Ryno expressed in a letter to one of his sisters ten days before their father's death seems genuine enough:

It will be extremely difficult for me to leave Baltimore at this time, but nothing shall keep me from the sick bed of the kindest, the best of fathers. . . . If my dear father, in his illness feel any solicitude about his family, tell him I would have him dismiss it all. . . . My home, my heart, and my purse will always be theirs, but I trust in Heaven that he may be long spared to us. Tell him that I ask his forgiveness for not having written to him so often as I should have done. It was not from any abatement of affection.[88]

In the end, Ryno was more actively involved in publishing than his father ever had been. When he moved to Baltimore, he founded and edited yet another journal, the *Baltimore Monthly Journal of Medicine and Surgery* (which also lasted only a year), and he was briefly co-editor of the *New York Medical Journal*. He contributed to still other publications,[89] and in 1829 he published *An Essay on the Diseases of the Middle Ear* (a translation from the French of a work by J. A. Saissy, "with a supplement of his own on diseases of the external ear").[90]

He was also rightly famed for having invented the lithotome, an instrument for performing vesical lithotomy. In the August 1835 issue of the *North American Archives of Medical and Surgical Science*, Ryno—an "[e]arly innovator in the surgical removal of the thyroid"—published a report of the first thyroidectomy ("Extirpation of the Thyroid Gland").[91] The great surgeon William Halstead said that Ryno's essay on the thyroid gland was a "modest and lucid report of a case, the importance of which he could hardly have comprehended."[92] His *Treatment of Fractures of the Lower Extremity by the Use of an Anterior Suspensory Apparatus*,[93] begun in the 1830s, did not appear until 1867, in part because Ryno continued experimenting with his invention—which he with some justification considered his major contribution to surgery—for more than thirty

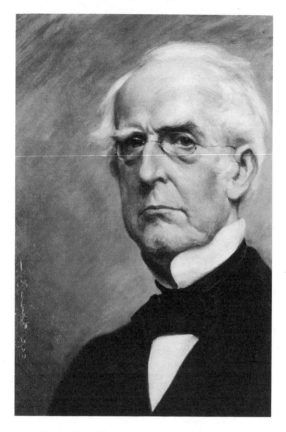

Nathan Ryno Smith, 1797–1877. Courtesy of the
Medical and Chirurgical Faculty of Maryland.

years.[94] By the end of his long life, he had "earned a world-wide reputation as a great teacher, practitioner, and operator, and added additional lustre to a name among the most distinguished in the medical annals of this country."[95] He taught at the University of Maryland from 1827 to 1867 and died in Baltimore a decade later.

On September 23, 1805, Nathan's third son, James Morven Smith, was born. (Prior to his birth, two daughters were born: Sarah Malvina, the one who died at sixteen; and Gratia Eliza.) In 1828 James, too, earned an M.D. from Yale. Ten years later he published "Cases of Necrosis illustrating the Practice of Exposing and Perforating the Diseased Bone at an early period in the progress of the malady" in the *American Journal of Medical Science*,[96] a paper explicitly based on his father's methods. No other record

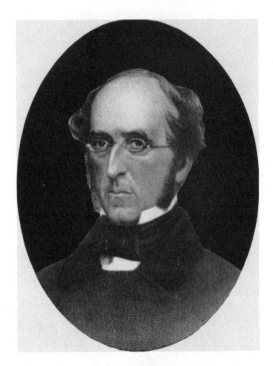

James Morven Smith, 1805–1853.
From Emily A. Smith's *Life & Letters of Nathan Smith*
(Yale University Press, 1914). Yale University, Harvey
Cushing/John Hay Whitney Medical Library.

of publications by James survives; he was not in his brother Ryno's class as a writer, though he also had a reputation as a skilled surgeon.

James's career was brought to an abrupt end in a New Haven Railroad accident that came to be known as the "Norwalk bridge disaster." This great tragedy in Norwalk, Connecticut, killed upwards of fifty people— among them several doctors returning from a medical meeting in New York City—on May 6, 1853. The catastrophe was front-page news in the New York papers the next day, and three days later the *New-York Daily Times* listed among the deceased "Dr. J. M. Smith" of Springfield, Massachusetts. The article[97] also quoted from the Springfield *Republican*:

The people of Springfield are called upon to mourn the loss of two of their most useful and honorable citizens, as victims of this terrible disaster. Dr. James M. Smith and Dr. James H. Gray are no more. Their sudden fall is regarded as a great public calamity by this whole community.

Dr. Smith was the leading physician, and one of the most experienced in this city—a man who was above reproach in his private character, and as high in pub-

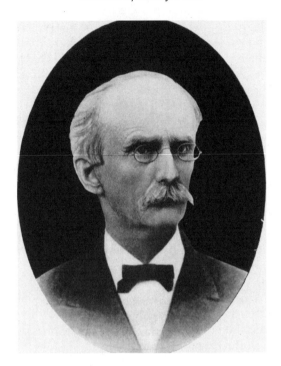

John Derby Smith, 1812–1884.
From Emily A. Smith's *Life & Letters of Nathan Smith*
(Yale University Press, 1914). Yale University, Harvey
Cushing/John Hay Whitney Medical Library.

lic esteem, as a man, as he was as a physician. He was the son of the late celebrated Dr. Nathan Smith of New-Haven, and leaves a wife and young family.

John Derby Smith, the youngest of Nathan Smith's four sons, born on
April 9, 1812, was ordained a Congregational minister and studied medicine only when he had to give up preaching because of throat trouble.
He earned an M.D. degree from the University of Maryland in 1846 and
served in the Civil War.[98] He did not, however, altogether give up on the
ministry, as a letter from his wife, Mary, to George Shattuck years later
makes evident: "Mr. Smith is now preaching at East Hampton, and we
hope the time is not far distant when he will find a place to settle where
he can be useful as a minister and receive a competent support for his
family."[99]

Mary's letter to Shattuck, like so many other Smith family letters to
that loyal friend, was full of talk about money. She went on to say: "The
sum you have so kindly and generously sent will enable us to meet all . . .

demands, and leave sufficient for the supply of our present wants." But this was not simply one more cry for financial help from the beleaguered Smiths; the connection between Shattuck and John Derby Smith was a special one. In the first place, John was Shattuck's godson; he had been named after the husband of Shattuck's "Aunt Derby" (aunt to Eliza Cheever Davis, who was Shattuck's wife[100]).

Secondly, it was Shattuck who had eased Nathan Smith's dying hours, not only by being present at his mentor's side as he lay dying, but by promising to make sure that young John's educational opportunities would not be curtailed as a result of his father's death. With help from Mrs. Derby (the Derbys—husband and wife—had been forever grateful to Nathan Smith for doing what he could to restore Mr. Derby's sight), Shattuck saw to it that John had every educational advantage. A long letter to Benjamin Silliman, written less than two weeks after Nathan's death, spells out the complex but exceedingly kind and generous provisions they had worked out.[101]

On the same day, Shattuck also wrote directly to John, explaining what they had done. In an understatement of staggering proportions, he signed himself "your father's friend, Geo. C. Shattuck."[102] That the rest of the family knew about the arrangement is evident from a letter Ryno wrote to Shattuck three months later:

I learned some time since, your benevolent intentions in [my brother John's] favour. I ought, before this to have expressed my gratitude for the respect & affection which you manifested toward our beloved parent in his last hours. Be assured it will be long remembered.[103]

The entire family benefited from the extraordinary and abiding friendship between George Cheyne Shattuck and Nathan Smith.

CHAPTER FIFTEEN

Epilogue

Dr. Smith was no ordinary man. . . . [H]e labored most assiduously during his whole life, not only to perform acceptably and beneficially the duties of a physician, but to diffuse among medical men, by his private intercourse with them and by his public instruction, correct notions of their profession.
—JONATHAN KNIGHT [1]

BY THE TIME Nathan Smith was in his early sixties, he had been famous and much in demand for many years. He was no doubt also vastly overextended; it is just as well that he finally gave up trying to teach at more than one institution. By 1826 he was, at last, Yale's alone.

A long and slow withdrawal from his labors, leading to pleasant years of a relaxing retirement, was not to be his, however. In the summer of 1828, shortly before he turned sixty-six, Smith had his first serious illness; the result was considerable weakness and relative incapacitation, which persisted for the next several months. In January of 1829, another episode (or series of episodes—probably cerebro-vascular accidents), cumulatively proved fatal. Smith's colleague Jonathan Knight, in his "Eulogium," gave voice to the depth of feeling occasioned by the older man's death. Stating first that all had hoped Smith might have many more years to continue his usefulness, Knight then exclaimed: "But alas! Our hopes are blasted. The last dread summons has reached him; his spirit has ascended to him who gave it, and his body must return to the dust from which it sprung."[2]

Quite apart from this pious commentary on death, Knight went on to give a poignant picture of just how great the loss was:

By this melancholy event, a bereaved family is called to mourn the loss of a kind and affectionate father, a tender, indulgent and well beloved parent; the institution with which he was connected, a chief pillar and support; the medical profession, a father and a friend; the poor, the sick and the distressed, a means of consolation and relief, and the community at large, a distinguished benefactor.

It is also to Knight that we owe the closest thing we have to an account of Smith's physical condition in the last months of his life:

About the middle of July last [1828], he was seized with a severe illness, which after a short continuance, left him, but in a very debilitated state. From this state his friends perceived with alarm that he did not entirely recover. He continued to be weak, with occasional attacks of illness, through the remainder of the summer and autumnal months. Though enfeebled in body, his mind retained its usual vigor and activity, and unwilling to yield to what he probably considered a trivial complaint, he continued, with the exception of a few days, his laborious employments. No considerable alteration in the state of his health appeared, until about four weeks since, when he was attacked with a severe influenza. This was accompanied and followed, by a painful and vertiginous affection of the head. By the use of remedies these symptoms were alleviated. On the evening of Tuesday, the 13th inst. [January 1829] he first perceived a slight numbness of the left hand, with a trifling indistinctness in his articulation. These symptoms of paralysis gradually increased, until the morning of the 26th inst. when the powers of life became exhausted, and at 6 o'clock, in the 67th year of his age, he slept the sleep of death.

That a contemporary—a close colleague and friend—should write with such sentimental tenderness about Smith's death and the shattered hopes of the various bereaved persons is hardly surprising. But it does not give us insight into the long-term significance of the man and his life, and it by no means fully reveals the richness of his legacy.

That legacy has three parts. The impressive array of Smith family doctors across the generations (well beyond the four sons; see Appendix B) is one. But while it is notable, it is hardly unique; many families in the annals of medical history have spawned numerous physicians.

Smith's legacy also includes the four medical schools he either founded or helped found. This unprecedented and unrepeatable feat created an enduring institutional testimony to Smith's dedicated interest in medical education.

The third and perhaps most important dimension of Smith's legacy is the most difficult to pinpoint. Exactly how much the force of his teaching affected the subsequent direction of therapeutics is impossible to say. What numbers of students—even many generations later—were taught *because of Nathan Smith* to pay closer attention to "patient inquiry," to make more systematic use of direct observation, above all to trust the *vis medicatrix naturae* rather than to rely on dogma and theory, is likewise impossible to say. What is undeniable is the unusually large number of physicians—many of them clinicians, surgeons, and medical teachers of great repute in their own right—who have paid tribute to Nathan Smith over the years, often long after his death. Even more than a century later, Dartmouth Medical School professors like Carleton P. Frost and Colin C. Stewart continued explicitly to perpetuate Nathan Smith's approach to

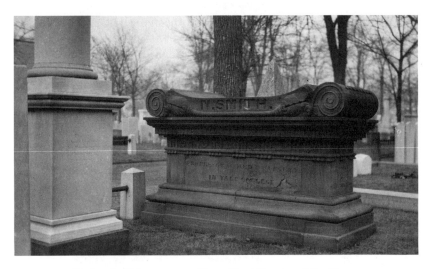

Nathan Smith's gravestone, Grove Street Cemetery, New Haven.
Courtesy of Yale University, Harvey Cushing/John Hay Whitney Medical Library.

medicine; they taught their students to love Smith and respect his judgment, to laugh at his jokes, and to adopt as their own his kindness and respect for patients.

Nor has it been only those associated with Dartmouth, Yale, Bowdoin, or UVM—or only physicians—who have admired Smith. Many distinguished individuals have, over the years, praised Smith's contributions. Alan Gregg, a Rockefeller Foundation vice president and great student of medical education, once referred to Nathan Smith as the "Johnny Appleseed of American medicine."[3] Henry I. Bowditch in 1851 said Smith's career was "brilliant," and that he "had more effect than any other man or set of men in bringing the pupil up to what he subsequently became . . . ."[4] Twenty years later, Oliver Wendell Holmes said much the same: "Nathan Smith . . . did a great work for the advancement of medicine and surgery in New England, by his labor as teacher and author,—greater, it is claimed by some, than was ever done by any other man."[5] When Oliver P. Hubbard gave a historical address on Dartmouth Medical School and Nathan Smith in 1879, his baseline was the presumption that Smith as a young man "had developed traits of character, patience, courage, industry, perseverance, self-reliance, and integrity, which . . . were to give him a decided superiority over his fellow-man . . . . Dr. Smith triumphed over difficulties which no other man would have dared to encounter . . . ."[6] Dartmouth physician John P. Bowler, at the centennial of Smith's death, commented on Smith having the "spirit of the pioneer, . . . zeal, resource-fulness, untiring energy and . . . a constant readiness for self-sacrifice, [making him] a chief among the frontiersmen of American medical teach-ing and practice."[7]

Hubbard's judgment and Bowler's observation are well supported by William Allen, who (though not a physician) knew Smith well as his pa-tient, friend, and academic colleague. "He had penetration," Allen said in his eulogy,

and a clear, accurate judgment. He was conversant with the experience of other men. He had large and long experience of his own. He was of ready memory and of present sagacity to apply his knowledge in any emergency. And he was cautious and considerate, far removed from hasty judgment and rash practice.[8]

Fully in consonance with that characterization was the tribute paid to Smith by one of modern medicine's greatest teachers, Harvey Cushing, in his celebrated 1928 address at Dartmouth, "The Medical Career":

Here, then, was a man who for Dartmouth men in particular may well serve as their ideal of a doctor. A man possessed of originality of thought, of energy, or re-sourcefulness, he became a brilliant surgeon in days when operations were beset with especial difficulties and hazards; an accurate and keen observer, he became an important contributor to medical literature; he had the courage to wage war-fare against the professional mountebanks that abounded in his day no less than in this; he had the sympathetic disposition and the generous spirit combined with common sense that made him sought after as a general practitioner; he had the sound judgment of a great teacher.[9]

Jonathan Knight had earlier spoken of Nathan Smith's "keen, discrim-inating inquisitiveness" and "highly retentive" memory, his "power of re-ducing all the knowledge, which he acquired, . . . to some useful practical purpose," and his "high degree" of "plain common sense." He rightly sin-gled out as significant Smith's habit of avoiding surgery where possible, but spoke also with admiration of Smith's ability to proceed "without re-luctance or hesitation" when he deemed surgery necessary. Smith was, Knight said, "calm, collected and cautious" when he operated, always es-chewing "useless parade."[10]

Another great physician and teacher, Samuel D. Gross, once said Smith was

[one] of the most extraordinary medical men whom this country has ever produced, whether we regard his great ability as a general practitioner, his skill and daring as a surgeon, or his versatility as a teacher of the different branches of medicine.[11]

William H. Welch echoed Gross, calling Smith "one of the most inter-esting and important figures in the history of American medicine" and proclaiming him as "a remarkable example of equal eminence in internal medicine and in surgery."[12] Elsewhere Welch elaborated thus:

Famous in his day and generation, he is still more famous today, for he was far ahead of his times, and his reputation, unlike that of so many medical worthies of the past, has steadily increased, as the medical profession has slowly caught up with him. . . . He was a man of high intellectual and moral qualities, of great originality and untiring energy, an accurate and keen observer, unfettered by traditions and theories, fearless, and above all blessed with an uncommon fund of plain common sense.[13]

At least indirectly related to what Cushing called Smith's "warfare against the professional mountebanks" was his deep commitment to improving medical education. As one writer has pointed out,

[h]is vision of the needs of the future was clear and his judgment sound, anticipating what is now generally accepted by modern educators, namely the need of a union of medical schools with established universities, in place of the proprietary medical colleges so common up to the end of the nineteenth century. Nathan Smith also demanded a higher education in medicine, and was an opponent of the superficial knowledge of his day and later.[14]

Smith's concern with, commitment to, and successes in medical education are so manifest that it is easy to forget how thin his own early education was. When one historian referred to "the formidable Harvard graduate Nathan Smith . . . [who] alone ably taught all the courses,"[15] he was using a turn of phrase that belies the simple background of the man, not a "Harvard graduate" in the sense of a college-educated man at all. Yet it was true that Smith was formidable. Another historian of medicine has pointed out that Nathan Smith "lectured on all the usual branches of medicine . . . a Herculean task, but he met it manfully, passing from one subject to another with astonishing ease. . . . [W]hen the history of our great men is written out, the enterprise, genius, perseverance, and success of Dr. Nathan Smith, will be remembered by every lover of science."[16]

Another commentator on Smith observed that his "ripe knowledge and keen observation, after a life of study and vast experience, had fitted him not only to become the leading physician and surgeon of his day but his rare talent for communicating his learning enabled him to instruct thousands of students in the medical schools to whose establishment he contributed so much."[17] And those thousands of students, as Jonathan Knight pointed out, gradually filled northern New England "with a race of young, enterprising, intelligent physicians, who all justly looked up to Dr. Smith as their friend and professional father."[18] Carleton B. Chapman, a former dean of Dartmouth Medical School, once said that students were "idolatrous in their praise of Smith . . . an accomplished and devoted teacher."[19]

One of the most successful efforts to sum up Smith's career was by the physician Warfield T. Longcope (a direct descendent of Smith):

[Smith's] writings attest the fact that he had a conception of disease which is eminently modern. In a day when the etiology of infectious diseases was unknown, when speculation as to the classification of disease processes was rife, and when doubt was being cast upon the specific nature of many diseases, he let no opportunity pass to emphasize his belief in their specific character. He dwelt with emphasis upon the necessity of accurate observation and the importance of factual experience as opposed to thin-spun theory. Elaborate hypotheses, not susceptible to practical test, aroused his sharp criticism, for he looked upon them as obscuring clear vision.[20]

Yet even this seems to fall short. The source of Smith's genius was kindness tempered by wisdom and an abiding concern for his patients' well being; he saw as his chief challenge the task of conveying to his students a passionate involvement in the great fight for the patient.

Smith's day books and letters provide evidence that his schedule was as crowded as that of any modern physician or surgeon. What does not show are the time-consuming horseback or coach rides to reach his patients, the need to improvise instruments before surgery could be carried out in kitchens abruptly re-arranged as operating rooms, the lack of anesthesia and modern diagnostic tests, the prolonged periods of careful watching at the bedside, the quick awareness when complications set in, and the prompt institution of countermeasures.

Smith in his person made thousands of people healthier; through his students he improved the health of two generations and more of New Englanders. His teaching brought instruction by case history into prominence. His use of cadaver operations to teach surgery and of postmortem evaluation of his cases helped replace the traditional (and dangerously inadequate) concentration on lectures and the printed works of the "authorities."

While Smith never categorically condemned venesection, blistering, purging, and the use of stimulants popular in his day, he did preach against the belief that physicians were necessarily reduced to choosing between stimulating and depleting therapies (or wildly combining them). His greatest gift to medical practice may have been his insistence that patients be given nothing until the need was absolutely clear: Do no harm; Give nature a chance; Make the patient comfortable; Be able to justify every drug used and then give the smallest doses that will be effective. In surgery Smith promoted a cautious and conservative approach as well: Avoid surgery whenever possible; Limit the surgery to the minimum; Use the procedures that are least painful for patients; Take advantage of the anatomy of ligaments, muscles, and bones to reduce pain for the patient and limit the damage done. These are the rules of medical and surgical practice by which Smith lived and worked; these are the lessons he taught.

By focusing so much of his attention on what was comfortable and beneficial for the patient, Smith introduced a new concern for the practical effect of medicine on patients—those whom doctors were supposed to assist. Indeed, as Jonathan Knight said, Smith "effected . . . a great and salutary change in the medical profession."[21] Nathan Smith's precepts remain today as important as they are basic.

APPENDIX

Chronology of Nathan Smith's Life and Career

1762	Born in Rehoboth, Mass.
1772	Smith family moves to Chester, Vt.
1784	Assists Dr. Josiah Goodhue in performing an amputation in Chester, Vt.
	Prepares for medical study with the Rev. Samuel Whiting in Rockingham, Vt.
1784–87	Apprentices with Dr. Goodhue in Putney, Vt.
1787	Begins medical practice in Cornish, N.H.
1789	Matriculates at Harvard Medical School
1790	Awarded M.B. degree by Harvard Medical School
1791	Marries Elizabeth Chase of Cornish (who dies, childless, in 1793)
1794	Marries Sarah Hall Chase (half-sister of first wife, Elizabeth) of Cornish
1795	David Solon Chase Hall Smith (first son) born
1796	Proposes a school of medicine and himself as the Professor of Theory and Practice of Medicine to the Board of Trustees at Dartmouth College, in Hanover, N.H.
	Sails for Scotland, to begin study abroad in Glasgow, Edinburgh, and London
1797	Elected Corresponding Member of the Medical Society of London
	Nathan Ryno Smith (second son) born
	Returns to Cornish from abroad
	Founds Dartmouth Medical School by giving first medical lectures at Dartmouth College
1798	Appointed Professor of Anatomy, Chemistry, Surgery, and Theory and Practice of Medicine at Dartmouth
	Awarded A.M. degree by Dartmouth College
1799	Sarah (Sally) Malvina Smith (first daughter) born
1801	Awarded M.D. degree by Dartmouth College
ca. 1801	Moves family to Windsor, Vt.
1802	Gratia Eliza Smith (second daughter) born
1803	Mary Amanda Smith (third daughter) born
ca. 1805	Moves family residence from Windsor to Hanover
1805	James Morven Smith (third son) born
1807	Catherine Camilla Smith (fourth daughter) born
1808	Invites Scottish anatomist Dr. Alexander Ramsey to join Dartmouth Medical School faculty
1809	New Hampshire Legislature votes $3,450 for a Medical Building at Dartmouth
	Laura Matilda Smith (fifth daughter) born

1811	New Medical House in Hanover completed
	Harvard converts M.B. degree to M.D.
1812	John Derby Smith (fourth son) born
1813	Resigns Dartmouth post
	Appointed Professor of Theory and Practice of Physic, Surgery, and Obstetrics—member of first faculty of the new Institute of Medicine at Yale College, in New Haven, Conn.
1815	Sarah (Sally) Malvina Smith (oldest daughter) dies
1816	Returns to Dartmouth to teach for one term
1817	Moves family residence from Hanover to New Haven
1819	Sarah Malvina Smith (sixth daughter) born
1821	Inaugurates medical instruction at Bowdoin College, in Brunswick, Me., thus helping to found the Medical School of Maine
	Helps found the Medical School of the University of Vermont, in Burlington, Vt.
	Teaches for the first time in Burlington
1825	Resigns appointment at Bowdoin College
	Teaches for the last time in Burlington
1829	Dies in New Haven and is buried in Grove Street Cemetery

The Generations of Smith Doctors

1st Generation   Nathan Smith (1762–1829)
                  M.B./M.D. Harvard, 1790/1811
                  M.D. (h.c.) Dartmouth, 1801

2nd Generation   David Solon Chase Hall Smith (1795–1859)
                  M.D. Yale, 1816

                  Nathan Ryno Smith (1797–1877)
                  M.D. Yale, 1820

                  James Morven Smith (1805–53)
                  M.D. Yale, 1828

                  John Derby Smith (1812–84)
                  M.D. University of Maryland, 1846

3rd Generation   Elisha Warfield Theobald (1818–51)
                  [married Sarah Frances Smith]
                  M.D. Transylvania, 1839

                  Berwick Bruce Smith (1826–60)
                  M.D. University of Maryland, 1849

                  Nathan Ryno Smith, Jr. (1831–56)
                  M.D. University of Maryland, 1855

                  Alan Penniman Smith (1840–98)
                  M.D. University of Maryland, 1861

                  Walter Prescott Smith (1842–63)
                  M.D. University of Maryland, 1863

                  Nathan Smith Lincoln (1828–98)
                  M.D. University of Maryland, 1852

                  David Paige Smith (1830–80)
                  M.D. Jefferson, 1853

4th Generation   Samuel Theobald (1846–1930)
                  M.D. University of Maryland, 1867

                  Elisha Warfield Theobald, Jr. (1850–77)
                  M.D. University of Maryland, 1875

                  Nathan R. Smith (1863–1938)
                  M.D. University of Maryland, 1886

Walter Prescott Smith [II] (1868–1902)
M.D. University of Maryland, 1890

Eugene McEvers Van Ness (1868–1938)
[married Eleanor McCulloh Smith]
M.D. University of Maryland, 1891

5th Generation   J. Whitridge Williams (1865–1931)
[married Caroline DeWolf Theobald]
M.D. University of Maryland, 1888

Warfield Theobald Longcope (1877–1953)
M.D. Johns Hopkins, 1901

6th Generation   Christopher Longcope (1928-)
M.D. Johns Hopkins, 1953

7th Generation   David Longcope (1967-)
M.D. University of Vermont, 1993

Notes

Author's Note

In the interest of completeness, I have written out in detail all information in the bibliography (e.g., I give full titles of journals). To tighten the endnotes, however, I have used abbreviations extensively; there, in addition to using standard short forms for journal titles, I have abbreviated names of publishers and of most libraries, and of a handful of people whose names occur most frequently. The list of these abbreviations appears below.

One note about those instances where citations of correspondence or other documents refer the reader both to the original and to a printed version in either James A. Spalding's book (JAS) or Emily A. Smith's book (EAS): Both Spalding and Smith treated the task of transcription casually; the result is that there may be discrepancies between the version I have used and one or another of the sources.

Abbreviations

JOURNALS

For the most part, the names of the journals will be self-evident or can be quickly deciphered; three possible exceptions are listed below. In addition, I always use *JAMA* (*Journal of the American Medical Association*) and *NEJM* (*New England Journal of Medicine*) rather than spelling them out, even in the bibliography.

Bull. NYAM	*Bulletin of the New York Academy of Medicine*
DMS Alum. Mag.	*Dartmouth Medical School Alumni Magazine*
DMS Qtly.	*Dartmouth Medical School Quarterly*

PUBLISHERS

CUP	Cambridge University Press
GPO	Government Printing Office
OUP	Oxford University Press
UPNE	University Press of New England

LIBRARIES AND OTHER INSTITUTIONS

BCL	Bowdoin College Library
B/HL	Bailey/Howe Library, University of Vermont
BRBML	Beinecke Rare Book and Manuscript Library, Yale University
CLM	Francis A. Countway Library of Medicine, Harvard University
C/WML	Cushing/Whitney Medical Library, Yale University
DCA	Dartmouth College Archives, Baker Library

DMS	Dartmouth Medical School
HMS	Harvard Medical School
M&A, YUL	Manuscripts and Archives, Yale Univerity Library
MHS	Massachusetts Historical Society
NHHS	New Hampshire Historical Society
NLM	National Library of Medicine
NYAML	New York Academy of Medicine Library
NYPL	The New York Public Library, Astor, Lenox and Tilden Foundations
UVM	University of Vermont
WIHM	Wellcome Institute for the History of Medicine, London

PERSONS

EDC	Ezekiel Dodge Cushing
JG	Josiah Goodhue
MO	Mills Olcott
EAS	Emily A. Smith
GCS	George Cheyne Shattuck
JAS	James A. Spalding
LS	Lyman Spalding
NS	Nathan Smith
NRS	Nathan Ryno Smith

Occasionally, in the references, the class year for graduates of Dartmouth College or Dartmouth Medical School is given as follows: A year in parentheses, e.g., "(1803)," indicates the college class; "(m1806)" means the medical school class of that year; and "(h1797)"—as for Nathan Smith—indicates an honorary degree.

All "YRG 47-J" references belong under the general heading of "Yale Lectures."

Chapter 1. The Early Years

1. *Complimentary Dinner Given to Professor S. D. Gross . . . April 10, 1879* (Philadelphia: J. M. Wilson, 1856), 13. Response of Samuel D. Gross to the first toast.

2. NS's gravestone in the Grove Street Cemetery in New Haven (see Herbert Thoms, "Nathan Smith," *Jrnl. Med. Ed.* 33, no. 12 [Dec. 1958]: 825) and most published accounts of his life say he was born on 30 Sept. 1762. This was clearly the family tradition. On the other hand, Richard LeBaron Bowen, in *Early Rehoboth: Documented Historical Studies of Families and Events in This Plymouth Colony Township*, 4 vols. (Rehoboth, Mass.: privately printed, 1946), 2:117, gives NS's birth date as 12 Sept. 1762, without any discussion that would indicate uncertainty on the point; similarly, James N. Arnold, in the earlier *Vital Record of Rehoboth, 1642–1896. Marriages, Intentions, Births, Deaths.* (Providence: Narragansett Hist. Publ., 1897), 745, gives 12 Sept. 1762 as NS's birthdate. Three writers—see the Putnam, Stone, and Williams entries in the Bibliography (pp. 347, 348, and 349)—follow Bowen and Arnold.

3. See Carl Bridenbaugh, *Cities in Revolt, Urban Life in America 1743–76* (New York: Knopf, 1955), 226–27, 232, 368–69, and 415, for insight into life in Newport and the vicinity in the colonial period.

4. George Dimmock to Gilman D. Frost, 22 Jan. 1920; Gilman Frost Gene-alogical Papers, DH-15, DCA.

5. Bernard Bailyn, Robert Dallek, David Brion Davis, et al., *The Great Republic: A History of the American People*, 3d ed. (Lexington, Mass.: Heath, 1985), 44.

6. Bowen, op. cit., 4; Land Records: Chester, Windsor County, Vt., Vol. B, p. 181.

7. See John Duffy, "Smallpox and the Indians of the American Colonies," *Bull. Hist. Med.* 25, no. 4 (July–Aug. 1951): 324–42, for a careful description and analysis of the waves of smallpox epidemics that swept the East Coast during a period of more than a century.

8. Richard N. Wilkie and Jack Tager, eds., *Historical Atlas of Massachusetts* (Amherst: Univ. of Mass. Press, 1991), 143.

9. Town Records: Chester, Windsor County, Vt., 1772–1775, Vol. A, pp. 19, 20, 22, 24, 26, 28, 31, 33, 35, 39, 40.

10. John Smith's gravestone in the Brookside Cemetery in Chester, Vermont, is inscribed as follows: "Here lies Buried Mr John Smeth Who died Janeury 13th 1775 In The 58th year of his age." Tradition has it that Smith died of a wilderness accident ("killed by the fall of a tree" is how it was put in JG to GCS, 4 Mar. 1829; Shattuck Papers, MHS), but there is no mention of such an accident in Chester Town Records. A notice in the Town Meeting Warning of 1 Feb. 1775 simply lets us know Smith had died by that time; one item of business was "To Choose an Overseer of the Poor in the Room of [in place of] Mr. John Smith, Decd." Town Records: Chester, Windsor County, Vt., 1772–1775, Vol. A, p. 42.

11. JG to GCS, 4 Mar. 1829; Shattuck Papers, MHS.

12. John F. Morse, "Introductory Lecture," *San Fran. Med. Press* 6, no. 16 (Jan. 1864): 169.

13. EAS, *The Life and Letters of Nathan Smith, M.B., M.D.* (New Haven: Yale Univ. Press, 1914), 5.

14. Samuel C. Harvey points out in "The Education of Nathan Smith," *Yale Jrnl. Biol. & Med.* 1, no. 5 (March 1929): 261, that the "physical prowess necessary for the discipline of adolescent boys was not less important than intellectual facility."

15. Vital Records: Chester, Windsor County, Vt., Vol. A, p. 141; Martha Mc-Danolds Frizzell, *A History of Walpole, New Hampshire*, 2 vols. (Walpole, N.H.: Walpole Hist. Soc., 1963), 2:224, cites a marriage between a Samuel Parker and Hannah Messer on 15 Apr. 1779, six months prior to the marriage of Samuel Parker and Elizabeth Smith noted in the Chester, Vt., Vital Records. No reference to this latter marriage—or to any other Samuel Parker—appears in Walpole town records. (The earlier town history, George Aldrich's *Walpole As it Was and As It Is, Containing the Complete Civil History of the Town From 1749 to 1879* [Claremont, N.H.: Claremont Manufacturing, Printer, 1880] also has nothing on a Samuel Parker.)

16. Land Records: Chester, Windsor County, Vt., Vol. B, p. 186 (12 Oct. 1779).

17. See, e.g., JG to GCS, 4 Mar. 1829; Shattuck Papers, MHS. EAS, op. cit., 4–5, and J[onathan] Knight, *An Eulogium on Nathan Smith, M.D.* (New Haven: Hezekiah Howe, 1829), reprinted in NRS, ed., *Medical and Surgical Memoirs, by Nathan Smith, M.D.* (Baltimore: Wm. A. Francis, 1831), 12–36. (All subsequent

references to Knight's "Eulogium" will be to the pages on which it is found in NRS, ed., *Memoirs*.)

18. EAS, op. cit., 4, quotes an unattributed source saying that NS "at one time 'narrowly escaped a bullet aimed at him by a son of the forest.'" She may have relied in part on Stephen W. Williams, "Dr. Nathan Smith," in his *American Medical Biography, or Memoirs of Eminent Physicians* (Greenfield, Mass.: L. Merriam, 1845), 525, for this tale—which Williams tells without giving a source. He does, at least, indicate general reliance on Knight, op. cit., and NRS, ed., op. cit.

19. EAS, loc. cit., goes on in the same paragraph to say that NS "was promoted from the ranks to a captaincy" at the age of eighteen (and other writers have clearly relied on her account). But see John E. Goodrich, *The State of Vermont Rolls of the Soldiers in the Revolutionary War 1775 to 1783* (Rutland, Vt.: Tuttle, 1904), 386, 533, 534. Those who credit NS with this promotion do not seem to have read Goodrich with sufficient care, apparently confusing the several different individuals by the name of "Nathan Smith"with each other.

20. JG to GCS, 4 Mar. 1829; Shattuck Papers, MHS. Written just six months before its author died at the age of seventy-one, this letter contains a number of anecdotes about Smith (and a poignant observation that there would be more to tell if Goodhue were not himself ill and thus finding it difficult to write), plus a confirmation of all Knight had said in his "Eulogium."

21. Williams, op. cit., 203. Williams says Kittredge was from "Fakesbury," but Thoms, op. cit., 817, says Dr. Thomas Kittredge was from Andover, thus making "Tewksbury"—a town bordering on Andover—a likely reading for the nonexistent "Fakesbury." But some confusion is understandable. There were "a dozen Dr. Kittredges practicing in New England" at the time; see JAS, *Life of Dr. Lyman Spalding* (Boston: W. M. Leonard, 1916), 43, n1. For more on Goodhue, see, e.g., Walter L. Burrage, "Goodhue, Josiah (1759–1829)," in Howard A. Kelly and Walter L. Burrage, eds., *American Medical Biographies* (Baltimore: Norman, Remington, 1920), 449.

22. Williams, op. cit., 204.

23. Burrage, op. cit., 449. Williams, loc. cit., says Kittredge had a medical library that "did not consist of more than half a dozen volumes." Whether Burrage confused the size of Kittredge's library with that of Goodhue, or whether it is true of each that (initially) only about six volumes were on hand, is not now clear. In any case, according to Burrage, op. cit., 450, when Goodhue could afford to buy books later in his career, he did so systematically, building a good medical library and making an effort to stay abreast of new information. Williams, op. cit., also stresses this, making the point twice; see pp. 204 and 209.

24. Williams, op. cit., 205; Burrage, op. cit., 449.

25. Oliver P. Hubbard, *Dartmouth Medical College and Nathan Smith: An Historical Discourse* (Concord, N.H.: Evans, Sleeper & Evans, 1879), 9, citing Henry I. Bowditch, *Memoir of Amos Twitchell, M.D.* (Boston: John Wilson and Son, 1851), 28, note.

26. Harvey Cushing, *The Medical Career: An Address on The Ideals, Opportunities, and Difficulties of the Medical Profession* . . . (Hanover, N.H.: Dartmouth College, 1929), 29.

27. EAS, op. cit., 5. Note that EAS uses precisely the same phrase Hubbard did: "without a tremor."

28. Thomas Francis Harrington, *The Harvard Medical School: A History,*

Narrative and Documentary, 1782–1905, 3 vols. (New York: Lewis Publ., 1905) 1:337.

29. Stephen W. Williams, "Dr. Josiah Goodhue," in his *American Medical Biography, or Memoirs of Eminent Physicians* (Greenfield, Mass.: L. Merriam, 1845), 206.

30. G. E. R. Lloyd, ed., *Hippocratic Writings* (London: Penguin, 1993), 67.

31. Stephen W. Williams, *A Biographical Memoir of Josiah Goodhue, M.D....* (Pittsfield, Mass.: Phineas Allen and Son, 1829), 11–12, quotes these words of JG's, saying they came from the latter's inaugural address as president of the Berkshire Medical Institution on 23 Dec. 1823. (This "Memoir," presented orally at the Berkshire Medical Institution on 20 Nov. 1829, shortly after JG's death, was the basis for Williams's article on JG in *American Medical Biography*; see *supra*, n29.) See also Peter D. Gibbons, "The Berkshire Medical Institution," *Bull. Hist. Med.* 38, no. 1 (Jan.–Feb. 1964): 45–64.

32. Knight, in NRS, ed., op. cit., 16.

33. Ibid., 16–17.

34. See Lyman Simpson Hayes, *History of the Town of Rockingham, Vermont, Including the Villages of Bellows Falls, Saxtons River, Rockingham, Cambridgeport, and Bartonsville, 1753–1907, with Family Genealogies* (Bellows Falls: Town of Rockingham, 1907), esp. pp. 123–26, for information on Samuel Whiting. See also Constance E. Putnam, "The Rockingham Roots of Dartmouth Medical School: Samuel Whiting and Nathan Smith" (unpublished mss.).

35. James R. Hadley, on the faculty at Yale at the time, in his journal for 5 Mar. 1843, claimed that William Tully (whom we will later meet) told him—*inter alia*—NS "was an illiterate man"; Laura Hadley Moseley, ed., *Diary (1843–1852) of James Hadley* (New Haven: Yale Univ. Press, 1951), 3. This is clearly false. Consider, for instance, NS's book-order account with Charles Spear, in Hanover, between 1811 and 1814. In addition to two books of poetry and a subscription to the *Dartmouth Gazette*, he purchased a copy of Homer's *Iliad* and a commentary on Homer—unlikely purchases for an illiterate; DA-3, Box 15 (S Folder), DCA. For comments on Hadley's report of Tully's assertion, see Oliver S. Hayward, "A Student of Dr. Nathan Smith," *Conn. Med.* 24, no. 9 (Sept. 1960): 555.

36. See Mary Cabot, *Annals of Brattleboro, Vt. 1681–1875* (Brattleboro: E. L. Hildreth, 1921), 1:208.

37. An item in the *[Brattleboro, Vt.] Reporter* 4, no. 160 (8 Mar. 1806): [2], attests to Dickerman's advanced ideas, in a report of his use of "Kine Pock" inoculations to ward off smallpox.

38. Receipts signed by JG, 20 July 1804 and 24 Sept. 1813; DA-3, Box 15 (G Folder), DCA.

39. JG to GCS, 4 Mar. 1829; Shattuck Papers, MHS.

40. For sample brief discussions of apprenticeship, see: Henry K. Beecher and Mark D. Altschule, *Medicine at Harvard: The First Three Hundred Years* (Hanover, N.H.: UPNE, 1977), 14–16; John Duffy, *From Humors to Medical Science: A History of American Medicine* (Urbana and Chicago: Univ. of Ill. Press, 1993), 130–31; Genevieve Miller, "Medical Apprenticeship in the American Colonies," *Ciba Symposium* 8, no. 10 (Jan. 1947): 502–10; and Carl J. Pfeiffer, *The Art and Practice of Western Medicine in the Early Nineteenth Century* (Jefferson, N.C.: McFarland, 1985), 111–12.

41. Charles Caldwell, *Autobiography* (Philadelphia: Lippincott, Grambo, 1855), 77. Quoted in William G. Rothstein, *American Physicians in the Nine-*

teenth Century: From Sects to Science (Baltimore: Johns Hopkins Univ. Press, 1985), 102.

42. Nathan S. Davis, *Contributions to the History of Medical Education and Medical Institutions in the United States of America 1776–1876* (Washington, D.C.: GPO, 1877), 241.

43. Daniel Drake, *Discourses, Delivered by Appointment, Before the Cincinnati Medical Library Association* (Cincinnati: Moore & Anderson, 1852), 55–56.

44. James Thomas Flexner, *Doctors on Horseback: Pioneers of American Medicine* (New York: Garden City Publ., 1939), 182–83.

45. Burrage, op. cit., 449.

46. Thomas Eaton Papers, Diary, 1791–1793; MS-387, DCA. Brief excerpts appeared in George Van Ness Dearborn, "Medical Practice in New England in 1792," *Boston Med. and Surg. Jrnl.* 196, no. 12 (24 Mar. 1927): 476–82.

47. Thirty-five years after NS's death, some thirty of his books (plus sixteen volumes of a London journal) were part of the Yale collection; see Frederick G. Kilgour, *The Library of the Medical Institution of Yale College and its Catalogue of 1865* (New Haven: Yale Univ. Press, 1960), 33–35, 39, 45, 47–50, 52, 54–55, 59–61, 66–67. By one hundred years after NS's death, it appears most of the books had been dispersed. A list prepared when the NS books then being kept on a special shelf in the "Medical Room" at Yale were scattered and shelved in the general collection included only eleven volumes, ranging from John Abernethy on surgery to two titles by Benjamin Rush. See Anne S. Pratt, to Samuel C. Harvey, 29 Jan. and 16 Feb. 1932; in files of C. E. Putnam, Concord, Mass.

48. Knight, "Eulogium," in NRS, ed., op. cit., 15.

49. This information and the two quotations that follow are from JG to GCS, 4 Mar. 1829; Shattuck Papers, MHS.

Chapter 2. Newly Minted Doctor

1. *The Works of Thomas Sydenham, M.D., on Acute and Chronic Diseases*, with notes by Benjamin Rush (Philadelphia: Benjamin & Thomas Kite, 1809), 362.

2. Nathan S. Davis, *Contributions to the History of Medical Education and Medical Institutions in the United States of America, 1776–1876* (Washington, D.C., GPO, 1877), 24.

3. JG to GCS, 4 Mar. 1829; Shattuck Papers, MHS.

4. Elijah W. Carpenter, "Lectures at New Haven on Surgery, Midwifery, Theory and Practice of Physic By Nathan Smith, M.D.," p. 50; YRG 47-J, M&A, YUL.

5. Wilder Dwight Quint, obituary notice on Samuel Powers, *Dart. Alum. Mag.* (Feb. 1930): 284–85; Samuel Powers (1874) Alumni File, DCA.

6. See, e.g., Virgina Reed Colby and James B. Atkinson, *Footprints of the Past: Images of Cornish, New Hampshire & the Cornish Art Colony* (Concord, N.H.: NHHS, 1996).

7. The two-volume "Journal of Dr. James Moore, 25 June 1790 — 2 Oct. 1794," comes to an abrupt end on p. 113 of vol. 2 (perhaps he left town). Account Books, Hanover, 39; Vault Mss., DCA. In *The Records of the Town of Hanover New Hampshire 1761–1818* (Hanover, N.H., 1905), 96 and 97, there are passing references to Dr. James More [sic] of Hanover as well as to Dr. George Eager in connection with a matter that came up in 1790. The latter had been in Hanover at

least since 1777, when he was "furnished" by Hanover to serve as a surgeon in the Revolutionary War; see *A History of Dartmouth College and the Town of Hanover New Hampshire,* by Frederick Chase (John K. Lord, ed.), 2 vols. (Cambridge: John Wilson and Son, 1891), 1:390. Thus we know there were at least these two physicians in the area.

8. This information, and much of what follows on the Chase family, is taken largely from Hugh Mason Wade, *A Brief History of Cornish 1763–1974* (Hanover, N.H.: UPNE, 1976), 18–19. See also entries under individual names in William H. Child, *History of the Town of Cornish, New Hampshire, with Genealogical Record, 1763–1918,* 2 vols. (Concord, N.H.: Rumford Press, [n.d.—probably 1911]).

9. See, e.g., NS Accounts, Beginning 1792, pp. 20 and 137; Vault Mss., DCA. Also see receipt from 10 Apr. 1806; DA-3, Box 15 (C Folder), DCA.

10. NS seems generally to have drunk alone. See, e.g., three separate charges to NS for a glass of brandy in Account Book of the Old Chase Tavern, Cornish, N.H., p. 187; Vault Mss., DCA. On the other hand, there is at least one account in NS's own hand of an occasion when he and several other physicians—following a medical meeting at Kimball's, in Charlestown, New Hampshire, "which was conducted with propriety & good order"—sat around and (not to put too fine a point on it) got drunk together. NS's account is both lighthearted and revealingly honest about this night on the town. NS to Benjamin Gilbert, 23 Aug. 1793; Mss. 793473, DCA.

11. Child, op. cit., 1:273.

12. See, in general, Cornish Town Records, Cornish, N.H.

13. Trinity Church Papers, Cornish Hist. Soc., Cornish, N.H., include documents of the "Episcopal Society of the Church of England" (e.g., 27 June 1800), "Trinity Church in Cornish" (e.g., 1 Aug. 1803), and "Protestant Episcopal Church" (e.g., 1 Nov. 1805). In this latter instance, Ithemer [sic] and Jonathan Chase were Wardens and Caleb Chase was Clerk. On 10 Apr. 1809, Lebbeus Chase, Caleb Chase, and Dr. Solomon Chase were all vestrymen. Most impressive, perhaps, was the roster of church officers on 7 Apr. 1806: Ithamar Chase, Moderator; Caleb Chase, Clerk; Jonathan Chase, Warden, and Dudley Chase and Dr. Solomon Chase, Vestrymen.

14. Child, op. cit., 2:335. The story was also recounted by Bela Bates Edwards in an asterisked note ("We remember to have heard an anecdote," with no indication as to what his source was), in his *Biography of Self-Taught Men,* 2 vols. (Boston: Benjamin Perkins & Co., 1846/7), 2:111–12.

15. NS Accounts, Beginning 1792, pp. 36, 18, 9, 17, 10, and 27 respectively; Vault Mss., DCA. Later account books and ledgers are, unfortunately, less informative with respect to what medical services NS performed; he tended to list only names, dates, and amounts charged.

16. Gordon A. Donaldson, "The Legacy of Nathan Smith," *Harvard Med. Alum. Bull.* 55, no. 1 (Feb. 1981): 22. Donaldson gave no source. We know NS sold his horse to go to England (NS to LS, 11 Dec. 1796; Mss. 796690, DCA—in JAS, *Life of Dr. Lyman Spalding* [Boston: W. M. Leonard, 1916], 7), which Donaldson also mentioned (24), though again without giving a source. To be sure, it is possible that NS resorted to this means of raising cash on both occasions, as A. W. Oughterson explicitly stated in "Nathan Smith and Cancer Therapy," *Yale Jrnl. Biol. & Med.* 12, no. 2 (December 1939): 125, 126. But Oughterson also gave no source for what he said.

17. JG reported that NS succeeded in raising the money to pay his tavern bill en route to his mother's by riding out to demand payment of an outstanding bill from an old patient who lived nearby. JG to GCS, 4 Mar. 1829; Shattuck Papers, MHS.

18. Henry K. Beecher and Mark D. Altschule, *Medicine at Harvard: The First Three Hundred Years* (Hanover, N.H.: UPNE, 1977), 29–30. See also the excellent account in Thomas Edward Moore, Jr., "The Early Years of the Harvard Medical School," *Bull. Hist. Med.* 27, no. 6 (Nov.–Dec. 1953): 530–61.

19. George E. Ellis, *Memoir of James Bigelow, M.D., LL.D.* (Cambridge, Mass.: J. Wilson, 1880), 15–16. Thomas Edward Moore, Jr., op. cit., 550–51, describes John Warren's approach to teaching in a way that gives plausibility to the idea that Warren influenced Smith considerably.

20. John B. Blake, *Benjamin Waterhouse and the Introduction of Vaccination: A Reappraisal* (Philadelphia: Univ. of Penn. Press, 1957), 12.

21. Beecher and Altschule, op. cit., 42, 44.

22. Benjamin Waterhouse to John Coakley Lettsom, 25 Nov. 1794, in Thomas Joseph Pettigrew, *Memoirs of the Life and Writings of the Late John Coakley Lettsom, M.D.*, 3 vols. (London: Longman, Hurst, Rees, Orme, and Brown, 1817) 2:464–65.

23. Beecher and Altschule, op. cit., 45. See also Francis D. Moore, "*In Medicina, Veritas*: The Birth and Turbulent Youth of the Faculty of Medicine at Harvard College," *NEJM* 307, no. 15 (7 Oct. 1982): 922–23.

24. Blake, op. cit., 74.

25. Oliver Wendell Holmes, *Address and Exercises at the One Hundredth Anniversary of the Foundation of the Medical School of Harvard University, October 17, 1883* (Cambridge, Mass.: John Wilson and Son, 1884), 6. The story is also told in Samuel C. Harvey, "The Education of Nathan Smith," *Yale Jrnl. Biol. & Med.* 1, no. 5 (March 1929): 263.

26. EAS, *The Life and Letters of Nathan Smith, M.B., M.D.* (New Haven: Yale Univ. Press, 1914), 10.

27. See *Harvard University: Quinquennial Catalogue of the Officers and Graduates, 1636–1930* (Cambridge, Mass.: Published by the University, 1930), 851. See also Thomas Francis Harrington, *The Harvard Medical School: A History, Narrative and Documentary, 1782–1905*, 3 vols. (New York: Lewis Publ., 1905) 1:335–54, where the entire ch. 13 ("Nathan Smith") is devoted to NS.

28. NS, "A dissertation on the causes and effects of spasm in fevers; pronounced by Mr. Nathan Smith, before the President, Medical Professors, and Governors of Harvard University, at Cambridge, July 5th, 1790, and dedicated to the Rev. J. Willard, S.T.D. Prof.," *Mass. Mag.* 3, no. 1 (Jan. 1791): 33–35; and 3, no. 2 (Feb. 1791): 81–83. Incidentally, one occasionally comes across references to NS having written a "graduation thesis" at Harvard on the circulation of the blood; see, e.g., [E. C. Kelly], "Bibliography of Nathan Smith's Writings," in *Medical Classics* 1, no. 8 (Apr. 1937): 775; Lee D. Van Antwerp, "Nathan Smith and Early American Medical Education," *Ann. Med. Hist.* 9, n.s. (Sept. 1937): 452; and Oliver P. Hubbard, *Dartmouth Medical College and Nathan Smith: An Historical Discourse* (Concord, N.H.: Evans, Sleeper & Evans, 1879), 10. But a carefully inserted handwritten note in the copy of Hubbard's essay in C. E. Putnam's possession (in the edition published the following year [Washington, D.C.: Globe, 1880]) on that same page says, "An error. V. p. 26"; a further handwritten notation on p. 26 draws attention to the fact that NS's "Dissertation on the causes and

effects of spasms in fevers" was his "Inaugural Dissertation," as we have already stated. These annotations appear to have been made either by the author of the essay (O. P. Hubbard) or by the librarian (M. D. Bisbee) in response to a letter to him from Hubbard. See O. P. Hubbard to M. D. Bisbee, 24 June 1897; Mss. 897374, DCA. No paper by NS on circulation of the blood has been found; neither has any reason (beyond the occasional undocumented claims) been found to support the idea that he wrote on the topic, as Hubbard makes clear in his letter to Bisbee.

29. A. Z., Note [to the editor], *Mass. Mag.* 3, no. 1 (Jan. 1791): 33.

30. Philozetemia, "Critique on Dr. Smith's Theory of Spasm," *Mass. Mag.* 3, no. 8 (Aug. 1791): 478–79; NS, "Dr. Smith's Reply," *Mass. Mag.* 4, no. 5 (May 1792): 314–15; Philozetemia, "Philozetemia's Reply to Dr. Smith," *Mass. Mag.* 4, no. 8 (Aug. 1792): 487–88; NS, "Dr. Smith's Replication to Philozetemia," *Mass. Mag.* 5, no. 4 (Apr. 1793): 218–21.

31. Philozetemia, "Reply," 487–88.

32. NS, "A dissertation," 34, 35, 81–83.

33. Beecher and Altschule, op. cit., 34, 35, 39; see also Edward Warren, *The Life of John Warren, M.D.* (Boston: Noyes, Holmes, 1874), 225–26.

34. Charles W. Turner, "Letters (1790–1800) of John Johnston, Rockridge Medical Student and Doctor," *Jrnl. Hist. Med. and Allied Sciences* 14, no. 2 (Apr. 1959): 193.

35. Oliver S. Hayward and Elizabeth H. Thomson, eds., *The Journal of William Tully, Medical Student at Dartmouth 1808–1809* (New York: Science History, 1977), 32.

36. Alton S. Pope and Raymond S. Patterson, "M. Appleton: Chronicler of Colonial Medicine," *Harvard Med. Alum. Bull.* 36, no. 4 (Spr. 1962): 19.

37. M[oses] Appleton, "Syllabus of a course of Anatomical Lectures delivered at Harvard University Oct. 1st 1794 by John Warren M.D."; CLM. The questions appear on ca. pp. 109–14 [no pg. nos. given]; they are quoted in Pope and Patterson, op. cit., 19, 21.

38. NS to Benjamin Waterhouse, 28 Dec. 1794, CLM. See also Francis D. Moore, op. cit., 922.

39. NS to John Warren, 2 Nov. 1790; J. C. Warren Papers, MHS.

40. NS to John Warren, 14 Feb. 1791; J. C. Warren Papers, MHS.

41. Compare this with the record we have of one John M. Martin having "Received for Dr Smith, of William Tully Twenty-five Dollars, in part his Bill for tuition"—quite independent of any board—on 4 Nov. 1809; DA-3, Box 15 (L–N Folder), DCA.

42. Benjamin Waterhouse to John Warren, [?] Feb. 1796; J. C. Warren Papers, MHS.

43. Benjamin Waterhouse to John Warren, 23 Apr. 1796; J. C. Warren Papers, MHS.

44. Benjamin Waterhouse to John Warren, 20 Feb. 1797 (emphasis in original); J. C. Warren Papers, MHS.

45. A draft memo (undated, but clearly from about this time) in John Warren's hand—giving his answers to Waterhouse's questions—indicates that his view of the affair was, indeed, more sympathetic to Smith than to Waterhouse; J. C. Warren Papers, MHS. See also John Warren's earlier affidavit in the Waterhouse affair, from [?] April 1795; J. C. Warren Papers, MHS.

46. The case of NS vs. Benjamin West, Trustee for Benjamin Waterhouse, hav-

ing first been decided in favor of NS, was appealed by Waterhouse and then continued to the May Term 1797, Superior Court, Keene, N.H. "The parties being three times solemnly called do not appear but make default. This action is therefore dismissed"; *Cheshire Records*, Vol. 4, p. 194.

47. NS to John Warren, 4 May 1797; J. C. Warren Papers, MHS.

48. Child, op. cit., 2:334. EAS, op. cit., 11, puts the date of death ten days earlier, on 14 April.

49. Years later, in a letter written to his close friend GCS, when *his* wife died, Smith expressed something of how he felt about his own first wife's death—one of the very few records we have in which NS shows any depth of emotion. NS to GCS, 3 July 1828; Shattuck Papers, MHS.

50. EAS, op. cit., 12.

51. Loc. cit.

52. Ibid., 13. But see EDC to Mehitable Cushing [mother], 15 Dec. 1809; EDC Papers (Folder 1), M&A, YUL.

53. EAS, op. cit., 21.

54. According to Louise Hubbard, intellectuals of the second half of the eighteenth century were "fond of reading poetry and the translations of the lays of Ossian were favorite pieces." See "Morven Got Its Name From an Ossian Lay," *Wash. Post* (7 July 1962): D10. In those "lays of Ossian," we can read such lines as "Did thy beauty last, O Ryno?" "Malvina is like the shower . . . They say that I am fair . . . ," and "[S]ons of cloudy Morven!" See James Macpherson, *Poems of Ossian*, 2 vols. (London: Printed for A. Strahan and T. Cadell, 1796), 2:187, 147, and 53 respectively. In a review of the most recent edition of Macpherson's work (Howard Gaskill, ed., *The Poems of Ossian and Related Works* [Edinburgh: Edinburgh Univ. Press, 1997]), Ossian's importance for late eighteenth- and early nineteenth-century readers and writers alike is repeatedly stressed. See Robert Crawford, "Post-Cullodenism," *London Rev. of Bks.* (3 Oct. 1996): 18.

55. NRS, ed., *Medical and Surgical Memoirs, by Nathan Smith, M.D.* (Baltimore: Wm. A. Francis, 1831), 9–12, 36–37.

56. Hayward and Thomson, eds., op. cit., 30.

Chapter 3. New Ventures

1. Composed (in Greek as well as in Latin) for students of the Classics at Montclair High School, Montclair, N.J., some time in the early part of the twentieth century. Translated by and in files of C. E. Putnam, Concord, Mass.

2. Cornish Town Records, Cornish, N.H., 30 Aug. 1790.

3. "As a result of differences of opinion, then everywhere prevailing, concerning inoculation and the fear that these [pest houses] might serve as centers of contagion, [they] were the subject of violent quarrels among citizens. . . ." Leon B. Richardson, *Fifty Years of Service: A History of the Mary Hitchcock Memorial Hospital.* (Hanover, N.H.: [no publ.] [1943]), 3.

4. NS to John Warren, 14 Feb. 1791; J. C. Warren Papers, MHS.

5. For entries on visits to Clark, Cady, and Dutton, see NS Accounts, Beginning 1792, pp. 27, 42, 63; Vault Mss., DCA. (Richard Lang's account with NS beginning 14 May 1801 [DA-3, Box 15 (L–N Folder), DCA] gives the balance in both dollars and pounds; hence we know $10 was equal to roughly £3 at that time.)

6. Account Book of the Old Chase Tavern, Cornish, N.H., 16 Nov. 1792, p.

187; Vault Mss., DCA. More often, as noted earlier, NS seems to have visited the tavern alone. In addition to the charges on that same page to NS for a glass of brandy (see *supra*, ch. 2, n10), he was charged on 6 May 1793, p. 195, for "1 mug Grog," then for "1 gill Rum," and finally "1 gill D°." He apparently enjoyed diverse libations. On 3 May 1792, he had half a mug of egg rum (p. 182), while later in that month—on one day—he had "3 glasses Rum in Toddy" (p. 183); in August, he had "1 Glass punch" (p. 184) and later "1 Glass Brandy Sling" (p. 185); in Feb. 1793 on one occasion he ordered "1 pt. wine" (p. 192). The list could easily be extended.

7. NS to John Warren, 30 Aug. 1791; J. C. Warren Papers, MHS.

8. Rufus Turner, ["Notebook of . . . , Medical Institution of Yale College 1813"], includes thirty pages of NS's remarks on midwifery and obstetrics along with his "Directions to the Accoucheur." Peter L. Woodbury, "Lectures on Theory and Practice of Medicine by Nathan Smith, M.D.," likewise includes "Directions to the Accoucheur" (pp. 173–96); both Turner's and Woodbury's notebooks are in YRG 47-J, M&A, YUL. Further evidence that NS regularly gave his lecture of advice to the accoucheur is that it appears in so many of the extant student notebooks. Among others are these: Worham L. Fitch, "Directions to the Accoucheur," in "Lectures on the Practice of Physic and Surgery by Nathan Smith . . . in the Medical Institution of Yale College, 1825," pp. 60–76; YRG 47-J, M&A, YUL. Avery J. Skilton, "Directions to the Accoucheur," pp. 149–52, in Eli Ives, "Lectures on the Diseases of Children"; MS F 12, NLM. See also Abraham Lines Smyth, "Directions to the Accoucher [sic]," in "Notes from Lectures [on the Theory and Practice of Physic] delivered in Yale College, New Haven, 1823"; NYAML (published with an introductory note in Gertrude L. Annan, "Advice of Nathan Smith, 1762–1829, on the Conduct of an Accoucheur," *Bull. NYAM* 12, no. 9 [Sept. 1936]: 528–34).

9. William C. Ellsworth, "Extracts from the lectures on the theory & practice of physic, as delivered in a course of lectures at Dartmouth College, Oct. 1, 1806 by Nathan Smith, M.D.," p. [14]; Vault Mss., DCA.

10. NS Daybook, Sept. 1797–Mar. 1801 [Day Book B], entries for 30 Jan. 1798 (p. 28) and 6 May 1798 (p. 56); Vault Mss., DCA.

11. See William F. Putnam (1930, m1932) to family members, 20 Jan. 1961, from Lyme, N.H.: "I have many beautiful vistas of the New Hampshire hills which are the beginning of the White Mountains. The bright snowcap on Moosilaukee, gleaming in the sun, contrasts with the somber, almost black dome of Smarts Mountain, while the nearer hills show their characteristic patches of snow, the dark green of the evergreens and the gray of the bare, deciduous trees, with the white lines of the birches frequently interspersed." In files of C. E. Putnam, Concord, Mass.

12. Dr. Garret K. Lawrence describes the local flora of upstate New York (not significantly different from that of northern New England) with specific reference to the medicinal properties such plants might offer in a letter to C. S. Rafinisque (author of *Medical Flora* [Philadelphia: Atkinson & Alexander, 1828]); see Alex Berman, "An Unpublished Letter from G. K. Lawrence to C. S. Rafinisque, October 8, 1828," *Bull. Hist. Med.* 34, no. 5 (Sept.–Oct. 1960): 461–70. The text of the letter itself appears on pp. 464, 467–68.

13. Nathan Noyes to Samuel and Rebecca Noyes [his parents], 16 Aug. 1798; Mss. 798466.1, DCA.

14. Jonathan Knight, "Eulogium," in NRS, ed., *Medical and Surgical Memoirs by Nathan Smith, M.D.* (Baltimore: Wm. A. Francis, 1831), 16.

15. Ibid., 17–18.

16. NS to John Warren, 2 Nov. 1790 and 30 Aug. 1791; J. C. Warren Papers, MHS.

17. Martin Kaufman, *American Medical Education: The Formative Years, 1795–1910* (Westport, Conn.: Greenwood, 1976), 30.

18. Cornish Town Records, Cornish, N.H., 8 Mar. 1796.

19. See the undated "Memorandum of books purchased by Newcomb A. Fairchild," which lists books ranging in price from "Barton on goitre" for $.50 and "Desault's surgery" at $2.50 to "Denman's Midwifery" at $4.00, "Physick's improved trephine" at $5.00, and "Burdin's medical Studies" for $7.50; DA-3, Box 15 (Accounts Relating to DMS Folder), DCA. (The last of these books was presumably Jean Burdin's *Course of Medical Studies* (London: Cuthnell and Martin, 1803), since that and Thomas Denman's *Introduction to the Practice of Midwifery*, 2^d ed. (London: J. Johnson, 1801) were both later among the books Smith gave Yale; see *supra*, ch. 1, n47.)

20. Account Books, Hanover 3: Jedediah Baldwin, Ledger, 1791–1811, Vol. 9, p. 49; DCA.

21. Later, when LS was assisting NS at Dartmouth (see ch. 4), LS's dissatisfaction with arrangements for his teaching responsibilities is a theme running through much of the correspondence; these letters are also our best source of information for NS's views on the subject. See, e.g., NS to LS, 8 Sept. 1800; LS Papers, NHHS. In JAS, *Life of Dr. Lyman Spalding* (Boston: W. M. Leonard, 1916), 48. Other relevant letters also in JAS, op. cit., are John Wheelock to LS, 9 Sept. 1800 (48–49); LS to William Woodward, 17 Sept. 1800 (49–50); and NS to LS, 30 Sept. 1800 (51).

22. Leon Burr Richardson, *History of Dartmouth College* (Hanover, N.H.: Dartmouth College Pubs., 1932), 236.

23. Ibid., 202–203; cf. Frederick Chase (John K. Lord, ed.), *A History of Dartmouth College and The Town of Hanover, New Hampshire*, 2 vols. (Cambridge, Mass.: John Wilson and Son, 1891) 1:615.

24. NS, "Proposal for [a] Medical Institution," Aug. 1796; Mss. 796490.2, DCA.

25. NS to Board of Trust, 25 Aug. 1796; Mss. 796475, DCA.

26. Extract from Minutes, Annual Mtg. of Board of Trustees (Dartmouth College), B. Woodward, secretary, Aug. 1796; Mss. 796490, DCA.

27. John Wheelock to the Rev. Samuel Peters, 7 Nov. 1796; Mss. 796607, DCA.

28. W. F. Bynum, *Science and the Practice of Medicine in the Nineteenth Century* (Cambridge: CUP, 1994), 4.

29. Tobias George Smollett, *The Expedition of Humphry Clinker* (New York: Century, 1907 [1770]), 243.

30. NS to LS, 19 Nov. 1796; Mss. 796619.1, DCA. In JAS, op. cit., 6. A memo with dates from 1796 to 1799 provides further evidence that the two men were working closely together during this period and that LS was probably serving as *locum tenens* for NS; certainly he was generally collecting bills on NS's behalf. See "Nathan Smith in account with Lyman Spalding"; DA-3, Box 15 (Accounts Relating to DMS Folder), DCA.

31. The lawyer (later judge) Sanford Kingsbury was a leading citizen (he often

held town office) of Claremont, New Hampshire. That he was relatively well-to-do is clear from the fact that he presented the Episcopal Church in Claremont with service of Holy Communion "of more valuable material" (probably silver—the service they had been using was of pewter); Otis F. R. Waite, *History of the Town of Claremont, New Hampshire for a period of One hundred thirty Years, From 1764 to 1894* (Manchester, N.H.: Town of Claremont, 1895), 100 (see also p. 446 for a summary account of Kingsbury's importance in town). Oliver P. Hubbard, *Dartmouth Medical College and Nathan Smith: An Historical Discourse* (Concord, N.H.: Evans, Sleeper & Evans, 1879), 12, note, tells us not only that NS "borrowed the money of Hon. Sanford Kingsbury," but that he repaid it. A note also exists in NS's hand (with no date and no addressee) that has to do with getting MO to help raise the money necessary to repay a loan from Judge Kingsbury; Mss. 001296, DCA. Further evidence of LS's involvement in NS's finances comes from a note dated 14 Feb. 1797 (thus while NS was abroad): "Borrowed of Colonel Spalding 1. 6. for Mrs Smith to go her journey which since paid"; Mss. 796103, DCA.

32. NS to LS, [?] Dec. 1796; Mss. 796690, DCA. In JAS, op. cit., 7 (there given with the date of 11 Dec.).

33. NS to LS, 11 Dec. 1796; Mss. 796661, DCA. In JAS, op. cit., 8 (there with no date given).

34. Dr. Bartlett lived in Boston. In referring to various transactions with Bartlett (see, e.g., NS to LS, 11 Sept. 1797, 17 Sept. 1800, and 30 Sept. 1800—all in JAS, op. cit., 10, 50, and 51–52 respectively), NS did not use Bartlett's first name. On the other hand, on his return from Europe, NS jointly with Thomas Bartlett and John Bellows of Boston signed two statements of money due to the United States (presumably customs charges) on 13 Sept. 1797, one due in eight months and one in ten (both are later marked "paid," apparently by Bartlett); see DA-3, Box 15 (Receipts and Oaths Folder), DCA. Two years later, on 17 Oct. 1799, a writ was issued against NS by Thomas Bartlett "apothecary of Boston" (the same person?) for failure to pay a bill that—with charges for damages and $.14 for the writ itself—came to $71.35 (again see DA-3, Box 15 [S Folder], DCA). Presumably NS eventually paid, though evidence he did so was not found.

35. EAS, *The Life and Letters of Nathan Smith, M.B., M.D.* (New Haven: Yale Univ. Press, 1914), 17.

36. Ibid., 19–20.

37. Robert E. Nye, Jr., "Nathan Smith's Trip to Edinburgh: A Waste of Time?" *DMS Alum. Mag.* [8, no. 1] (Fall 1983): 27.

38. Ibid., esp. 41. See also Nye to Oliver S. Hayward, 5 Nov. 1982; personal communication. In the files of C. E. Putnam, Concord, Mass.

39. NS to John Warren, 4 May 1797; J. C. Warren Papers, MHS.

40. EAS, op. cit., 18.

41. Bynum, op. cit., 4.

42. EAS, op. cit., 18.

43. William Quynn letters home, 12 Nov. 1783 and 15 Dec. 1783, quoted in Dorothy Mackay Quynn and William Rogers Quynn, "Letters of a Maryland Medical Student in Philadelphia and Edinburgh (1782–1784)," in *Maryland Hist. Mag.* 31, no. 3 (Sept. 1936): 196. A contemporary of Quynn's had the following to say about the university in Edinburgh: "[A]ll the chairs are ably filled; those in particular which relate to the study of medicine, as is evident from the number of ingenious physicians, *élèves* of this university, who prove the abilities of their mas-

ters." Thomas Pennant, *A Tour in Scotland*, 3d ed. (Warrington: Printed by W. Eyres, 1774 [1769]), 56–57.

44. Stephen Jacyna, "Theory of Medicine, Science of Life: The Place of Physiology Teaching in the Edinburgh Medical Curriculum, 1790–1870," in Vivian Nutton and Roy Porter, eds., *The History of Medical Education in Britain* (Amsterdam: Rodopi, 1995), 144.

45. Ibid., 146.

46. Stephen W. Williams, "Dr. Nathan Smith," in his *American Medical Biography, or Memoirs of Eminent Physicians* (Greenfield, Mass.: L. Merriam, 1845), 529.

47. NS Passport, 25 Apr. 1797; Mss. 797275.1, DCA.

48. Oliver S. Hayward and Elizabeth H. Thomson, eds., *The Journal of William Tully, Medical Student at Dartmouth 1808–1809* (New York: Science History, 1977), 30.

49. Worham L. Fitch, op. cit., and his "Extracts from Lectures on Surgery at the Medical Institution at New Haven by Nathan Smith, 1824," together show Cullen being mentioned more frequently than any other physician; only one of NS's twenty-four references to Cullen in Fitch's notes is favorable.

50. See William H. McMenemey, "Alexander Philips Wilson Philip (1770–1847), Physiologist and Physician," *Jrnl. Hist. Med. and Allied Sciences* 13, no. [3] (July 1958): 289–328, for a good discussion of Wilson Philip's developing interests, experiments, and career.

51. EAS, op. cit., 20.

52. J. Johnston Abraham, *Lettsom, His Life, Times, Friends and Descendants* (London: Wm. Heinemann Medical Books, 1933), 365.

53. Council of the Medical Society of London, Minutes, 22 May 1797; microfilm copy in WIHM Library. See Robert E. Nye, Jr., "Nathan Smith's Time in London: A Better Investment?," *DMS Alum. Mag.* [10, no. 1] (Fall 1985): 14, and Nye to Oliver S. Hayward, 14 Sept. 1983; personal communication. In the files of C. E. Putnam, Concord, Mass.

54. In a mid-April (presumably of 1811) letter to GCS, NS commented on having received a package with, *inter alia*, a diploma from the Medical Society of London—apparently a duplicate of the one he said he had received "from the same Society" in 1797; in EAS, op. cit., 63.

55. Henry R. Viets, *Medical History, Humanism, and the Student of Medicine* (Hanover, N.H.: Dartmouth Pubs., 1960), 26.

56. Ibid., 27. Viets was apparently relying on Abraham, op. cit., in making these assertions. What Abraham's authority for the claim was, however, is by no means clear; see Robert E. Nye, Jr., "London," 14.

57. Daniel Adams, "An Inaugural Dissertation on the Principle of Animation . . ." (Hanover, N.H.: Moses Davis, 1799), [3], and Cyrus Perkins, "An Inaugural Dissertation on Fever . . ." (Boston: E. Lincoln, 1802), [3], both spelled out their version of the affiliation, as "Corresponding Member of the London Medical Society"—though Adams abbreviated the last three words to "L.M.S." Avery Skilton, op. cit., was one of several students who headed their lecture notes with NS's name followed by "C.S.M.S. Lond." or just "C.S.M.S." That same sequence of letters appeared after NS's name on his article in *Amer. Med. Rev. and Jrnl.* 2, no. 1 (Sept. 1825): 140. Properly abbreviated, "Corresponding Member, Medical Society of London" should of course read "C.M.M.S.L." No one seems to have written it that way.

58. NS to LS, 11 Sept. 1797; in JAS, op. cit., 11.

59. NS's comment, quoted in EAS, op. cit., 20.

Chapter 4. The Founding of Dartmouth Medical School

1. C. Plini Secundi [Pliny the Elder] (Carolus Mayhoff, ed.), *Naturalis Historiae Libri XXXVII* 2, Liber VII, 1 (Lipsiae: Teubneri, 1875), 2. C. E. Putnam, trans.

2. See Leon Burr Richardson, *History of Dartmouth College* (Hanover, N.H.: Dartmouth College Pubs., 1932), 204–09.

3. Timothy Dwight, *Travels in New-England and New-York*, 4 vols. (New Haven: Timothy Dwight, 1821) 2:115, referring to his visit sometime between 18 and 28 Sept. 1797.

4. Rufus Graves, of whom we will shortly hear more, was a useful man; he ran a General Store in Hanover—complete with a Tannery—where he sold, among other things, hay and liquor.

5. NS Daybook, Sept. 1797–Mar. 1801 [Day Book B], 27 Feb. 1798, p. 35; Vault Mss., DCA.

6. NS to LS, 24 Jan. 1808; in EAS, *The Life and Letters of Nathan Smith, M.B., M.D.* (New Haven: Yale Univ. Press, 1914), 38, and in JAS, *Life of Dr. Lyman Spalding* (Boston: W. M. Leonard, 1916), 143.

7. LS to Samuel Brown, 1 Apr. 1799; Mss. 799251.1, DCA. Given LS's explicit report to Brown about how he assisted in NS's lectures in the autumn of 1797, this letter—though not written until eighteen months after the fact—has been seen as critical evidence that medical lectures took place in Hanover at that time. Important though this has seemed to Dartmouth people, the letter does not appear in JAS, op. cit. (In fact, Samuel Brown appears there only in notes—on pp. 10 and 54, where JAS tells us that Brown was "hooted" out of Boston, and on p. 55, where JAS says he does not know why—though the 12 Sept. 1800 letter from Benjamin Waterhouse to LS that JAS quotes there gives a hint; see also John B. Blake, *Benjamin Waterhouse and the Introduction of Vaccination: A Reappraisal* [Philadelphia: Univ. of Penn. Press, 1957], 16–17, for a discussion of Brown's less-than-honorable role in the vaccination business.)

There are other pieces of evidence to support the 1797 claim. One is to be found in LS to Benjamin Waterhouse, 12 July 1798; in JAS, op. cit., 22 (handwritten copy, attested, at CLM). In a postscript to that letter, LS wrote: "Sir, we have just completed our second course of medical lectures." If the spring 1798 lectures were the second course, the first has to have been no later than autumn 1797 (and it cannot have been earlier, since we know NS was out of the country from Dec. 1796 to Sept. 1797).

Finally, Oliver P. Hubbard, *Dartmouth Medical College and Nathan Smith: An Historical Discourse* (Concord, N.H.: Evans, Sleeper & Evans, 1879), 14, in a note, quotes a letter from NS to his wife, 20 Nov. 1797: "I am so much engaged here, and the time for beginning my business is so near, that I cannot come to Cornish till I begin my lectures" (Hubbard gives no indication where the original of this important letter is)—and NS himself wrote, years later, "Respecting the origin of the medical school in this place [Hanover], I gave the first course of Med. Lectures in 1797, begun in Nov. . . ." NS to GCS, 20 [sic: postmarked 15] Apr. 1811; Mss. 811265, DCA. Phineas Sanborn Conner likewise quoted NS to Sally Smith, 20 Nov. 1797. See typescript of Conner's "Address" on the medical school's first hundred years, p. 3; Vault Mss., DCA. See also the longer version of his "Address": Dartmouth Medical College, *Centennial Exercises* ([Hanover, N.H.: Dartmouth Press, 1907]), 5–6. There Conner says the date of the first lecture is uncertain, but he acknowledges that "Chase in his history of the College says November 22 was the date." Ibid., 6.

8. Jo Gallup was born on 30 Mar. 1769 and died on 12 Oct. 1849; see *Dartmouth College and Associated Schools General Catalogue, 1769–1940* (Hanover, N.H.: Dartmouth College Pubs., 1940), 837. For more on Jo Gallup, see ch. 7, *infra.*

9. Levi Sabin was born on 16 Jan. 1764 and died 30 Oct. 1808; see *Dartmouth College*, 837. See also Robert Graham, "A Firm Foundation," *Dartmouth Medicine* 16, no. 1 (Fall 1991): 15.

10. See Dartmouth College Trustees, Records and Charter, Vol. 1 (July 1770–Aug. 1812), 22 Aug. 1798, p. 222; Vault Mss., DCA. LS was also granted an M.B.; this was clearly meant as an honorary degree, since his Harvard M.B. was noted.

11. Hubbard, op. cit., 33, quotes Edward E. Phelps, a student of NS's at Yale (in 1825) who was later on the faculty at Dartmouth: NS's "reading of cases at the bedside . . . was most remarkable for its accuracy." Jonathan Knight in his "Eulogium" said NS's ability to cut to the "important and essential phenomena" in cases was a "process so rapid, as to resemble . . . intuition"; in NRS, ed., *Medical and Surgical Memoirs, by Nathan Smith, M.D.* (Baltimore: Wm. A. Francis, 1831), 27. William Allen, too, spoke of NS's "apparently intuitive knowledge of disease"; *An Address Occasioned by the Death of Nathan Smith, M.D. . . .* (Brunswick, Me.: G. Griffin, Printer, 1829), 17.

12. This is on the hypothesis that the money paid to Sanford Kingsbury in 1817 was, indeed, connected with debts incurred by the trip abroad.

13. LS to Samuel Brown, 1 Apr. 1799; Mss. 799251.1, DCA.

14. For this and the following two quotations, see Dartmouth College Trustees, Records and Charter, Vol. 1 (July 1770–Aug. 1812), 23 Aug. 1798, pp. 222–23, and 28 Aug. 1798, p. 229; Vault Mss., DCA. (The vote to award NS an M.D. degree is recorded in the same volume, on [25] Aug. 1801, p. 246.) That the initiative in founding the medical school came from NS is clear. Even so, one historian wrote that the "establishment of the Dartmouth Medical School in 1797 brought to the community Dr. Nathan Smith . . . ," giving NS short shrift indeed. Leon B. Richardson, *Fifty Years of Service: A History of the Mary Hitchcock Memorial Hospital* (Hanover, N.H.: [no publ., 1943]), 1. The truth is quite the other way around: NS brought the medical school to the community.

15. NS to LS, 24 Jan. 1801; LS Papers, NHHS. In JAS, op. cit., 80.

16. See Dartmouth College Trustees, Records and Charter, Vol. 1 (July 1770–Aug. 1812), 28 Aug. 1798, pp. 227–29; Vault Mss., DCA.

17. NS to GCS, [?] Nov. 1808; in EAS, op. cit., 42–43 (copy in Shattuck Papers, MHS).

18. The evidence is in a charge to Noyes for the course of lectures. See NS Daybook, Sept. 1797–Mar. 1801 [Day Book B], 30 Dec. 1797, p. 20; Vault Mss., DCA.

19. Nathan Noyes to Samuel and Rebecca Noyes [his parents], 16 Aug. 1798; Mss. 798466.1, DCA.

20. See Dartmouth College Trustees, Records and Charter, Vol. 1 (July 1770–Aug. 1812), 28 Aug. 1799, p. 232; Vault Mss., DCA.

21. Ibid., 29 Aug. 1799, p. 233; Vault Mss., DCA.

Chapter 5. The Heart of the Matter

1. Alexander Gordon, *A Treatise of the Epidemic Puerperal Fever of Aberdeen* (London: J. Robinson, 1795), 59. Quoted in Irvine Loudon, "Medical Education and Medical Reform," in Vivian Nutton and Roy Porter, eds., *The History of Medical Education in Britain*, (Amsterdam: Rodopi, 1995), 232.

2. See William Osler, "A Rhode Island Philosopher (Elisha Bartlett)," *Trans. R.I. Med. Soc.* 6 (1899): 15–46; and Seebert J. Goldowsky, *Yankee Surgeon: The Life and Times of Usher Parsons (1788–1866)* (Boston: Countway Library, 1988), 194, n33.

3. Elisha Bartlett, *An Essay on the Philosophy of Medical Science* (Philadelphia: Lea & Blanchard, 1844), 180.

4. Oliver S. Hayward and Elizabeth H. Thomson, eds., *The Journal of William Tully, Medical Student at Dartmouth 1808–1809* (New York: Science History, 1977), 52–53.

5. NS, "Introductory Lecture on the progress of medical Science" [n.d.]; BRBML. In EAS, *The Life and Letters of Nathan Smith, M.B., M.D.* (New Haven: Yale Univ. Press, 1914), 179 (the lecture is on pp. 169–79).

6. EAS, op. cit., 26. NS's manuscript notebook containing the "Heads of Lectures on Anatomy" is in the BRBML.

7. A. T. Lowe to Oliver P. Hubbard, 7 Apr. 1879; Mss. 879257, DCA.

8. EDC to Nathaniel Cushing, 22 Jan. 1811; EDC Papers (Folder 4), M&A, YUL.

9. Isaac Patterson to Oliver P. Hubbard, 13 Oct. 1879; Mss. 879563, DCA.

10. Jonathan Knight, "Eulogium," in NRS, ed., *Medical and Surgical Memoirs, by Nathan Smith, M.D.* (Baltimore: Wm. A. Francis, 1831), 28.

11. NS, *A Practical Essay on Typhous Fever* (New York: E. Bliss & E. White, 1824), 82–85; in NRS, ed., op. cit., 94–96.

12. Ebenezer Adams to GCS, 6 Dec. 1809; Shattuck Papers, MHS.

13. Hayward and Thomson, eds., op. cit., 32.

14. Samuel Farnsworth, "Lectures by Dr Smith Dartmouth University [sic] Oct. 20th AD 1812," p. 28; Vault Mss., DCA. Also J. S. Goodwin, "Extracts from Lectures delivered at Dartmouth . . . 1812, 1813," pp. 70–71; Vault Mss., DCA.

15. Rufus Turner, [Notebook of . . . , Medical Institution of Yale College 1813], n.p. [final entries]; YRG 47-J, M&A, YUL. These case reports appear at the end of Turner's notebook, making it appear they may have been notes of what NS informally recounted to some students about house calls rather than formal lecture notes.

16. Isaac Patterson to Oliver P. Hubbard, 13 Oct. 1879; Mss. 879563, DCA.

17. Peter Murray Jones, "Reading Medicine in Tudor Cambridge," in Nutton and Porter, eds., op. cit., 157.

18. Alton S. Pope and Raymond S. Patterson, "M. Appleton: Chronicler of Colonial Medicine," *Harvard Med. Alum. Bull.* 36, no. 4 (Spr. 1962): 18, conclude that Appleton copied his notes years later into the neat notebook they analyzed.

19. Avery J. Skilton, "Lectures on the Theory and Practice of Physic by Nathan Smith, M.D., C.S.M.S. Lond, Professor of the Theory and Practice of Physic in the Medical Institution of Yale College" (1826–27), pp. 122, 136, in Eli Ives, "Lectures on the Diseases of Children"; MS F 12, NLM. Judging from the content of some notes, Skilton was already in practice when he attended these lectures by NS.

20. See Worham L. Fitch, "Lectures on the Practice of Physic and Surgery by Nathan Smith . . . in the Medical Institution of Yale College, 1825," p. 249; YRG 47-J, M&A, YUL (see also Oliver S. Hayward, "The History of Oncology: III. America, and the Cancer Lectures of Nathan Smith," *Surgery* 58, no. 4 [Oct. 1965]: 748 [esp. Fig. 4]). The last page of at least one other student's notes also appears to have been signed and dated by NS at the end of the course, as if he had checked the notes. See Elijah W. Carpenter, "Lectures at New Haven on Surgery, Midwifery, Theory and Practice of Physic By Nathan Smith, M.D.," p. 175 ("March 5th 1814"); YRG 47-J, M&A, YUL. How often NS made such notations is difficult to guess.

21. William G. Rothstein, *American Physicians in the Nineteenth Century: From Sect to Science* (Baltimore: Johns Hopkins Univ. Press, 1985), 90–91.

22. Daniel Drake (Henry D. Shapiro and Zane L. Miller, eds.), *Physician to the West* (Lexington: Univ. of Kentucky Press, 1970), 153.

23. Rothstein, op. cit., 91.

24. Marie-François-Xavier Bichat (Constant Coffyn, trans.), *General Anatomy Applied to Physiology and the Practice of Medicine*, 2 vols. (London: Printed for S. Highley, 1824) 1:xiv.

25. William C. Ellsworth, "Extracts from the lectures on the theory & practice of physic, as delivered in a course of lectures at Dartmouth College, Oct. 1, 1806, by Nathan Smith, M.D.," Lecture 1st [n.p.] in Smith, Nathan, "William C. Ellsworth . . ."; Vault Mss., DCA.

26. David Shelton Edwards, "Theory & Practice of Physic by Nathan Smith MD [1815]," Lecture 1st [n.p.], in NS, "Lectures on the Theory and Practice of Physic"; MS C 300, NLM.

27. Farnsworth, op. cit., 39.

28. EAS, op. cit., 26–27, 169.

29. Skilton, op. cit., 43.

30. Ibid., 44.

31. Despite the apparent care with which he took notes, Fitch seems to have slipped when it came to dating his two notebooks. The second, his "Extracts From Lectures on Surgery Delivered at the Medical Institution at New Haven by Nathan Smith 1824" (YRG 47-J, M&A, YUL), has "1824" as part of its title. The notes themselves begin on 12 Nov. 1825 and end 9 May 1826, however, and on the inside cover of that notebook is written "No. 2"—which makes "1825" a more plausible part of the title. The other notebook—"Lectures," op. cit. (see *supra*, n20)—*does* have the date "1825" as part of its title, but those lectures also purport to begin on 12 Nov. 1825 and to end on 16 Feb. *1825*. Thus the opening date on "Extracts" probably should have been 12 Nov. *1824*, just as the date in the title should have been "*1824*." Fitch appears to have inadvertently reversed the dates in the titles of the two notebooks; the content, of course, is unaffected.

32. The name "Worham L. Fitch" does not appear in the *Catalog of the Officers and Graduates of Yale University in New Haven Connecticut* (New Haven: Publ. by the Univ., 1824), though he is listed in a folder labeled "Yale School of Medicine Graduates and non-Graduates" (in the office of the Medical Historical Librarian at C/WML). Coupled with the dates on Fitch's notebooks, this leads to the conclusion that the young man attended Yale for two courses of medical lectures in 1824–26 but never earned a Yale degree. See also Alfred Minot Copeland, ed., *Our County and Its People: A History of Hampden County, Massachusetts*, 3 vols. (Boston: Century Memorial Publ., 1902) 1:344.

33. Another extremely rich source is the two-volume set of notes taken by Peter L. Woodbury, "Medical Institution of Yale College, Lectures on Theory and Practice of Medicine, and on Surgery and Midwifery, by Nathan Smith, M.D. November 26, 1813–14"; YRG 47-J, M&A, YUL. The Woodbury notes are also available on microfilm in the C/WML.

34. Fitch, "Extracts," 15–16.

35. Ibid., 23–24.

36. Goldowsky, op. cit., 58 (emphasis in original); for a brief discussion of the point, see also pp. 60–61.

37. Fitch, "Extracts," 30.

38. Ibid., 421–22.

39. Fitch, "Lectures," 242–43.

40. Ibid., 210.

41. Ibid., 345. NS's confusion about whether dysentery was contagious—by no means a simple question—went back at least as far as his "Dissertation" at Harvard; that contained a convoluted paragraph in which he concluded dysentery, like influenza, is "often produced by a contagion arising from the putrefaction of vegetable matter" (NS, "A dissertation on the causes and effects of spasm in fevers," *Mass. Mag.* 3, no. 2 [Feb. 1791]: 82). In its vague abstraction, this is all too much like his later remark that scrofula "depends on a particular condition of the digestive organs" (Fitch, "Lectures," 404). By the time NS was lecturing at Yale, he was devoting more time to the discussion of dysentery (the quoted passage comes in the midst of several pages on the topic in Fitch's notes; see "Lectures," 334–48). Despite NS's expressed confidence and his long list of proposed remedies, we have no evidence that he grasped the true complexity of the issue: "Dysentery" might mean any one of a number of things. In any case, it is clear today that his understanding of whatever was meant by "dysentery" was not so good as his understanding of many other diseases and conditions.

42. Fitch, "Extracts," 35–36.

43. Fitch, "Lectures," 102.

44. Fitch, "Extracts," 337.

45. Ibid., 11.

46. Ibid., *passim.*

47. Skilton, op. cit., 3–39 (Ives), 137–44 (Smith), and 155–69 (Knight).

48. Cf. Skilton, op. cit., 149–52, and Fitch, "Lectures," 60–76. NS's "Directions to the Accoucher [sic]," as taken down by his Yale student Abraham Lines Smyth (with the somewhat puzzling notation "Not given in his lectures"), was published posthumously in *Bull. NYAM*, 2d series, 12, no. 9 (Sept. 1936): 529–34, in Gertrude L. Annan, "Advice of Nathan Smith, 1762–1829, on the Conduct of an Accoucheur"—which consisted of Smyth's version of NS's remarks prefaced by an introductory note by Annan on pp. 528–29. This lecture is the one block of instructive material that most frequently appears, intact, in extant student notebooks. Roger S. Skinner's "Notes on the lectures of Nathan Smith, M.D., professor of surgery, theory and practice of physic, and midwifery, at Yale college, New Haven" [n.d.], M&A, YUL, also contains the notation "Not given in his lectures." One wonders whether NS handed out printed copies—but if he did, none seems to have survived.

49. John Ayrton Paris, *The Elements of Medical Chemistry* (London: W. Phillips, 1825), ix, x–xi.

50. George Washington Corner, *Two Centuries of Medicine: A History of the*

School of Medicine, University of Pennsylvania (Philadelphia: J. B. Lippincott, 1965), 70–71.

51. *The Med. Repository* 2 (1799): 337. The ad reads, in part, "This institution was established in August, 1798." Of course that was strictly true, if one dates from the Board of Trustees' formal approval. But as we know, NS had begun teaching (with LS's help) in 1797; see *supra*, ch. 4, n7.

52. JAS, *The Life of Dr. Lyman Spalding* (Boston: W. M. Leonard, 1916), 3, 11 (plus note on that page).

53. LS, *A new nomenclature of chemistry, proposed by Messers. de Morveau, Lavoisier, Berthollet, and Fourcroy; with additions and improvements* (Hanover, N.H.: Moses Davis, 1799).

54. LS to NS, 14 Oct. 1800; LS Papers, NHHS. In JAS, op. cit., 52.

55. Abraham Hedge to LS, 18 Nov. 1800; in JAS, op. cit., 65.

56. NS to LS, 12 Feb. 1809; Mss. 809162, DCA. In JAS, op. cit., 156.

57. Daniel Adams, *An Inaugural Dissertation on the Principle of Animation . . .* (Hanover, N.H.: Moses Davis, 1799): "To Nathan Smith, A.M., Professor of Medicine at D. University, and Corresponding Member of the L.M.S., this Dissertation is Respectfully inscribed, by his Much Obliged and Grateful Pupil, The Author," [p. 3]. Cf. LS, *An Inaugural Dissertation on the Production of Animal Heat . . .* (Walpole, N.H.: David Carlisle, Jun. 1797): "To Nathan Smith, M.B. This Dissertation is Respectfully Inscribed by His Grateful Pupil, The Author," [p. 3]. LS's dedication of his thesis to NS is also mentioned in JAS, op. cit., 10.

58. LS to Daniel Adams, 24 Oct. 1799; in JAS, op. cit., 24.

59. Daniel Adams to LS, 14 Nov. [1799]; CLM. In JAS, op. cit., 25.

60. Hayward and Thomson, eds., op. cit., 53.

61. Ibid., 58.

62. Andrew Mack, "Journal Kept during a course of chemical Lectures D[artmouth] College Oct. 4, 1810, by Dr Smith"; Vault Mss., DCA.

63. Isaac Patterson to Oliver P. Hubbard, 13 Oct. 1879; Mss. 879563, DCA.

64. EDC to Nathaniel Cushing, 30 Oct. 1809; EDC Papers (Folder 1), M&A, YUL.

65. Hayward and Thomson, eds., op. cit., 76.

66. Harvey Cushing, *The Medical Career: An Address on The Ideals, Opportunities, and Difficulties of the Medical Profession . . .* (Hanover, N.H.: Dartmouth College, 1929), 36, 38.

67. Knight, in NRS, ed., op. cit., 27.

68. EAS, op. cit., 32–33. EAS acknowledges that she gets the anecdote from Oliver P. Hubbard—though, as is her wont, she neither gives the precise citation (*Dartmouth Medical College and Nathan Smith: An Historical Discourse* [Concord, N.H.: Evans, Sleeper, & Evans, 1879], 14–15) nor tells us she is quoting a note of Hubbard's (from his p. 15) when she informs us that Isaac Patterson confirmed the event occurred some time in 1810. Hubbard does say he is quoting the letter from Patterson (Isaac Patterson to Oliver P. Hubbard, 13 Oct. 1879; Mss. 879563, DCA).

69. Hayward and Thomson, eds., op. cit., 43, 45.

70. We know NS often gave conservative advice in his lectures: "owing to the constant nausea which generally attends on this disease [enteritis] little can be done by medicines given by the mouth"; "Physicians are apt to crowd medicines too fast in this disease [colic]"; "I put him into a tub of warm water and washed off the ointment and then put him into bed" (Fitch, "Lectures," 157, 328, 436–

37). A lovely passage in which Thomas Jefferson urged what amounts to watchful waiting is quoted by Rothstein, op. cit., 43, who goes on to acknowledge that few physicians used such strategies. NS was unusual.

71. NS, *Typhous*, 56–57 (in NRS, ed., op. cit., 78). This is but one of several places in the essay on typhous fever where Smith advised waiting and watching with patients, leaving them to get well without the burden of further—or any—medication.

72. Jacob Bigelow's *Discourse on Self-limited Diseases* (Boston: N. Hale, 1835), was a protest against therapeutic excess. For a brief comment on Bigelow's role, see Rothstein, op. cit., 61–62.

73. Hayward and Thomson, eds., op. cit., 76.

74. Thomas Francis Harrington, *The Harvard Medical School: A History, Narrative and Documentary, 1782–1905*, 3 vols. (New York: Lewis Publ., 1905), 1:448–50, prints John Warren's address. See especially some of the central passages on p. 449 for harbingers of NS's remarks.

75. William C. Ellsworth, "Chemical Lectures As Delivered in a Course of Lectures at Dartmouth College . . . ," [29–31], in Smith, Nathan, "William C. Ellsworth . . ."; Vault Mss., DCA.

Chapter 6. Trouble in the Anatomy Department

1. From Thomas Hood, "Mary's Ghost—A Pathetic Ballad," in his *Complete Poetical Works*, Walter Jerrold, ed. (London: Henry Frowde, OUP, 1906), 77. Quoted (without attribution) in James Thomas Flexner, *Doctors on Horseback* (New York: Garden City Publ., 1939), 18–19. Ruth Richardson helped track this down.

2. Buckminster Brown, "John Warren, 1753–1815," in Samuel D. Gross, ed., *Lives of Eminent American Physicians and Surgeons* (Philadelphia: Lindsay & Blakiston, 1861), 91, 98.

3. Henry K. Beecher and Mark D. Altschule, *Medicine at Harvard: The First Three Hundred Years* (Hanover, N.H.: UPNE, 1977), 33; see also Edward Warren, *The Life of John Warren* (Boston: Noyes, Holmes, 1874), 225–26, and *The Harvard Medical School 1782–1906* [Boston: HMS, 1906], 1, 2.

4. Suzanne M. Schultz, *Body Snatching: The Robbing of Graves for the Education of Physicians in Early Nineteenth Century America* (Jefferson, N.C.: McFarland & Co., 1992), 30.

5. Worham L. Fitch, "Extracts From Lectures on Surgery Delivered at the Medical Institution at New Haven by Nathan Smith, 1824," p. 389; YRG 47-J, M&A, YUL.

6. Twentieth-century followers of Smith's precepts have also understood that permission to do autopsies can be obtained in most cases (even in general practice), that this is one of the best ways to answer questions about diagnosis and treatment, and that it is one of the most important tools physicians have for learning from their own mistakes. See William F. Putnam, "Post-Mortem Examination in Rural General Practice," *NEJM* 224, no. 8 (20 Feb. 1941): 324–28.

7. Giovanni Battista Morgagni, *On the Seats and Causes of Diseases*, 2d Amer. Ed. (Printed in E. Walpole, N.H., 1808), 396. A translation of Morgagni's *De sedibus et causis morborum per anatomen indigatis* (Venetiis: Ex typographia Remondiniana, 1761) had already appeared in 1774, published in Rivington, N.Y.

8. J. F. Payne, *Thomas Sydenham* (London: T. Fisher Unwin, 1900), 232. Payne said this remark appeared in a projected treatise by Sydenham and John Locke, "still extant in MS in the Shaftesbury Papers." Elsewhere (p. 70) Payne said Sydenham "never attached much importance to this department [anatomy] of medical training."

9. John P. Kimball, "Lectures on Surgery, Delivered at Newhaven . . . 1819," p. 301; CLM.

10. NS, "On Amputation at the Knee-joint," *Amer. Med. Rev. and Jrnl.* 2, no. 2 (Dec. 1825): 370.

11. Fitch, op. cit., 146, 220, 423.

12. EDC to Nathaniel Cushing, 27 Dec. 1809; CLM.

13. Abraham Hedge to LS, 18 Nov. 1800; in JAS, *The Life of Dr. Lyman Spalding* (Boston: W. M. Leonard, 1916); 65.

14. Why Augustus Torrey, who is listed in the class of 1801, was given a ticket permitting him to attend NS's fifth course of lectures beginning 1 Oct. 1800 *gratis* is not clear (see Mss. 800551, DCA); it may be he had already attended and paid for two courses but had not yet taken his exam.

15. See Seebert J. Goldowsky, *Yankee Surgeon: The Life and Times of Usher Parsons (1788–1866)* (Boston: Countway Library, 1988), 179, for an account of the same thing happening in Providence in 1823.

16. Charles Adams to Joseph Wheeler, 8 Nov. 1812; Mss. 812608, DCA.

17. See Thomas Bartholinus, *De anatomica practica, ex cadaveribus morbosis adornada consilium* [*Advice on Practical Anatomy, Prepared from Diseased Cadavers*] (Hafniae: sumptibus P. Hauboldi, 1674).

18. Antonio Benivieni, *De Abditis nonnullis ac mirandis morborum et sanationum* [*On the Hidden Causes of Diseases . . .*] (Florence: Phillipus Giunta, 1507). For a very brief discussion of Benivieni's contribution, see Knut Haeger, *The Illustrated History of Surgery* (Gothenburg, Sweden: Nordbok, 1988), 95–96. A more extensive analysis, "Antonio Benivieni and His Contribution to Pathological Anatomy" by Esmond R. Long, appears in the reprint edition of Benivieni's work (Springfield, Ill.: Charles C Thomas, 1954), xvii–xlvi.

19. For a discussion of Morgagni's role, see Paul Klemperer, "Morbid Anatomy Before and After Morgagni," *Bull. NYAM* 37, no. 11 (Nov. 1961): 741–60.

20. William G. Rothstein, *American Physicians in the Nineteenth Century: From Sects to Science* (Baltimore: Johns Hopkins Univ. Press, 1985), 90.

21. Lois N. Magner, *A History of Medicine* (New York: Marcel Dekker, 1992), 163. Vesalius's work was originally published as *De humani corporis fabrica* (Basileae: [Ex officina Joannis Oporini, 1543]).

22. W. F. Bynum, *Science and the Practice of Medicine in the Nineteenth Century* (Cambridge: CUP, 1994), 93.

23. Ruth Richardson, *Death, Dissection, and the Destitute* (London: Routledge, 1987), 7.

24. David Charles Sloane, *The Last Great Necessity: Cemeteries in American History* (Baltimore: Johns Hopkins Univ. Press, 1991), 75.

25. Times have changed. For a look at current attitudes on this subject in, e.g., Britain, see Ruth Richardson and Brian Hurwitz, "Donors' attitudes towards body donation for dissection," *Lancet* 346, no. 8970 (July 29, 1995): 277–79.

26. Goldowsky, op. cit., 182. Here Goldowsky quotes an anecdote from Charles W. Parsons, *The Medical School Formerly Existing in Brown University, Its Professors and Graduates* (Providence: S. S. Rider, 1881), 38–39, that vividly

illustrates why anatomy courses—or the activities of anatomy students—were so often notorious. See also Beecher and Altschule, op. cit., 38.

27. This letter is of some added interest in that it was written by NS's son NRS, while he was teaching in Baltimore, and it was addressed to a former colleague of NS's at Bowdoin. NRS to Parker Cleaveland, 25 Sept. 1830; Parker Cleaveland Papers, Special Collections, BCL. As early as the 1820s, in fact, the medical school at Maryland had such a supply of cadavers—thanks to a small fine being the only punishment for robbing graves—"that it was able to sell its surplus to colleges as far away as Maine." F. L. M. Pattison, *Granville Sharp Pattison: Anatomist and Antagonist, 1791–1851* (Tuscaloosa, Ala.: Univ. of Alabama Press, 1987), 115.

28. Henry I. Bowditch, *Memoir of Amos Twitchell* (Boston: John Wilson and Son, 1851), 37.

29. NS to GCS, 14 May 1810; BRBML. In EAS, *The Life and Letters of Nathan Smith, M.B., M.D.* (New Haven: Yale Univ. Press, 1914), 51–52.

30. NS to LS, 12 Feb. 1809; Mss. 809162, DCA. In JAS, op. cit., 156.

31. NS to MO, 10 July 1819; Mss. 819410, DCA.

32. Schultz, op. cit., 46–47. See also the New Haven, Conn. *Pilot* 3, no. 122 (15 Jan. 1824): [3], under the headline "Another Grave-yard Plundered." The story was also carried in the *Connecticut Herald* 21, no. 15 (13 Jan. 1824), under the headline "A Shameful Outrage." Another Connecticut paper, the *Columbian Register* (on 17 Jan. 1824) gave the news item the simple headline "Robbery of a Grave."

33. Abel Lawrence Peirson, John C. Warren, William Ingalls, et al., *Address to the Community on the Necessity of Legalizing the Study of Anatomy, By Order of the Massachusetts Medical Society* (Boston: Perkins & Marvin, 1829), [3]. A sympathetic review of this *Address* appeared in the *N.Y. Med. and Physical Jrnl.* 2, no. 2, n.s. (Jan. 1830): 342–50. Signed "B," it was probably written by John Beck, a former editor of the journal.

34. Richardson, op. cit., 65, 66; Schultz, op. cit., 69, 77, *et passim*.

35. See Bynum, op. cit., 12; Margaret M. Coffin, *Death in Early America: The History and Folklore of Customs and Superstitions of Early Medicine, Funerals, Burials, and Mourning* (Nashville/New York: Thomas Nelson, 1976), 191. For an excellent discussion with a very different take from NS's on the issue of using criminals' and paupers' bodies for dissection purposes, see not only Richardson, op. cit., in general (esp. pp. 163, 175, 187), but also her "'Trading assassins' and the licensing of anatomy" in Roger French and Andrew Wear, eds., *British Medicine in an Age of Reform* (London/New York: Routledge, 1991), 74–91.

36. Carl Bridenbaugh, "Dr. Thomas Bond's Essay on the Utility of Clinical Lectures," *Jrnl. Hist. Med. and Allied Sciences* 2, no. 1 (Winter 1947): 13–14.

37. NS Daybook, Sept. 1797–Mar. 1801 [Day Book B], 22 Apr. 1798, p. 52; Vault Mss., DCA.

38. William Frederick Norwood, *Medical Education in the United States Before the Civil War* (New York: Arno, 1971 [1944]), 218 (where Norwood misidentifies Ramsay as Irish); see also G. P. Bradley, "Biographical Sketch of Alexander Ramsay, M.D., of Parsonsfield," *Maine Med. Assoc. Trans.* 8, no. 1 (1883): 170, 171, 174. Robert E. Nye, Jr., "Nathan Smith's Time in London: A Better Investment?," *DMS Alum. Mag.* [10, no. 1] (Fall 1985): 14–15, gives information on Ramsay missing from other sources.

39. Bynum, op. cit., 12, 13.

40. Bradley, op. cit., 161, apparently quoting Samuel L. Knapp, *American Biography* (New York: Conner & Cooke, 1833), 269—though he does not say so explicitly here. Henry R. Viets, "Ramsay, Alexander (1754?–Nov. 24, 1824)," in Dumas Malone, ed., *Dictionary of American Biography* 15:337, attributes this view to Bradley—almost certainly a misreading.

41. Whitfield J. Bell, Jr., *The Colonial Physician & Other Essays* (New York: Science History, 1975), 228, quoting James Rush.

42. Oliver S. Hayward and Elizabeth H. Thomson, eds., *The Journal of William Tully, Medical Student at Dartmouth 1808–1809* (New York: Science History, 1977), 66–67.

43. Bradley, loc. cit.

44. Norwood, op. cit., 218; he is probably citing (without attribution) JAS, "Ramsay, Alexander (1754–1824)," in Howard A. Kelly and Walter L. Burrage, eds., *American Medical Biographies* (Baltimore: Norman, Remington, 1920), 952—who in turn was no doubt relying on the remark in Knapp, loc. cit. (quoted by Bradley, op. cit., 163), that Ramsay "declared he was among Hottentots or brutes" if he was not the center of attention.

45. Bradley, loc. cit., again quoting Knapp, op. cit., 270. JAS, in "Ramsay," op. cit., 953, says that "Ingalls of Boston" was also able to "manage" Ramsay.

46. Alexander Ramsay, "Certificate" in response to request from LS, 7 Feb. 1818; CLM. In JAS, *Life*, 287–88. JAS, in "Ramsay," loc. cit., points out that "charming letters of recommendation" from Alexander Ramsay belie his reputation for hating all doctors; apparently LS was not the only young doctor for whom Ramsay wrote such a "Certificate."

47. James A. Spalding, "Ramsay, Alexander (1754–1824)," in Howard A. Kelly, ed., *Cyclopedia of American Medical Biography*, 2 vols. (Philadelphia: W. B. Saunders, 1912), 2:304.

48. Goldowsky, op. cit., 4.

49. NS to LS, 9 Oct. 1808; Mss. 808559, DCA. In JAS, *Life*, 150.

50. NS to LS, 8 Nov. 1808; Mss. 808608, DCA. In JAS, *Life*, 151.

51. B. C. Lister, "Ramsay, Alexander" in Martin Kaufman, Stuart Galishoff, and Todd L. Savitt, eds., *Dictionary of American Medical Biography* (Westport, Conn.: Greenwood, 1984), 622.

52. JAS, "Ramsay," in Kelly and Burrage, eds., op. cit., 953. In a surviving draft of a letter, LS expressed his disappointment that Ramsay ran afoul of just about everyone at Fairfield; he had thought, he said, that he was doing the institution a favor by recommending Ramsay. LS to James Hadley, 10 Dec. 1817; draft of letter at CLM. (Not in JAS, *Life*.)

53. Hayward and Thomson, eds., op. cit., 67.

54. Ibid., 69.

55. On 4 Oct. 1808, NS borrowed $200 from MO for the purpose. Account Books, Hanover, 41: MO Accounts of his law practice, 1800–1840, Vol. 2, 1807–1825, p. 9, DCA. In Aug. 1809, MO charged NS $10 interest on that bill; p. 108 of the same account book. (MO recorded at the same time $100 owed him by NS with *no* interest to be charged, "money [NS] sent to Europe for an apparatus.") On 3 Nov. 1808, Robert Bradley received $1,000 on Ramsay's behalf from NS; see receipt in DA-3, Box 15 (Accounts Relating to DMS Folder), DCA.

56. NS to LS, 22 Sept 1808; LS Papers, NHHS. In JAS, *Life*, 149–50. Apropos the medals, a charge from "30 [sic] Feb. 1809" in the account book of Jedediah Baldwin (the Hanover silversmith) is entered as follows: "To two Medals for Dr

Ramsay $17.00"; Account Books, Hanover, 3: Jedediah Baldwin post office and tinkering ledger, Jan. 1806-Mar. 1811, Vol. 7, p. 37, DCA. (A bill confirming the $17.00 charge is in DA-3, Box 15 [A–B Folder], DCA.) But see also John Bontell to Andrew Mack, 22 Mar. 1809 (Mss. 809222, DCA), which tells us the medals were "drawn by Wales" (even though Ramsay himself was a skilled draughtsman; see *infra*, n67). A search for one of these medals, which Ramsay seems to have awarded wherever he taught, has so far been in vain.

57. The ad appeared (with slight alterations in the text and corrections in spelling and punctuation), in the *Portsmouth [N.H.] Oracle* 19, no. 52 (1 Oct. 1808): [3]. A year later NS again had ads placed in the *Oracle* (whether with LS's help is not known), though only in the form of simple course announcements; Ramsay, after all, had left. See *Portsmouth [N.H.] Oracle*, as follows: 20, no. 49 (9 Sept. 1809): [3]; no. 50 (16 Sept. 1809): [4]; no. 51 (23 Sept. 1809): [5]; and no. 52 (30 Sept. 1809): [5].

58. Interestingly enough, it was another controversial Scot who—in a career that overlapped with the last years of Ramsay's life—next had the reputation for being the "best anatomist" around. At the height of his career, Granville Sharp Pattison was "widely considered—particularly in the United States—the best lecturer in anatomy then living"; Pattison, op. cit., 220.

59. Ramsay arrived in the United States in 1805 for a lecture tour (Bradley, op. cit., 162, relying on Knapp, op. cit., 269), so it is possible Smith had heard him either in this country or during his own time abroad.

60. NS to LS, 9 Oct. 1808; Mss. 808559, DCA. In JAS, *Life*, 150. These are the "particular specimens" referred to earlier (see *supra*, n49).

61. NS to LS, 8 Nov. 1808; Mss. 808608, DCA. In JAS, *Life*, 151.

62. NS to GCS, [?] Nov. 1808; BRBML (copy in Shattuck Papers, MHS). In EAS, op. cit., 43.

63. LS to William Neil, 28 Nov. 1808; Mss. 808628.2, DCA. (Not in JAS, *Life*.)

64. NS to GCS, 28 Nov. 1808; BRBML (copy in Shattuck Papers, MHS). In EAS, op. cit., 45.

65. NS to LS, 9 Oct. 1808; Mss. 808559, DCA. In JAS, *Life*, 150.

66. "Communication of Alex. Ramsay, M.D., . . . To . . . medical practitioners . . ."; Mss. 819374.2, DCA.

67. Some of Ramsay's original anatomical drawings (complex flap-anatomies devised for his lectures) are at the CLM. See also "Alexander Ramsay," in K. B. Roberts and J. D. W. Tomlinson, *The Fabric of the Body* (Oxford: Clarendon Press, 1992), 498–501, for a brief discussion and reproduction of drawings of the heart by Ramsay. At the WIHM Library there is a printed copy of Ramsay's *Anatomy of the Heart, Cranium, Brain . . .* (Edinburgh: Arch. Constable; London: Longman, Hurst, Rees, Orme, and Brown, 1813) with a series of fifteen colored plates drawn by Ramsay; five of the plates in this publication have cut-outs and flaps to show successive layers as dissection proceeds. Another copy of this splendid volume is at the NLM.

68. John Bontell to Andrew Mack, 22 Mar. 1809; Mss. 809222, DCA.

69. Bradley, op. cit., 171, quoting from an address Ramsay delivered in New York in 1818.

70. NS to GCS, 31 Dec. 1808; BRBML (copy in Shattuck Papers, MHS). In EAS, op. cit., 45–46.

71. Bell, op. cit., 217.

72. See, e.g., the letters to and from EDC at the CLM and in the EDC Papers, M&A, YUL. There are also Cushing papers at the MHS.

73. EDC to Nathaniel Cushing, 2 Dec. 1809; EDC Papers (Folder 4), M&A, YUL.

74. NS to LS, 13 Feb. 1810; Mss. 810163, DCA. In JAS, *Life*, 186.

75. Ebenezer Adams to GCS, 6 Dec. 1809; Shattuck Papers, MHS.

76. EDC to Mehitable Cushing [mother], 15 Dec. 1809; EDC Papers (Folder 1), M&A, YUL.

77. See Account Books, Hanover, 41: MO Accounts of his law practice, 1800–1840, Vol. 2, 1807–1825, p. 9, DCA.

78. EDC to Nathaniel Cushing, 22 Jan. 1811; EDC Papers (Folder 4), M&A, YUL.

79. EDC to Mehitable Cushing [sister], 11 Feb. 1810; CLM.

80. Deposition of EDC, 18 Nov. 1810; Shattuck Papers, MHS.

81. GCS to EDC, 4 Dec. 1810; EDC Papers (Folder 3), M&A, YUL. We know GCS was in touch with EDC more than once; the latter wrote home that he had had "two very polite letters from Dr. Shattuck." EDC to Nathaniel Cushing, 27 Dec. 1810; CLM.

82. EDC to Nathaniel Cushing, 27 Dec. 1809; CLM.

83. EDC to Nathaniel Cushing, 23 May 1810; CLM.

84. EDC to Nathaniel Cushing, 7 Oct. 1810; CLM.

85. EDC to Nathaniel Cushing, 28 Nov. 1810; CLM.

86. Carleton B. Chapman, *Dartmouth Medical School: The First 175 Years* (Hanover, N.H.: UPNE, 1973), 38.

87. *Concord [N.H.] Gazette* 3, no. 37 (13 Feb. 1810): [3].

88. NS to GCS, 14 May 1810; BRBML. In Chapman, op. cit., 21–22; in EAS, op. cit., 51–52.

89. NS to GCS, 20 Dec. [1811?]; BRBML. In EAS, op. cit., 71.

90. NS to GCS, [?] May 1819; Mss. 819340.2, DCA. NS's added comment that "the one [cadaver] brought by T. was excellent" supports Bowditch's claim that NS relied heavily on Amos Twitchell in this business; see *supra*, n28.

91. NS to LS, 6 Mar. 1818; Mss. 818206.3, DCA. In JAS, *Life*, 293.

92. NS to MO, 30 Jan. 1824 and 28 Feb. 1824; MS-436, Box 4 (Folder 62), DCA. This is the incident alluded to *supra*, n32.

93. See, e.g., Charles B. Johnson, "Getting My Anatomy in the Sixties," *Bull. Soc. of Med. Hist. of Chicago* 3, no. 1 (1923): 109–15, for a vivid description of what was still involved in obtaining cadavers for medical students a full half-century later.

Chapter 7. *Students, Colleagues, and Friends*

1. Samuel Elder, fragment of undated letter (addressee unknown); Mss. 000676, DCA.

2. Oliver S. Hayward and Elizabeth H. Thomson, eds., *The Journal of William Tully, Medical Student at Dartmouth 1808–1809* (New York: Science History, 1977), 72.

3. Alexander Boyd to William Boyd, 26 Nov. 1810; Mss. 810626.2, DCA.

4. Hayward and Thomson, eds., op. cit., 54.

5. Ibid., 21, 30.

6. Ibid., 48.

7. Ibid., 68. A year later Alexander Boyd, whose comments on trouble-making students we just read, expressed (in that same letter) essentially the identical sentiment: "The more I become acquainted with Doct. Smith the more I have reason to esteem him." Alexander Boyd to William Boyd, 26 Nov. 1810; Mss. 810626.2, DCA.

8. Hayward and Thomson, eds., op. cit., 74–75.

9. Much of the information about Tully can be found in greater detail in Oliver S. Hayward, "Essay on William Tully," in Hayward and Thomson, eds., op. cit., xiii–xxiv (see esp. p. xxi); and in Oliver S. Hayward, "A Student of Dr. Nathan Smith," *Conn. Med.* 24, no. 9 (Sept. 1960): 553 *et seq.* See also Frederick Clayton Waite, *The First Medical College in Vermont: Castleton 1818–1862* (Montpelier, Vt.: Vermont Hist. Soc., 1949), 77, and John S. Billings, "Literature and Institutions," in Edward H. Clarke, Henry J. Bigelow, Samuel D. Gross, et al., *A Century of American Medicine 1776–1876* (Philadelphia: Henry C. Lea, 1876), 303–304.

10. William Tully, *Materia Medica or Pharmacology and Therapeutics* (Springfield, Mass.: Jefferson Church, 1857).

11. Frederick Clayton Waite, *The Story of a Country Medical College: A History of the Clinical School of Medicine and the Vermont Medical College, Woodstock, Vermont 1827–1856* (Montpelier, Vt.: Vermont Hist. Soc., 1945), 46. In general, the information about Gallup that follows comes either from this book or from Oliver S. Hayward, "Jo Gallup, New England Epidemiologist (1769–1849)," *NEJM* 269, no. 19 (7 Nov. 1963): 1015–18. See also Waite, *First Medical College*, 76, 77.

12. Joseph Gallup, *Sketches of Epidemic Diseases in the State of Vermont from Its First Settlement to the Year 1815* . . . (Boston: T. B. Wait, 1815).

13. Noah Webster, *A Brief History of Epidemic and Pestilential Diseases* . . . (Hartford, Conn.: Hudson & Goodwin, 1799).

14. William Frederick Norwood, review of Waite, *Story, Jrnl. Hist. Med. and Allied Sciences* 1, no. 2 (Apr. 1946): 343–44.

15. Recall JG to GCS, 4 Mar. 1829; Shattuck Papers, MHS.

16. EDC to Nathaniel Cushing, 30 Oct. 1809; EDC Papers (Folder 1), M&A, YUL.

17. EDC to Mehitable Cushing [mother], 15 Feb. 1809; EDC Papers (Folder 1), M&A, YUL.

18. EDC to Mehitable Cushing [sister], 3 Aug. 1810; EDC Papers (Folder 3), M&A, YUL.

19. EDC to Mehitable Cushing [mother], 15 Dec. 1809; EDC Papers (Folder 1), M&A, YUL.

20. EDC to Nathaniel Cushing, 30 Oct. 1809; EDC Papers (Folder 1), M&A, YUL.

21. Stephen W. Williams, "Dr. Ezekiel Dodge Cushing," in his *American Medical Biography, or Memoirs of Eminent Physicians* (Greenfield, Mass.: L. Merriam, 1845), 118.

22. Henry I. Bowditch, *Memoir of Amos Twitchell* (Boston: John Wilson and Son, 1851), 15.

23. Ibid., 83.

24. Oliver P. Hubbard, *Dartmouth Medical College and Nathan Smith: An Historical Discourse* (Concord, N.H.: Evans, Sleeper, & Evans, 1879), 8, makes

this claim, saying that Twitchell had made the observation to his student Dr. H. F. Crain, who in turn passed the remark on to Hubbard.

25. Bowditch, op. cit., 50.

26. Bowditch, op. cit., 44–45, 48. This memoir is full of rich detail on Twitchell.

27. See the letter by Henry O. Smith (1886), in *Dartmouth Alum. Mag.* 32, [no. 5] (Feb. 1940): 7; Amos Twitchell (1802, m1805) Alumni File, DCA.

28. H. O. Smith, in the letter already cited (*supra*, n27), says Twitchell turned down positions at Dartmouth, Bowdoin, and the University of Vermont; Bowditch, op. cit., 88 and 90, mentions those three plus Vermont Academy of Medicine and Castleton (two incarnations of the same institution); Oliver S. Hayward once wrote (though without supporting documentation) of Twitchell that "it is said . . . he was offered professorships in twelve different medical schools" (Hayward, "Essay," xix).

29. Amos Twitchell to Francis Brown, 28 June 1819; Mss. 819378, DCA. Some question has been raised about President Brown's motive in offering the position to Twitchell—as has the possibilty that Twitchell was being disingenuous in his expressed reasons for turning it down; see Robert E. Nye, Jr., "Cyrus Perkins, M.D., (1778–1849)," *DMS Qtly.* 3, no. 2 (Autumn 1966): 34. For Ramsay's plans, see Alexander Ramsay to Francis Brown, 24 June 1819; Mss. 819374.2, DCA.

30. Bowditch, op. cit., 66 *et seq.*

31. Ibid., 75.

32. See Amos Twitchell (1802, m1805) Alumni File, DCA.

33. ØBK, *Records* (1787–1813), 23 May 1799, p. 105; DCA.

34. See esp. JAS, "The Friendship of Dr. Nathan Smith and Dr. Lyman Spalding," *Bull. Amer. Acad. Med.* 7, no. 9 (Oct. 1906): 714–34. JAS in an undated latter to "Doctor Lane" speaks of two trips NS and LS made together to Cambridge, and in a memo ("Human touches in the lives of Dr. Nathan Smith and my Grandfather Dr. Lyman Spalding"), also undated, he wrote "Dr. Smith came on horseback to Harvard to hear Grandfather defend his thesis in 1797. They rode back to Cornish on horseback"—a strong sign of loyal friendship; letter and memo in files of C. E. Putnam, Concord, Mass.

35. LS to William Woodward, 17 Sept. 1800; NS to LS, 30 Sept. 1800; LS to John Wheelock, 1 Oct. 1800. See JAS, *The Life of Dr. Lyman Spalding* (Boston: W. M. Leonard, 1916), 48–52, where this is discussed and these three letters— among others—are quoted.

36. There is disagreement. JAS, in "Friendship," says "three terms" (p. 3), and in the undated memo already quoted (see *supra*, n34) he says LS boarded with NS "in 1797, 1798, and 1799 during the Lecture terms." NS could not recall whether it was one term or two ("a course . . . in 1801 or 1802"—he was wrong about the dates and probably the number as well). See NS to GCS, 20 [sic: postmarked 15] Apr. 1811; Mss. 811265, DCA. In EAS, *The Life and Letters of Nathan Smith, M.B., M.D.* (New Haven: Yale Univ. Press, 1914), 63. LS's letter of resignation was in October 1800, just when the fourth year's courses should have been starting—making it probable that three is the correct number of terms. (That, however, is on the assumption there was only one term a year; he may have taught even more, as there were probably two terms a year. See the letter from LS to Benjamin Waterhouse cited *supra*, ch. 4, n7.)

37. LS to NS, 14 Oct. 1800; LS Papers, NHHS. In JAS, *Life*, 52.

38. JAS, *Life*, 58, speculates that LS resigned in part because Waterhouse

urged him to devote himself to a vaccination campaign that would be hampered were he to return to Dartmouth. See Benjamin Waterhouse to LS, 25 Sept. 1800; in JAS, *Life*, 57–58. See also the draft of a letter, LS to Benjamin Waterhouse, Aug./Sept. 1800; CLM. One can imagine that having Waterhouse engaged in business with LS would have needled NS, helping explain the uncharacteristically brisk and somewhat formal tone in his letters to LS at the time. See, e.g.: NS to LS, 8 Sept. 1800; LS Papers, NHHS (in JAS, *Life*, 48), and NS to LS, 24 Jan. 1801, LS Papers, NHHS (not in JAS, *Life*).

39. See correspondence files at DCA, CLM, and NHHS. The single best collected source of these letters is JAS, *Life* (see index entry "Smith, Nathan," p. 377). See also JAS, "Friendship," *passim*.

40. Jane W. Dieffenbacher, *This Green and Pleasant Land: Fairfield, New York* (Fairfield, N.Y.: Town of Fairfield, 1996), 226. For more on LS's role at Fairfield, see generally pp. 225–29 and 235–36.

41. LS, *An Address delivered at Fairfield, VII December MDCCCXIII at the inauguration of the officers of the College of Physicians & Surgeons, of the Western District of the State of New York* (New York: Wm. Treadwell, 1814), 11.

42. Advertisement in *NEJM & Surg.* 5 (1816): 108.

43. NS to LS, 6 Mar. 1818; Mss. 818206.3, DCA. In JAS, *Life*, 293–95.

44. See JAS, *Life*, 267.

45. "Historical Introduction," *The Pharmacopoeia of the United States of America 1820* (Boston: Wells and Lilly, for Charles Ewer, 1820), 5. The Introduction, though unsigned, was presumably written at least in part by LS. But even JAS in his laudatory account of his grandfather's role does not make this explicit: "It opened with a brief Historical Introduction stating Dr. Spalding's original suggestion for the work, the recommendations of the New York County Medical Society, and the formation of four District Medical Conventions to be followed by a National Convention"; JAS, *Life*, 360. The same uncertainty attends the "Preface" to the work.

46. "Preface," *The Pharmacopoeia*, op. cit., 3.

47. See, e.g., LS to Jacob Bigelow, 22 Feb. 1820, 1 Mar. 1820, and 10 May 1820; all CLM.

48. See Lloyd G. Stevenson, "Putting Disease on the Map: The Early Use of Spot Maps in the Study of Yellow Fever," *Jrnl. Hist. Med. and Allied Sciences* 20, no. 3 (July 1965): 243, for a detail of the spot map of the East River dock area in Felix Pascalis's "Statement on the Occurrences during Malignant Yellow Fever in the City of New York," *Med. Repository* 5, n.s. (1820): 229–56 (map opp. p. 229).

49. LS, *Reflections on Yellow Fever Periods; or, A particular investigation of the long contested question, whether the yellow fever can originate from abroad* (New York: C. Turner, 1819). A letter to LS from E. W. King (Chr., New York City Board of Health), dated 14 Sept. 1819 (two days after the talk was given), has an outline of the talk on the back, perhaps the basis of the subsequently published abstract of it; CLM. Carefully pasted into LS's "Medical Portfolio" on p. 264 is the newspaper clipping with the printed abstract of his "Reflections" as published in the *Commercial*, 16 Sept. 1819 [n.p.]; CLM. LS's interest in the subject is well attested; on pp. 272 and 273 of the same "Portfolio" are letters to the editor (from what publication is unclear) on yellow fever, over the name of Felix Pascalis.

50. Bernard Bailyn, Robert Dallek, David Brion Davis, et al., *The Great Republic: A History of the American People* (Lexington, Mass.: Heath, 1985), 302.

51. JAS, *Life*, 366.

52. JAS, "Friendship," 733.

53. Dieffenbacher, op. cit., 235–36, mentions—for example—Josiah Noyes, George Cheyne Shattuck, and James Hadley, Sr., along with Reuben Dimond Mussey (and in addition to LS, who—though not a Dartmouth graduate—certainly counts as a "Dartmouth doctor," given his role in the early years and his honorary M.B.).

54. "Smith, Ashbel (1805–1886)," in Howard A. Kelly and Walter L. Burrage, eds., *American Medical Biographies* (Baltimore: Norman, Remington, 1920), 1065.

55. R. D. Mussey to John Mussey [father], 31 May 1803; Mss. 803331, DCA.

56. Kenneth C. Cramer, "Dusting the DMS Archives," *DMS Alum. Mag.* [7, no. 1] (Fall 1982): 29.

57. Thomas Chadbourne to Samuel Fletcher, 23 July 1838; Mss. 838423, DCA.

58. NS to Daniel Webster, 31 July 1805; Mss. 805431, DCA.

59. William Osler, "Men and Books: Nathan Smith," *Canad. Med. Assoc. Jrnl.* 4, no. 12 (1914): 1110.

60. GCS's generosity to Dartmouth was quite extraordinary. President Nathan Lord, in his July 1853 report to the Board of Trustees, referred to purchases GCS had already made for the observatory, on which ground was to be broken the following September; see Mss. 853440, DCA. In his report from the previous year, in July 1852, Lord wrote of "the liberality of Dr. George C. Shattuck . . . [who] has deposited one thousand Doll. for the purchase of books," and the College librarian, O. P. Hubbard, in his 1851–52 report to the Board of Trustees similarly wrote of "valuable donations" by GCS; see Mss. 852440, DCA, and Mss. 852900.4, DCA, respectively. Hubbard's 1854 report to the Board refers to five paintings presented to the library by GCS; see Mss. 854426, DCA.

61. This information on GCS comes from Brenda M. Lawson, "Manuscripts on the History of Medicine at the Massachusetts Historical Society," in *Proceedings MHS* 103 (1991): 168–70, and Henry K. Beecher and Mark D. Altschule, *Medicine at Harvard: The First Three Hundred Years* (Hanover, N.H.: UPNE, 1977), 58, 74–75, 107.

62. NS "Certificate" for GCS, 16 Oct. 1806; Shattuck Papers, MHS. On the same date, a letter generally recommending GCS was jointly signed by John Wheelock, John Smith, John Hubbard, Roswell Shirtliff [later "Shurtleff"], and NS—in other words, the entire Dartmouth faculty; Shattuck Papers, MHS.

63. NS to GCS, 22 June 1806/1807 (both dates appear in the letter—one inside and one outside); M&A, YUL. In EAS, op. cit., 35 (she dates it 22 Jan. 1806).

64. GCS not only won three times in two years—submitting papers on both contest topics in 1807, he won both—but collected the essays and published them in a slim volume: *Three Dissertations on Boylston Prize Questions for the Years 1806 and 1807* (Boston: Farrand, Mallor; [also] Hastings, Etheridge, & Bliss, 1808). (He sent a copy to President Thomas Jefferson, with a charming cover letter, saying the book was sent out of "the great respect [the] author feels for the man who has so successfully cultivated physical science" [GCS to Thomas Jefferson, 28 Oct. 1808; Jefferson Papers, MHS].) Thus it is no surprise that NS should have wanted help from GCS.

65. NS to GCS, 28 Nov. 1808; BRBML (copy in Shattuck Papers, MHS). In EAS, op. cit., 43–46. The topic on which NS wanted to write—"On the Diagnostics of Scirrhous and Cancerous Tumors with the comparative advantages of ex-

tirpation by the knife and by caustic"—was announced in the newspaper. See the announcement (clipped and mounted, with no way to tell what newspaper or which page it came from) in LS, "Medical Portfolio," p. 185; CLM. We will return to a discussion of NS's work on this subject in ch. 14.

66. NS to GCS, 31 Dec. 1808; BRBML (copy in Shattuck Papers, MHS). In EAS, op. cit., 46.

67. NS to GCS, [?] Oct. 1809; a second letter with no day indicated, [?] Oct. 1809 (but after 4 Oct., when he also wrote); and 12 Sept. 1809; all BRBML. In EAS, op. cit., 47, 49–50, and 42 respectively (she erroneously dates this last letter 15 Sept. 1807).

68. NS to GCS, 10 Dec. 1809; BRBML (copy in Shattuck Papers, MHS). Smith did business with McKinstry later, anyway, as a promissory note to "Smith & Perkins" from Nathan McKinstry of Newbury, dated 2 Aug. 1811 indicates; DA-3, Box 15 (L–N Folder), DCA. Presumably it was also the same "Dr. McKinstry of Newbury, Vt." who organized the dissection of the corpse after Grafton County (N.H.) carried out its first execution. See Maurice Bear Gordon, *Aesculapius Comes to the Colonies* (Ventnor, N.J.: Ventnor Publ., 1949), 132.

69. Lawson, *op. cit.*, pp. 168–70.

70. The Dutch doctor and chemist Hermann Boerhaave (1668–1738) is generally considered the leading internist of his day, "probably the most influential physician of the eighteenth century." Lois N. Magner, *A History of Medicine* (New York: Marcel Dekker, 1992), 226. See generally pp. 226–27.

71. Ebenezer Adams to GCS, 6 Dec. 1809; Shattuck Papers, MHS.

72. NS to GCS, 11 July 1810; Shattuck Papers, MHS.

73. NS to GCS, 3 July 1828; Shattuck Papers, MHS.

74. Edward H. Leffingwell, for example, served as a physician in Peru from 1825 to 1834; *General Catalogue of Bowdoin College and the Medical School of Maine: A Biographical Record of Alumni and Officers 1794–1950* (Brunswick, Me.: Pub. by the College, 1950), 439. See also *Dartmouth College and Associated Schools General Catalog, 1769–1940* (Hanover, N.H.: Dartmouth College Pubs., 1940), 837–38. Information is given in these pages on where thirty-seven of the sixty-two students who received medical degrees from 1797 to 1812 settled to practice; all but five of those appear to have been located at one time or another in small towns and villages.

Chapter 8. Assuring the Medical School's Future

1. William Allen, *An Address Occasioned by the Death of Nathan Smith, M.D. . . .* (Brunswick, Me.: G. Griffin, Printer, 1829), 7–8.

2. See receipt signed by Benjamin Hall for money received of "Nathan Smith School Committee," 12 Apr. 1793, and receipt signed by "Nathan Smith School Committee" for Nathaniel Hall's payment of school tax (for 1793), 8 Apr. 1794; DA-3, Box 15 (H Folder), DCA.

3. Note of 1 Aug. 1803, in Trinity Church Papers, Cornish Hist. Soc., Cornish, N.H.

4. An inventory of items costing a total of £100-11-6, charged (we do not know whether by NS or by Sally) on 28 May 1800 and paid by NS on 7 June 1800, can be seen in DA-3, Box 15 (C Folder), DCA.

5. See will of Jonathan Chase, 15 Jan. 1801; Mss. 801115, DCA.

6. Mss. 801155, DCA.

7. 1 Dec. 1802; DA-3, Box 15 (W–Z Folder), DCA.

8. Receipt dated 2 July 1804; DA-3, Box 15 (H Folder), DCA.

9. NS to GCS, 12 July 1804; Shattuck Papers, MHS. In EAS, *The Life and Letters of Nathan Smith, M.B., M.D.* (New Haven: Yale Univ. Press, 1914), 32.

10. Dartmouth College Trustees, Records and Charter, July 1770-Aug. 1812, Vol. 1, p. 249 (28 Aug. 1801) and p. 260 (27 Aug. 1802); Vault Mss., DCA.

11. Dartmouth College Trustees, Records and Charter, July 1770–Aug. 1812, Vol. 1, pp. 265–66 (26 Aug. 1803); Vault Mss., DCA. See also Mss. 803490.1, DCA.

12. Dartmouth College Trustees, Records and Charter, July 1770–Aug. 1812, Vol. 1, p. 279 (28 Aug. 1804); Vault Mss., DCA.

13. EDC to Mehitable Cushing [mother], 15 Dec. 1809; EDC Papers (Folder 1), M&A, YUL.

14. See Richard Lang's running account with NS from late 1798 through 1803 (on two sheets); DA-3, Box 15 (L–N Folder), DCA.

15. Account Books, Hanover, 3: Jedediah Baldwin, Accounts of his jewelry shop ledger, 1791–1811, Vol. 9, p. 49; DCA. That Baldwin took the chemistry course is clear from a $5 charge in NS Daybook, Sept. 1797-Mar. 1801 [Day Book B], 30 Dec. 1797, p. 18; Vault Mss., DCA.

16. Thomas Stokes & Co., New York, 28 Apr. 1804, to Jed Baldwin; Mss. 001152, DCA.

17. See, e.g., the bill from William Tuttle, Lebanon, N.H., to NS, for deliveries on 31 May, 23 July, and 4 Nov. 1806, and on 2 July 1807; DA-3, Box 15 (T–V Folder), DCA.

18. NS Certificate, 28 Nov. 1808; Mss. 808628.1, DCA.

19. Asa Porter to MO, ["Monday evening"; no day or month given] 1801; MS-436, Box 1 (Folder 4), DCA.

20. NS to MO, 16 Mar. 1802; Mss. 802216, DCA.

21. NS to MO, 9 July 1803; Mss. 803409.1, DCA.

22. See "Sketches of Alumni of Dartmouth College," in *The New Hampshire Repository, Devoted to Education, Literature and Religion,* conducted by William Cogswell, (Gilmanton, N.H.: Alfred Prescott, Printer, 1846), 1:270–71, for a brief account of MO's life.

23. NS to MO, 15 Oct. 1826; Mss. 826265, DCA.

24. See Account Books, Hanover, 41; MO Accounts of his law practice, 1800–1840, Vol. 1, 1800–1807, 7 Aug. 1802 (first mention of a charge to NS) and 13 Nov. 1804 ("I am to make no charge for the above"), p. 42; DCA. See also, e.g., the following: NS to MO, 7 July 1823 (request to take care of James Morven Smith); MS-436, Box 4 (Folder 59). NS to MO, 29 Feb. 1824 ("I shall see you in the month of June & will then pay you for all expenses etc."); MS-436, Box 4 (Folder 65). Six letters in 1827 from NS to MO about the latter's son Charles Olcott (boarding with NS) and his drinking; MS-436, Box 4 (Folder 70). All DCA.

25. NS to John Warren, 2 Nov. 1790; J. C. Warren Papers, MHS.

26. A receipt is extant, for example, for payments "To advertising Medical Lectures" in the Windsor paper for the years 1801–04; also, *inter alia,* for the *New Hampshire Gazette* for 27 Sept. 1808, and for the *New Hampshire Patriot,* 3 Oct. 1809; DA-3, Box 15 (Accounts Relating to DMS Folder), DCA. Quoted is one such ad as it appeared in the *Dartmouth Gazette* 8, no. 371 (3 Oct. 1806): [1].

27. Account with Joseph Nancrede, 10 Feb. 1803; DA-3, Box 15 (N–Perkins Folder), DCA.

28. *Journal of the Honorable Senate* [of the State of New Hampshire], June Session — 1803, Friday June 19th, p. 49; State Archives, Concord, N.H.

29. Dartmouth College Trustees, Records and Charter, July 1770-August 1812, Vol. 1, p. 300 (29 Aug. 1806); Vault Mss., DCA.

30. NS to LS, 24 Jan. 1808; in JAS, *The Life of Dr. Lyman Spalding* (Boston: W. M. Leonard, 1916), 143.

31. For an analysis of NS's political abilities and achievements, see Oliver S. Hayward, "Nathan Smith (1762–1829), Politician," *NEJM* 263, no. 24 (15 Dec. 1960): 1235–43; and 263, no. 25 (22 Dec. 1960): 1288–91.

32. NS to GCS, 31 Dec. 1808; BRBML (copy in Shattuck Papers, MHS). In EAS, op. cit., 46.

33. NS to LS, 21 May 1809; LS Papers, NHHS. In JAS, op. cit., 159.

34. NS to LS, 22 June 1809; LS Papers, NHHS. In JAS, op. cit., 145 (he dates the letter 1808—surely an error, given the timing of the events in question).

35. NS petition of 14 June 1809; LS Papers, NHHS.

36. The chronology of events spelled out in what follows is taken largely from a letter to the editor signed by "Z" and headlined "Falsehoods Detected," in the *Concord [N.H.] Gazette* 3, no. 37 (13 Feb. 1810): [2]. The letter was reprinted in the *Dartmouth Gazette* on 21 Feb. 1810. For additional details—beyond those explicitly cited *infra* in n37 and n38—see *Journal of the House of Representatives of the State of New-Hampshire*, June Session — 1809, Wednesday June 14th, (Concord: Geo. Hough, August 1809), 29, 64, and 87, where the various stages of legislative action from committee referral to final passage in the House can be found.

37. See *Journal of the House*, p. 38, and *Journal of the Honorable Senate of the State of New-Hampshire*, June Session — 1809, Wednesday June 14th (Concord: Geo. Hough, August 1809), p. 24; NH State Archives, Concord, N.H.

38. For the roll-call vote and passage in the House on 20 June 1809, see *Journal of the House*, pp. 73–75; for the roll-call vote and passage in the Senate on 22 June 1809, see *Journal of the Honorable Senate*, p. 71. For the text of the Act as it was finally enacted on 23 June 1809, see "An Act appropriating three Thousand four Hundred and Fifty dollars . . . ," in *Laws of New Hampshire* 7:813–14; see also Mss. 809372.2, DCA. Most of the text of the Act was printed a few months later in the *Concord [N.H.] Gazette* 3, no. 39 (27 Feb. 1810): [3], under the headline "Dr. Smith's Medical School," with an accompanying letter (signed "No Party-Man"); see *infra*, n40.

39. NS to GCS, [?] Oct. 1809; BRBML. In EAS, op. cit., 50.

40. See, again, "Falsehoods Detected" by "Z," in the *Concord [N.H.] Gazette* (see *supra*, n36). The chief point of the letter was to show that—whatever the project's merits—the opposition had been nonpartisan. Two issues later, the letter signed "No Party-Man" made the same point; the *Concord [N.H.] Gazette* 3, no. 39 (27 Feb. 1810): [3].

41. John Duffy, *From Humors to Medical Science*, 2^d ed. (Urbana, Ill.: Univ. of Ill. Press, 1993), 24. See also Carl Bridenbaugh, *Cities in Revolt: Urban Life in America 1743–76* (New York: Knopf, 1955), 131–32.

42. Charles E. Rosenberg, *The Care of Strangers: The Rise of America's Hospital System* (New York: Basic Books, 1987), 21.

43. NS to GCS, 20 [sic: postmarked 15] Apr. 1811; Mss. 811265, DCA. In EAS, op. cit., 63.

44. NS to Benjamin Silliman, 6 Aug. 1814; Silliman Family Papers, M&A, YUL.

45. NS to GCS, [?] Apr. 1811; in EAS, op. cit., 65.

46. NS to GCS, 26 June 1812; BRBML (copy in Shattuck Papers, MHS). In EAS, op. cit., 73.

47. NS to MO, 28 Jan. 1817; Mss. 817128, DCA.

48. The order was issued 22 Feb. 1817. See "Orders on the treasurer by the Governor of New Hampshire from June 5th 1816 to June 2^{d} 1819" [in Gov. Plumer's handwriting], p. 28; Mss. 816355, DCA.

49. NS to GCS, 2 May 1811; BRBML (copy in Shattuck Papers, MHS). In EAS, op. cit., 67.

50. Ruggles Sylvester to EDC, 3 Mar. 1811; EDC Papers (Folder 4), M&A, YUL.

51. Lemuel Cook receipt, 29 June 1811; DA-3, Box 15 (C Folder), DCA.

52. Lemuel Cook receipt, 9 July 1811; DA-3, Box 15 (Accounts Relating to DMS Folder), DCA.

53. Lemuel Davenport bill, for July–Oct. 1811; DA-3, Box 15 (Accounts Relating to DMS Folder), DCA. Errors in the arithmetic of the original have not been corrected.

54. Long & Clement bill, for Oct.–Nov. 1815; DA-3, Box 15 (L–N Folder), DCA. A similar, unsigned, bill was tendered to NS again for work done on 21 Sept. and 4 Oct. 1816 "To repairing the medical house"; DA-3, Box 15 (Accounts Relating to DMS Folder), DCA.

55. It was also, by a few days, the *first* purpose-built "Medical House" in the country. Nicholas Romayne, having resigned his position at Columbia's College of Physicians and Surgeons in New York, undertook to start a new medical school in 1811 (called "The Medical Institution of the State of New York"). He was largely responsible for raising the money, etc., for a "new three-story building, especially built" and "completed and ready for the winter session." Lectures in New York began on 4 Nov. 1811. See Thomas Gallagher, *The Doctors' Story* (New York: Harcourt, Brace & World, 1967), 155–56. This was a few days after the October 1811 opening of the term at Dartmouth.

56. Nehemiah Cleaveland, *History of Bowdoin College* (Boston: James Ripley Osgood, 1882), 138, comments that his friendship with Wheelock caused NS to be sad for the troubles at Dartmouth "though [he was] no partisan." Quoted in EAS, op. cit., 112.

57. Certainly in later years, as the College vs. University controversy warmed up, this seems to have been true. See Robert E. Nye, Jr., "Cyrus Perkins, M.D., (1778–1849)," *DMS Qtly.* 3, no. 2 (Autumn 1966): 34.

58. ØBK, *Records* (1787–1813), 4 Apr. 1799, p. 93; DCA.

59. See Oliver S. Hayward and Elizabeth H. Thomson, eds., *The Journal of William Tully, Medical Student at Dartmouth, 1808–1809* (New York: Science History, 1977), 72, for a full description of an episode that reduced Smith and students alike to tears.

60. ØBK, op. cit., 26 Aug. 1807, p. 187; DCA.

61. Dartmouth College Trustees, Records and Charter, July 1770–Aug. 1812, Vol. 1, p. 240 (29 Aug. 1800); Vault Mss., DCA.

62. Dartmouth College Trustees, Records and Charter, July 1770–Aug. 1812, Vol. 1, p. 340 (25 Aug. 1809) and p. 348 (24 Aug. 1810); Vault Mss., DCA.

63. Oliver Wendell Holmes, *Addresses and Exercises at the One Hundredth Anniversary of the Foundation of the Medical School of Harvard University, October 17, 1883* (Cambridge, Mass.: John Wilson and Son, University Press, 1884), 6. The remark is so often quoted—almost always about Smith, but generally with no more than a vague attribution (see, e.g., the version in EAS, op. cit., 77)—that it has gone into medical folklore. George Washington Corner, in *Two Centuries of Medicine: A History of the School of Medicine, University of Pennsylvania* (Philadelphia: J. B. Lippincott, 1965), for example, refers on p. 23 to "the ancient jest" about faculty members occupying "not chairs but settees" without a hint of awareness that Holmes said it, never mind about whom. The only specific citation found was correct as to the location of Holmes's remark (see *supra*, beginning of this note), but inexplicably misstated the object of the encomium; Thomas Edward Moore, Jr., in "The Early Years of the Harvard Medical School," *Bull. Hist. Med.* 7, no. 6 (Nov.–Dec. 1953): 542, said Holmes made the remark about John Warren, at Harvard. The citation Moore himself gave, however, provides evidence that the remark was not about Warren but about von Haller, who—besides holding the three professorships mentioned—carried on investigations in and wrote about physiology; he was also a poet, no doubt a further factor in winning the admiration of Holmes—himself a poet. Regardless of whether Holmes ever made the quip about NS, it fits no one in this country more aptly.

64. Dartmouth College Trustees, Records and Charter, July 1770–Aug. 1812, Vol. 1, p. 348 (24 Aug. 1810); Vault Mss., DCA.

65. *Dartmouth Gazette*, 16 Oct. 1811, p. 1.

66. Memorandum [n.d.]; DA-3, Box 15 (Accounts Relating to DMS Folder), DCA. The partnership had originally been announced in the *Dartmouth Gazette* on 25 Sept. 1810, p. 1, and again on 3 Oct. 1810, p. 1.

67. Nye, op. cit., 28–34—on which much of what is said here relies heavily—helpfully gathers in one place most of what we know about Perkins. Phineas Sanborn Conner confirmed that—even in 1897—information on Perkins was hard to find. See typescript of his "Address" on the medical school's first hundred years, p. 14; Vault Mss., DCA.

68. Cyrus Perkins, *An Inaugural Dissertation on Fever . . .* (Boston: E. Lincoln, 1802), [3].

69. NS gave a note to Cyrus Perkins for $951.00 on 28 Oct. 1813, in what was apparently a final settlement of the assets of the partnership; DA-3, Box 15 (N–Perkins Folder), DCA. On the back of the note is a record of payments NS made, totaling $637.00; when or whether the balance was paid is not to be found there. On the other hand, a memo from 26 Nov. 1816 headed "Dr. Nathan Smith in account with Cyrus Perkins, Dr" (also in the N–Perkins Folder) gives evidence that the two men were still doing business with each other at that late date; payments are noted for legal charges, ads for the *Oracle*, and four loads of manure!

70. William Barlow and David O. Powell, "Student Views of the Medical Institution at Dartmouth in 1813 and 1814," *Historical New Hampshire* 31, no. 3 (Fall 1976): 103, quoting Simon Woodward to Ezra Bartlett, 28 Oct. 1814, and 105, quoting Malthus A. Ward to Ezra Bartlett, 19 Nov. 1814.

71. Ibid., 98.

72. Nye, op. cit., 31.

73. The obituary notice in the *New-York Daily Tribune* 9, no. 14 (25 Apr. 1849): [3], consisted of a single sentence announcing that Cyrus Perkins had died.

Chapter 9. Nathan Smith's Medical Practice

1. Moses Maimonides (Suessman Muntner, ed.), *The Medical Writings of Moses Maimonides: Treatise on Asthma* (Philadelphia: Lippincott, 1963), 84–85.

2. Carl J. Pfeiffer, *The Art and Practice of Western Medicine in the Early Nineteenth Century* (Jefferson, N.C.: McFarland and Co., 1985), 103.

3. William G. Rothstein, *American Physicians in the Nineteenth Century: From Sects to Science* (Baltimore: Johns Hopkins Univ. Press, 1985), 41.

4. John Henry Warner, "American Doctors in London During the Age of Paris Medicine," in Vivian Nutton and Roy Porter, eds., *The History of Medical Education in Britain* (Amsterdam: Rodopi, 1995), 359.

5. Ibid., 358.

6. See, generally, W. F. Bynum, *Science and the Practice of Medicine in the Nineteenth Century* (Cambridge: CUP, 1994).

7. Editorial, *Mass. Physician* 29, no. 7 (July 1970): 6.

8. John Armstrong, *Practical Illustrations of Typhus Fever, of the Common Continued Fever, and of Inflammatory Diseases, &c. &c.*, 1st Amer. ed. from the 3d Eng. ed.), with notes by Nathaniel Potter (Philadelphia: James Webster, 1821), 222. See, too, Thomas Beddoes, *Researches Anatomical and Practical Concerning Fever* (London: Longman, Hurst, Reed, and Orme, 1807), 167–69, where the story is also quoted from Thomas Dovar [sic], *Ancient Physician's Legacy . . .* (London: Printed for the relict of the late R. Bradley, 1733), 67. Beddoes (p. 167) calls Dover a "buccaneer and physician" and observes that "this simple narrative" has a "somewhat ludicrous air [that] carr[ies] . . . its own evidence."

9. For a rollicking good story of nineteenth-century adventurism and the man who "gave quinine to the world" (p. xii), see Gabriele Gramiccia, *The Life of Charles Ledger (1818–1905): Alpacas and Quinine* (London: Macmillan, 1988).

10. NS, *A Practical Essay on Typhous Fever* (New York: E. Bliss & E. White, 1824), 51. In NRS, ed., *Medical and Surgical Memoirs, by Nathan Smith, M.D.* (Baltimore: Wm. A. Francis, 1831), 74.

11. See William Cullen, *First Lines of the Practice of Physic* (Edinburgh: C. Elliot, 1786), 2 vols., e.g., I, part I, ch. VI, sect. I, "Of the Cure in Continued Fevers," pp. 180–254. See also NS, op. cit., e.g., 52, 58, 61, 71–72, and 81–83. In NRS, ed., op. cit., 75–76, 78–79, 81, 88–89, and 94–96. A version of this chart originally appeared in Oliver S. Hayward, "Nathan Smith's Medical Practice or Dogmatism versus Patient Inquiry," *Bull. Hist. Med.* 36, no. 3 (May–June, 1962): 265–67.

12. See, e.g., Worham L. Fitch, "Lectures on the Practice of Physic and Surgery by Nathan Smith . . . in the Medical Institution of Yale College, 1825," p. 126, and his "Extracts From Lectures on Surgery Delivered at the Medical Institution at New Haven by Nathan Smith, 1824," p. 427; YRG 47-J, M&A, YUL. Bell was especially interested in technique and in the use of simpler instruments wherever possible—as evidenced in his 1784 encyclopedia *System of Surgery*, according to Knut Haeger, *The Illustrated History of Surgery* (Gothenburg, Sweden: Nordbok, 1988), 171.

13. See, e.g., Fitch, "Lectures" and "Extracts," *passim*. See also Oliver S. Hay-

ward, "The Basis in Sydenham, Rush, and Armstrong for Nathan Smith's Teaching," *Ann. of Intern. Med.* 56, no. 2 (Feb. 1962): 346.

14. Hippocrates (Wesley D. Smith, ed. and trans.) Vol. 7, *Epidemics* 6, sect. 5 (Cambridge, Mass.: Harvard Univ. Press, 1994), 254 (Greek), 255 (English).

15. EAS, *The Life and Letters of Nathan Smith, M.B., M.D.* (New Haven: Yale Univ. Press, 1914), 26–27, and 175.

16. Benjamin Rush, *The Works of Thomas Sydenham, M.D., on Acute and Chronic Diseases* (Philadelphia: Benjamin & Thomas Kite, 1809), 97–98, 172.

17. NS, "A dissertation on the causes and effects of spasm in fevers . . . ," *Mass. Mag.* 3, no. 1 (Jan. 1791): 35.

18. Fitch, "Lectures," pp. 173–74.

19. James Thomas Flexner, *Doctors on Horseback: Pioneers of American Medicine* (New York: Garden City Publ., 1939), 65.

20. Rush, op. cit., 14 n3, and 126 note.

21. Cullen, op. cit., lv.

22. Cullen, op. cit., xxii–xxiii.

23. Cullen, op. cit., xxv.

24. Whitfield J. Bell, Jr., "Medical Practice in Colonial America," *Bull. Hist. Med.* 31, no. 4 (Sept.–Oct. 1957): 444. According to Bell, this 4 Apr. 1794 letter is in the Miller Collection, Richmond, Va., Academy of Medicine.

25. Irvine Loudon, "Medical Education and Medical Reform," in Nutton and Porter, eds., op. cit., 232.

26. NS, "A Nosological Arrangement of Diseases," in Alexander Philips Wilson Philip (NS, ed.), *A Treatise on Febrile Diseases, Including the Various Species of Fever and All Diseases Attended with Fever*, 2d Amer. ed., from the 3d London ed. 1813, 2 vols. (Hartford, Conn.: Cooke & Hale, 1816) 1:29.

27. Loc. cit.

28. Ibid., 30–31.

29. Ibid., 33.

30. David Shelton Edwards, "Doct. N. Smith Nosological Arrangement of diseases Nov. 1815" [n.p.], in NS, "Lectures on the Theory and Practice of Physic"; MS C 300, NLM.

31. NS to GCS, 22 June 1806/1807 (both dates appear in the letter—one inside and one outside); M&A, YUL. In EAS, op. cit., 35–36 (she dates it 22 Jan. 1806).

32. NS to LS, 7 Mar. 1813; Mss. 813207, DCA. In JAS, *The Life of Dr. Lyman Spalding* (Boston: W. M. Leonard, 1916), 270.

33. NS to LS, 6 Mar. 1818; Mss. 818206.3, DCA. In JAS, op. cit., 294.

34. Fitch, "Lectures," 30–31.

35. NS, *Typhous*, 51. In NRS, ed., op. cit., 74.

36. Cullen, op. cit., 124–26.

37. NS, *Typhous*, 22. In NRS, ed., op. cit., 55.

38. William Osler, "Some Aspects of American Medical Bibliography," *Aequanimitas*, 3d ed. (New York: McGraw-Hill, [n.d]), 302–303.

39. William H. Welch, "Introduction," in EAS, op. cit., [v]; see also his "The Relation of Yale to Medicine," *Yale Med. Jrnl.* 8, no. 5 (Nov. 1901): 142.

40. NS, *Typhous*, 15–16, 18, 19, 21. In NRS, ed., op. cit., 50–55.

41. Ibid., 43, 45–49, 51, 53–54 (or NRS, ed., op. cit., 69–78).

42. Knut Haeger, op. cit., 9.

43. Samuel Foote, "The Devil Upon Two Sticks, a Comedy in Three Acts," in his *English Plays 1778* (London: Printed by T. Sherlock, for T. Cadell, 1778), 61.

44. John Collop, "Against Phlebotomy to a Leech" and "For Phlebotomy," in his *Poesis Rediviva* (London: Printed for Humphrey Moseley, 1655), 48–49. Collop wrote many poems on medical subjects and persons. In the same volume, see, e.g., "Of the Blood" (p. 46), "On the Humours" (p. 48), "The Sequesterd Priest pidling [i.e., working at in a trifling way] in Physick" (p. 53), "On Doctor Harvey" (pp. 57–58). Somewhat more accessibly, these same poems can be found in Conrad Hilberry, ed., *The Poems of John Collop* (Madison, WI: Univ. of Wisconsin Press, 1962), 89 *et seq.*

45. It was not until the French physician Pierre-Charles-Alexandre Louis published his comparative study *Recherches anatomique, pathologiques et thérapeutique sur la maladie connue sous les noms de fièvre typhoide, putride . . .* in 1828 and (even more influentially) his *Recherches sur les effets de la saignée dans quelques maladies inflammatoires . . .* in 1835 (see "Louis, Pierre-Charles-Alexandre," in *Nouvelle Biographie Générale*, 46 vols. [Paris: Firmin Didot Frères, 1862], 31:1047) that the idea of evaluating the efficacy of a treatment by keeping accurate records and then analyzing the data statistically began to gain currency. Only then could the rationale for bleeding finally begin to be laid to rest. See Robert E. Nye, Jr., "Nathan Smith's Time in London: A Better Investment?," in *DMS Alum. Mag.* [10, no. 1] (Fall 1985): 15; see also Seebert J. Goldowsky, *Yankee Surgeon: The Life and Times of Usher Parsons (1788–1868)* (Boston: Countway Library, 1988), 133. For a brief look at Louis's influence on one young American physician, see Oliver Wendell Holmes, "Some of My Early Teachers," in *Medical Essays* (Boston: Houghton Mifflin, 1883), 431–34.

46. Fitch, "Extracts," 460–68.

47. Ibid., 52.

48. Fitch, "Lectures," 220. At other points, too, he commended venesection. For example, in a lecture on how to treat "Injuries of the Brain," he also said that in "dangerous" cases where "a fracture is combined with an injury of the external parts"—after the operation—"bleeding is necessary." Fitch, "Extracts," p. 51.

49. Avery J. Skilton, "Lectures on the Theory and Practice of Physic by Nathan Smith, MD, C.S.M.S. Lond . . . ," p. 102, in Eli Ives, "Lectures on the Diseases of Children"; MS F 12, NLM.

50. Fitch, "Extracts," 401.

51. Martin Kaufman, *The University of Vermont College of Medicine* (Hanover, N.H.: UPNE, 1979), 26, 27. Kaufman's sweeping generalization about Smith seems to have been based on his reading of a single set of student notes, which he says were taken by Isaiah Whitney in 1822 at UVM. (Librarians at UVM were unable to locate—or even confirm the existence of—any such set of notes, nor does a student by that name appear in the university records. Queried in March 1997, Kaufman himself said simply he knew nothing of the whereabouts of the notes and could not help.) In the brief aside that is all Kaufman devotes to NS in his book, he ignores the significance of repeated cautions from NS when recommending bleeding (like "we have regard to the state of the pulse and general appearance of the patient"; Fitch, "Lectures," p. 110). NS did *not* recommend dogmatic and mindless venesection in the manner of Rush; indeed, William H. Welch went so far as to say that NS did more "than any other man" to do away with the "indiscriminate use" of the lancet. See Welch, "The Relation of Yale to Medicine," *Yale Med. Jrnl.* 8, no. 5 (Nov. 1901): 142.

52. Fitch, "Lectures," 1.

53. Asa Porter to MO, ["Monday evening"; no day or month given] 1801; MS-436, Box 1 (Folder 4), DCA.

54. NS to LS, [probably 20 Sept. 1800; see *infra*, ch. 10, n82]; Mss. 000645, DCA. In JAS, op. cit., 91. NS to LS, 25 Aug. 1809; Mss. 809475, DCA. In JAS, op. cit., 89. (The date on this letter is smudged. JAS read it as "1801" but acknowledged in a footnote that date had to be incorrect; internal evidence confirms the letter was written later, and in the DCA it has been catalogued—surely correctly—as dating from 1809).

55. Nathan Noyes to LS [n.d.]; in JAS, op. cit., 71. Noyes received his M.B. degree in 1799; see Mss. 799490, DCA.

56. One of those in attendance was Dr. Torrey, of Windsor—Erastus Torrey (m1805), younger brother of the Augustus Torrey (m1801) for whom NS had written a letter of recommendation on 19 May 1804; Mss. 804319, DCA. There he stated that the older Torrey, as a student, had "exhibited a good genius" (the same phrase used, as we have seen, to describe GCS and many others) and that on "examination for a medical Degree he was found well qualified." One hopes the professor had general confidence in the younger Torrey as well, even though his skill in this case was deemed insufficient.

57. Mary Pepperrell Sparhawk Cutts, *The Life and Times of Hon. William Jarvis of Weathersfield, Vermont* (New York: Hurd and Houghton, 1869), 316–17.

58. NS to GCS, 2 May 1811; BRBML (copy in Shattuck Papers, MHS). In EAS, op. cit., 66.

59. NS, *Typhous*, 76, 77, 78. In NRS, ed., op. cit., 91, 93, 95.

60. See NS, Accounts, Beginning 1792, for references to drug usage: e.g., p. 15 (peppermint), p. 18 (Bal. Copaiva, castor), p. 19 (bitters), p. 21 (rad. Valerian), p. 28 (guiac), p. 36 (opium); Vault Mss., DCA. For a general discussion of NS's use of drugs, see Oliver S. Hayward, "Medical Practice," 260–67.

61. Fitch, "Lectures," 297. The second remark is quoted by Bryce A. Smith, "Notes on the Materia Medica of Nathan Smith," *Yale Jrnl. of Biol. and Med.* 11, no. 3 (Jan. 1939): 194, from Dan King, "Notes from the Lectures on the Theory & Practise of Physic given at the Medical College New Haven 1814. 15. by Nathan Smith, M.D. C.S.M.S."; M&A, YUL.

62. Bryce A. Smith, op. cit., 201.

63. Fitch, "Lectures," 445–46.

64. Ibid., 99–100.

65. Ibid., 423.

66. Ibid., 369, 372.

67. Skilton, op. cit., p. 101, under the heading "Phthisis Pulmonalis."

68. G. E. R. Lloyd, *Hippocratic Writings* (London: Penguin Books, 1983), 222.

69. Fitch, "Lectures," 274.

70. Ibid., 282, 283, 284.

71. Ibid., 285.

72. Ibid., 157.

73. See Benjamin Waterhouse's rather whining letter to John Coakley Lettsom, 25 Nov. 1794, quoted in Thomas Joseph Pettigrew, *Memoirs of the Life and Writings of the Late John Coakley Lettsom, M.D.*, 3 vols. (London: Longman, Hurst, Rees, Orme, and Brown, 1817) 2:464–65.

74. Elisha Bartlett, *An Essay on the Philosophy of Medical Science* (Philadel-

phia: Lea & Blanchard, 1844), 206–207. Quoted by William B. Bean, "Elisha Bartlett — His Views of Benjamin Rush," *Arch. Intern. Med.* 116, no. 3 (Sept. 1965): 321–22.

75. Fitch, "Lectures," 79.

76. NS, "Observations on the Pathology and Treatment of Necrosis," in NRS, ed., op. cit., 116.

77. NS, *Typhous*, 81. In NRS, ed., op. cit., 94.

78. Fitch, "Lectures," 287.

79. See index under "domestic medicine," in Dorothy Porter and Roy Porter, *Patients' Progress* (Cambridge: Polity Press, 1989), 290.

80. NS, *Typhous*, 83, 84, 85. In NRS, ed., op. cit., 95–96. NS made similar remarks in his notes on Wilson Philip, op. cit.; see, e.g., 1:217.

Chapter 10. *Nathan Smith's Surgical Practice*

1. Attributed to Cato by St. Jerome, *Epistula* LXVI, 9, in *Sancti Eusebii H. Epistulae* (Vindobonae: F. Tempsky, 1910), Vol. 54 of *Corp. Script. Eccl. Lat.* (I. Hilberg, ed.), 659. C. E. Putnam, trans.

2. See Martin S. Pernick, *A Calculus of Suffering: Pain, Professionalism, and Anesthesia in Nineteenth-Century America* (New York: Columbia Univ. Press, 1985), 3 *et passim*, for a discussion of William T. G. Morton's demonstration of his "Letheon Gas" in the now-famous operation performed by surgeon John Collins Warren at Massachusetts General Hospital, on 16 Oct. 1846—the first use of anesthesia in surgery.

3. William Cheselden (1688–1752)—Knight misspelled the name—was the pre-eminent British surgeon of his day, famed among other things for the speed of his operations (especially lithotomy); see Knut Haeger, *The Illustrated History of Surgery* (Gothenburg, Sweden: Nordbok, 1988), 145–48.

4. Jonathan Knight, *An Eulogium on Nathan Smith, M.D.* (New Haven: Hezekiah Howe, 1829), reprinted in NRS, ed., *Medical and Surgical Memoirs by Nathan Smith, M.D.* (Baltimore: Wm. A. Francis, 1831), 35–36; Knight may have been relying here on a statement NS himself made in lecture. See, e.g., Worham L. Fitch, "Extracts From Lectures on Surgery Delivered at the Medical Institution at New Haven by Nathan Smith 1824," pp. 96–97; YRG 47-J, M&A, YUL.

5. William Allen, *An Address Occasioned by the Death of Nathan Smith, M.D....* (Brunswick, Me.: G. Griffen, Printer, 1829), 8.

6. Ibid., 74.

7. NS to MO, 15 Jan. 1817; Mss. 817115, DCA.

8. For insight into one period of the Yale years, for example, see 145 pages of NS's notes on visits to patients in New Haven and vicinity—with names, treatment, and charges—that appear at the back of his notebook (turned upside down to reverse the reading direction) labeled "Introductory Lecture on the progress of medical Science"; BRBML.

9. See NS Daybook, Sept. 1797–Mar. 1801 [Day Book B], *passim*; Vault Mss., DCA.

10. NS to EDC, 13 Aug. 1820; EDC Papers (Folder 7), M&A, YUL.

11. EDC to Nathaniel Cushing, 30 Oct. 1809; EDC Papers (Folder 1), M&A, YUL.

12. See, e.g., NS Daybook, Sept. 1797–Mar. 1801 [Day Book B], 15 Feb. 1798, p. 32 *et passim*; Vault Mss., DCA.

13. NS to MO, [?] Sept. 1817; Mss. 817540.2, DCA.

14. NS to LS, 13 Feb. 1810; Mss. 810163, DCA. In JAS, op. cit., 186.

15. NS to GCS, 5 May 1823; in EAS, op. cit., 123.

16. Fitch, op. cit., 70.

17. NS to MO, [?] Oct. 1819; Mss. 819590, DCA.

18. R. K. French, *The History and Virtues of Cyder* (New York: St. Martin's Press, 1982), 15; see also the chapter "Cyder and medicine," 51–69.

19. Oliver S. Hayward's files indicate this wonderful anecdote could be found in the notebook Samuel Elder kept while he was a student at Dartmouth (Vault Mss., DCA). In fact, it does not appear in that notebook—nor has diligent searching turned it up in any of the other notebooks in the DCA kept by NS's students. Nonetheless, Hayward's careful transcription of the story makes it clear he found it somewhere during his researches, and it seemed too delightful to omit.

20. A. T. Lowe to Oliver P. Hubbard, 16 Apr. 1879; Mss. 879266, DCA.

21. Fitch, op. cit., 9.

22. Ibid., 67.

23. Ibid., 117.

24. Ibid., 247, 249.

25. Ibid., 296.

26. Ibid., 6.

27. Ibid., 6–7.

28. Ibid., 78–79.

29. G. E. R. Lloyd, *Hippocratic Writings* (London: Penguin, 1983), 291–302 *inter alia*.

30. Fitch, op. cit., 7–8, 9.

31. Ibid., 10–11, 70.

32. Ibid., 54–55, 57–59.

33. Ibid., 30–31.

34. Ibid., 38.

35. Ibid., 40–41.

36. Ibid., 44–45.

37. Ibid., 49–50.

38. A rare instance of someone else being called in after NS had failed to cure was noted by Elias Frost: "Doct. Harroon[,] ol['] Dr Lewis and the very greatly Celebrated Nathan Smith Lecturer of Dartmouth College had visited her and all announced her case a consumption and beyond any medical aid. In this situation I was called." Elias Frost, "Chronicle of the Frost Family with Anecdotes and Notices Illustrative of Individual Characters with an Autobiography of the Compiler" (Meriden, N.H., 10 May 1853), 77; Mss. 853310, DCA. For a discussion of Frost's chronicle that puts the reference to NS in context, see Walter A. Backofen, "Elias Frost, M.D., and His Strategy for Being Remembered" (unpublished mss., 23 pp.).

39. Fitch, op. cit., 178–79.

40. Ibid., 184.

41. Oliver P. Hubbard, *Dartmouth Medical College and Nathan Smith: An Historical Discourse* (Concord: Evans, Sleeper, & Evans, 1879), 29, quoting Professor A. S. Packard.

42. NS to GCS, 18, 21, and 28 Mar. 1811; BRBML. In EAS, op. cit., 54–59.

43. NS to GCS, 19 May 1811; BRBML. In EAS, op. cit., 69.

44. NS to MO, [?] Sept. 1817; Mss. 817540.2, DCA.

45. Alexander Boyd to William Boyd, 26 Nov. 1810; Mss. 810626.2, DCA.

46. Fitch, op. cit., 100–11, 222–26, 275–76.

47. John Stevenson's *On the Morbid Sensibility of the Eye* . . . was written from "Great Russell-Street, Bloomsbury, October 1, 1810" and published in England in 1810. NS's endorsement, dated 10 Jan. 1815 and printed on the back cover of the American edition (Hartford, Ct.: Horatio G. Hale, 1815), was clearly intended to boost sales in a country where Stevenson was not known.

48. Samuel Elder, "Medical Notebook, containing notes of lectures by Nathan Smith . . . ," 3 Dec. [1811], p. [18]; Vault Mss., DCA.

49. Fitch, op. cit., 311, 319. At least some of what NS said in the lectures Fitch attended seems to have come quite directly from the paper he wrote in 1808 for the Boylston Prize competition, "Dissertation on scirrhous & Cancerous Affections"; BRBML (a typed copy is at the CLM). For further discussion of this paper—which appears never to have been published—see *infra*, n56 and n57, and ch. 14.

50. Fitch, op. cit., 264.

51. Ibid., 274.

52. Ibid., 323–24.

53. Ibid., 290–93.

54. Ibid., 340, 340–41.

55. NS to LS, 25 Aug. 1809 (see *supra*, ch. 9, n54); Mss. 801474.1, DCA. In JAS, op. cit., 89.

56. In his unpublished "Dissertation on scirrhous & Cancerous Affections," NS reported on some two dozen cases. This will be discussed *infra*, ch. 14.

57. See, e.g., NS Daybook, Sept. 1797–Mar. 1801 [Day Book B], *passim*; Vault Mss., DCA. For an excellent—albeit brief—overview of the history of cancer therapy, with particular reference to NS's cancer practice, see A. W. Oughterson, "Nathan Smith and Cancer Therapy," *Yale Jrnl. Biol. & Med.* 12, no. 2 (Dec. 1939): 122–36. (Disappointingly, the author did not bother with footnotes, thus making it difficult to track his quotations; some are from the already-mentioned manuscript NS wrote on scirrhous and cancerous affections, but Oughterson used other sources as well.) For NS on cancer, see also Oliver S. Hayward, "The History of Oncology: III: America, and the Cancer Lectures of Nathan Smith," *Surg.* 58, no. 4 (Oct. 1965): 745–57.

58. Fitch, op. cit., 96–97.

59. Ibid., 449.

60. Ibid., 83.

61. Ibid., 134.

62. Ibid., 140–42.

63. Ibid., 160–63. NS learned about spines at least in part by dissections; see Samuel Farnsworth, "Lectures by Dr Smith Dartmouth University Oct 20th AD 1812," p. 3; Vault Mss., DCA.

64. Fitch, op. cit., 17–18.

65. Ibid., 358.

66. Ibid., 359–60.

67. Ibid., 394, 399. NS had extensive experience and a considerable reputation on the subject of how to treat dislocations. He published one article ("Case of Dislocated Humerus reduced ten and a half months after the Displacement,"

Phila. Monthly Jrnl. of Med. and Surg. 1, no. 5 [Oct. 1827]: 214–17—which was also translated into German; see bibliography, p. 338). His son NRS earlier wrote up for publication another of his father's cases ("Reduction of a Shoulder which had been dislocated seven months"), which appeared in the same journal, vol. 1, no. 3 (Aug. 1827): 128. NS was interested in all kinds of dislocations; see ch. 14 for an account of his role as an expert witness in a court case involving a possible dislocation of the hip.

68. Fitch, op. cit., 425–27.

69. Ibid., 435, 437.

70. Ibid., 438.

71. NS, "Observations on Fractures of the Femur, with an account of a new splint," *Amer. Med. Rev., and Jrnl.* 2, no. 1 (Sept. 1825): 140–50 (reprinted in NRS, ed., op. cit., 129–41) and NS, "Observations on Fractures of the Leg, with an account of a new support," *Amer. Med. Rev., and Jrnl.* 2, no. 2 (Dec. 1825): 355–58.

72. NRS, ed., op. cit., 37.

73. See C. E. Putnam, "What Happened to Nathan Smith's 'New Splint'?" read at MEPHISTOS Conference, Harvard University, Cambridge, Mass., Feb. 1994 (unpublished mss.).

74. NS, "Observations on the Pathology and Treatment of Necrosis," *Phila. Monthly Jrnl. of Med. and Surg.* 1 (1827): 11–19, 66–75; reprinted in NRS, ed., op. cit., pp. 97–121.

75. See, e.g., Beecher and Altschule, op. cit., 58; Gordon A. Donaldson, "The First All-New England Surgeon," *Am. Jrnl. Surg.* 135, no. 4 (April 1978): 476; Herbert Thoms, "Nathan Smith," *Jrnl. of Med. Ed.* 33, no. 12 (Dec. 1958): 825; and William H. Welch, in his introduction to EAS, op. cit., [v–vi]. Thomas Francis Harrington, in his *Harvard Medical School: A History, Narrative and Documentary, 1782–1905*, 3 vols. (New York: Lewis Publ., 1905), 1:352, says that NS brought "truth and progress" to the surgeon, showing in his necrosis essay the "power of accurate description, and a method of treatment which seems to have anticipated modern surgery." (Harrington was almost certainly relying on Welch —"admirable description of symptoms, and the introduction of methods of treatment which anticipated modern surgery"—without attribution; see Welch, "The Relation of Yale to Medicine," *Yale Med. Jrnl.* 8, no. 5 [Nov. 1901]: 142.)

76. Fitch, op. cit., 366.

77. NS, "Necrosis," in NRS, ed., op. cit., 118–19.

78. Fitch, op. cit., 366.

79. LeRoy S. Wirthlin, "Nathan Smith (1762–1828[sic]): Surgical Consultant to Joseph Smith," *Brigham Young University Studies* 17, no. 3 (Spring 1977): 320, 321. In this and a later article—"Joseph Smith's Boyhood Operation: An 1813 Surgical Success"—in the same journal, vol. 21, no. 2 (Spring 1981): 131–54, Wirthlin tells the story in more nearly the detail it deserves; his accounts have been heavily relied on here. His quotations both from Smith's "Necrosis" paper and from lecture notes taken by J. S. Goodwin, at Dartmouth, in 1812 ("Extracts from Lectures Delivered at Dartmouth Medical Theatre . . ."; Vault Mss., DCA)—thus at just the time of Joseph Smith's operation (his family lived in Lebanon from 1811 to 1813)—further enhance the discussion. A rather different account of how the episode unfolded, and of research into the matter, appears in Seymour E. Wheelock, "The Prophet, the Physicians and the Medical School," *DMS Alum. Mag.* [9, no. 2] (Spring 1984): 25–27. William D. Morain, in his

Sword of Laban: Joseph Smith, Jr., and the Dissociated Mind (Washington, D.C.: Amer. Psychiatric Press, 1998) explores the Freudian implications (for young Joseph) of the episode.

80. Gilman Kimball, "The President's Annual Address: A Biographical Sketch of Dr. Nathan Smith, Founder of the Dartmouth Medical College," *Gyn. Trans.* 8 (1883): 35. Quoted in EAS, *The Life and Letters of Nathan Smith, M.B., M.D.* (New Haven, Conn.: Yale Univ. Press, 1914), 115. In the "Report of the morning session (19 Sept. 1883) of the Eighth Annual Meeting of the American Gynecological Society," *Medical News* 43, no. 12 (Sept. 22, 1883): 324–25, an exchange relevant to this whole issue is recorded: "Dr. Kimball again alluded to Dr. Smith's performance of the operation of ovariotomy, and claimed that Dr. Smith was entitled to the same honors as had been bestowed on McDowell.

"Dr. S. D. Gross said that he had thought that Dr. Smith had performed his operation with the knowledge that it had been previously performed by McDowell . . . ." Gross went on to insist that it was unlikely NS did not see the published account of McDowell's operation—to which Kimball responded thus: "[I]ntercourse between the east and west was at this time very difficult . . . . I fully believe that he knew nothing of McDowell's case."

81. Isaac Patterson to Oliver P. Hubbard, 13 Oct. 1879; Mss. 879563, DCA.

82. NS to LS, [probably 20 Sept. 1800]; Mss. 000645, DCA. In JAS, *The Life of Dr. Lyman Spalding* (Boston: W. M. Leonard, 1916), 91. (On p. 90, JAS observes that this letter is "undated, but probably written in September 1801"; 1800 seems more likely, given the content.)

83. [John Talbott], Editorial, "Nathan Smith of Dartmouth (1762–1829)," in JAMA 199, no. 2 (9 Jan. 1967): 159.

84. NS, "Observations on the Pathology and Treatment of Necrosis," in NRS, ed., op. cit., 116, 121.

85. Surprisingly, however, even in an article on Smith as a surgeon—"Yale's first professor of surgery: Nathan Smith, M.D. (1762–1829)," *Surgery* 64, no. 2 (Aug. 1968): 524–28—Gustaf E. Lindskog recounts the story in a mere two sentences buried in a general paragraph. How NS presented this famous case orally can be found in his students' lecture notes. See, e.g., John P. Kimball, "Lectures on Surgery, Delivered at Newhaven, Connecticut, By Nathan Smith . . . ," p. 295 *et seq.*; CLM. See also Avery J. Skilton, "Ovarian Dropsy" (in his "Lectures on the Theory and Practice of Physic by Nathan Smith MD, C.S.M.S. Lond . . . ," p. 122 *et seq.*, in Eli Ives, "Lectures on the Diseases of Children"; MS F 12, NLM. An imaginative version of the story (based on historical documents but fleshed out with invented conversation) appears in Seymour E. Wheelock, "A First-Rate Tale," *Dartmouth Medicine* 15, no. 1 (Fall 1990): 48–51. Wheelock concludes that NS must have know about McDowell's successes and that he simply did not want to acknowledge he was not the first.

86. NS, "Case of ovarian dropsy, successfully removed by a surgical operation," *Amer. Med. Recorder* 5 (1822): 124–26. Reprinted in NRS, ed., *Medical and Surgical Memoirs, by Nathan Smith, M.D.* (Baltimore: Wm. A. Francis, 1831), 227–30, and in two foreign journals; see Bibliography, p. 338.

87. NRS, ed., op. cit., 36, 233. A. Scott Earle is more cautious than Wheelock, op. cit., but he too thinks it improbable that NS was unaware of McDowell's pioneering work. See Earle's "Nathan Smith and his contributions to surgery," in *Surgery* 54, no. 2 (Aug. 1963): 415. Recall also the discussion between Gilman Kimball and S. D. Gross, *supra*, n80. Leslie T. Morton in his *Medical Bibliogra-*

phy . . . , 3d ed. (Philadelphia: J. B. Lippincott, 1970), 699, also says NS apparently did not know about McDowell's priority.

88. James Thomas Flexner, *Doctors on Horseback* (New York: Garden City Publ., 1939), 150–51; Editorial, "Ephraim McDowell (1771–1830)—Kentucky Surgeon," *JAMA* 186, no. 9 (30 Nov. 1963): 862. See also Henry K. Beecher and Mark D. Altschule, *Medicine at Harvard: The First Three Hundred Years* (Hanover, N.H.: UPNE, 1977), 58. McDowell's paper, "Three Cases of Extirpation of Diseased Ovaria," appeared in the *Eclectic Repertory & Analyt. Rev.* 7, no. 2 (April 1817): 242–44; two years later he published "Observations on Diseased Ovaria" in the same journal, vol. 9, no. 4 (Oct. 1819): 546–53.

89. Flexner, op. cit., 152; see pp. 121–62 for the whole dramatic story. See also Herbert Thoms, "Nathan Smith and Ovariotomy," *Intern. Abstr. Surg.* 48 (Apr. 1929): 305–307, and the complete text of "Ephraim McDowell" (see *supra*, n88), 861–62, for a brief account of this pioneer physician's career.

90. Robert Houstoun, "An Account of a Dropsy in the left Ovary of a Woman, aged 58. Cured by a large Incision made in the Side of the Abdomen," *Phil. Trans* 33 (1724, 1725): 15, London, 1726. Flexner, op. cit., 131, mentions three other early physicians who are on record as having at least *considered* the possibility that extirpating an ovarian tumor might be beneficial: Theodore Schorkopoff in 1685, Ehrenfried Schlenker in 1712, and John Hunter in 1787.

91. Lawrence D. Longo, "Classic pages in Obstetrics and Gynecology," *Am. Jrnl. Ob. and Gyn.* 126, no. 4 (Oct. 15, 1976): 506. NS himself, in a lecture at Yale, said he did not think it "of much consequence to have a ligature that could not be taken out or that will be absorbed as it is said that leather will"; see Fitch, op. cit., 80.

92. NS, "Ligature of the External Iliac Artery, for the Cure of Aneurism," in NRS, ed., op. cit., 237.

93. Fitch, op. cit., 191.

94. Worham L. Fitch, "Lectures on the Practice of Physic and Surgery by Nathan Smith . . . in the Medical Institution of Yale College 1825," pp. 87, 337, 431; YRG 47-J, M&A, YUL.

95. Fitch, "Extracts," 59–60.

96. Gilman Kimball, op. cit., 35, reports it "is claimed, and justly, I suppose, that he was the first to perform staphylorrhaphy in this country"—and this is quoted (among other places) in EAS, op. cit., 115. A brief anonymous biographical commentary on NS in which the same claim is made—perhaps relying on one or the other of these sources—appeared in *Amer. Jrnl. Surg.* 16, no. 3 (June 1932): 539. But Samuel D. Gross, in his essay "Surgery," in Edward H. Clarke, Henry J. Bigelow, Samuel D. Gross, et al., *A Century of American Medicine 1776–1876* (Philadelphia: Henry C. Lea, 1876), 177, mentions what he considers the first three American surgeons to do the procedure, and NS is not one of them.

97. NS to LS, 7 Mar. 1813; Mss. 813207, DCA. In JAS, op. cit., 270. See also NS, "Femur," 140. NS's son NRS further claimed that his father "devised and introduced a mode of amputating the thigh, which . . . is sufficiently original to bear his name"; NRS, ed., op. cit., 37.

98. Gross, op. cit., 162, *does* mention this as a first for NS. Morton, op. cit., 514, likewise says NS performed the "first amputation of a knee joint in America." See also NS's own account, "On Amputation at the Knee-joint," *Amer. Med. Rev., and Jrnl.* 2, no. 2 (Dec. 1825): 370–71.

99. See NS, "Description of a New Instrument for the Extraction of Coins &

Other Foreign Substances from the Oesophagus," *Amer. Med. Rev. and Jrnl.* 2, no. 1 (Sept. 1825): 168–69 (reprinted in NRS, ed., op. cit., 239–40); see also Fitch, "Extracts," pp. 232–34.

100. Fitch, "Extracts," p. 234–36.

101. See NS, "Necrosis," in NRS, ed., op. cit., 110–11. See also Fitch, "Lectures" and "Extracts," *passim*. Further, see NS to GCS, 11 July 1810; Shattuck Papers, MHS.

102. Alexander Boyd to William Boyd, Jr., 26 Nov. 1810; Mss. 810626.2, DCA.

103. Fitch, "Extracts," 175.

104. Ibid., 179.

105. NS to LS, 25 Aug. 1801; in JAS, op. cit., 90.

106. Welch, "Relation," 141; quoted in Beecher and Altschule, op. cit., 59.

107. NS to MO, 20 Jan. 1814; Mss. 814120, DCA.

Chapter 11. A New Challenge

1. Henry Bond to Nathaniel Wright, 11 July 1813; Mss. 813411, DCA. William H. Welch corroborated Bond's sentiments seventy years later, saying that "Nathan Smith shed undying glory upon the Yale Medical School"; Welch, "The Relation of Yale to Medicine," *Yale Med. Jrnl.* 8, no. 5 (Nov. 1901): 141. Quoted in Henry K. Beecher and Mark D. Altschule, *Medicine at Harvard: The First Three Hundred Years* (Hanover, N.H.: UPNE, 1977), 59.

2. Dartmouth College Trustees, Records, Aug. 1813–July 1840, Vol. 2, p. 3 ([24] Aug. 1813); Vault Mss., DCA.

3. Ernest I. Kohorn, "The Department of Obstetrics and Gynecology at Yale: the First One Hundred Fifty Years, from Nathan Smith to Lee Buxton," *Yale Jrnl. Biol. & Med.* 66, no. 2 (Mar.–Apr. 1993): 86, n1.

4. William Frederick Norwood, *Medical Education in the United States Before the Civil War* (New York: Arno, 1971), 195, cites Welch, op. cit., 137–38 *et seq.*, crediting Dwight. Harold Saxton Burr, in "The Founding of the Medical Institution of Yale College," *Yale Jrnl. Biol. & Med.* 6, no. 3 (Jan. 1934): 336–37, gives a brief discussion of the way the negotiations between the Society and the University went.

5. Jean-François Coste (trans. Anthony Pelzer Wagener, with intro. and notes), "The Adaptation of the Ancient Philosophy of Medicine to the New World," *Jrnl. Hist. Med. and Allied Sciences* 7, [no. 1] (Winter 1952): 45.

6. Dartmouth College Trustees, Records and Charter, July 1770–Aug. 1812, Vol. 1, [25] Aug. 1801, p. 246.

7. See, e.g., Yale University Corporation Minutes, 12 Sept. 1810, p. 130; 10 Sept. 1811, p. 132; 29 April 1812, p. 137; 31 Aug. 1813, p. 149.

8. Ibid., 12 Sept. 1810, p. 130.

9. Ibid., 10 Sept. 1811, p. 132.

10. Walter Ralph Steiner, "Historical Address: The Evolution of Medicine in Connecticut, with the Foundation of Yale Medical School as its Notable Achievement," in the *Memorial of the Centennial of the Yale Medical School, 1814–1915* (New Haven: Yale Univ. Press, 1915), 24.

11. Herbert Thoms, *The Doctors of Yale College 1702–1815 and The Found-*

ing of the Medical Institution (Hamden, Conn.: The Shoe String Press, 1960), 59; also 57.

12. Kohorn, op. cit., 87.

13. Burr, op. cit., 338–40. See also Burr's earlier "Jonathan Knight and the Founding of the Yale School of Medicine," *Yale Jrnl. Biol. & Med.* 1, no. 6 (1928–29): 338; further, Stephen W. Williams, "Dr. Mason Fitch Cogswell," in his *American Medical Biography, or Memoirs of Eminent Physicians* (Greenfield, Mass.: L. Merriam, 1845), 108.

14. Welch, op. cit., 141.

15. Timothy J. Gridley to Jonathan Knight, 20 Nov. 1810. The next passage quoted comes from this same letter. Oliver S. Hayward's notes indicated he saw this letter at Yale; recent efforts to locate it were unsuccessful.

16. Here is evidence that NS was not oblivious to, or so thick-skinned as to be unaffected by, negative public opinion and publicity. He wrote this letter a few weeks after the "angry letter" in the *Concord [N.H.] Gazette* that was quoted earlier; see *supra*, ch. 6, n87.

17. NS to GCS, 14 May 1810; BRBML. In Carleton B. Chapman, *Dartmouth Medical School: The First 175 Years* (Hanover, N.H.: UPNE, 1973), 21–22; also in EAS, *The Life and Letters of Nathan Smith, M.B., M.D.* (New Haven: Yale Univ. Press, 1914), 51–52.

18. Benjamin Silliman to Jonathan Knight, 22 Dec. 1812; C/WML.

19. "Infidelity" was used by Congregationalists to describe what they perceived as the too-casual attitude toward religion sometimes exhibited by Episcopalians even while in good standing in their own churches. It could also refer to the deism, agnosticism, or atheism of free thinkers of the Tom Paine variety.

20. William Allen, *An Address Occasioned by the Death of Nathan Smith, M.D.* . . . (Brunswick, Me.: G. Griffin, Printer, 1829), 21, 22–23.

21. Benjamin Silliman to Jonathan Knight, 22 Dec. 1812; C/WML. The letter from NS to Benjamin Silliman to which Silliman refers was written on 2 Sept. 1813; in EAS, op. cit., 88.

22. Benjamin Silliman to Jonathan Knight, 22 Dec. 1812; C/WML.

23. NS to GCS, [?] Oct. 1809; BRBML. In EAS, op. cit., 50.

24. Timothy J. Gridley to Jonathan Knight, 20 Nov. 1810. See *supra*, n15.

25. At the time of Dwight's death, NS wrote with feeling: "I doubt if any man since Genl. Washington has died in the United States, who has been more universally lamented than Dr. Dwight." NS to MO, [?] Jan. 1817; Mss. 817115, DCA. The same would not be said when John Wheelock died.

26. Moses Porter (Coös Bank), to MO, [?] Aug. 1808; MS-436, Box 2 (Folder 23), DCA. Porter said he was enclosing $700, but—given subsequent court action—it is clear this was an error. He meant $600, as a later receipt makes clear; see *infra*, n27.

27. The receipt for payment by NS on 28 Apr. 1813 was signed by Wm. H. Woodward; DA-3, Box 15 (W–Z Folder), DCA.

28. NS to LS, 20 July 1809; LS Papers, NHHS. In JAS, *Life of Dr. Lyman Spalding* (Boston, Mass.: W. M. Leonard, 1916), 163.

29. MO memorandum, 27 Oct. 1813; DA-3, Box 15 (N–Perkins Folder), DCA.

30. James Hillhouse mortgage contract, 29 Dec. 1814, Hartford, Conn.; DA-3, Box 15 (H Folder), DCA.

31. NS to the President and Board of Trust (Dartmouth College), 12 July 1813; Mss. 813413, DCA.

32. NS to LS, 16 Nov. 1813; LS Papers, NHHS. In JAS, op. cit., 272; he quotes only part of the letter, omitting these details: "[I] have commenced my surgical courses in the new Medical Institution. We have about forty pupils."

33. NS to MO, 3 Dec. 1813; Mss. 813653, DCA.

34. NS to MO, 20 Jan. 1814; Mss. 814120, DCA.

35. NS to Benjamin Silliman, 31 Mar. 1813; in EAS, op. cit., 86 (who reports that this letter as well as the 2 Sept. 1813 one already cited [see *supra*, n21] was— in 1914—in the possession of NS's great-grandson, Samuel Theobald).

36. NS to GCS, 22 June 1806/1807 (both dates appear in the letter—one inside and one outside); M&A, YUL. In EAS, op. cit., 36 (she dates it 22 Jan. 1806).

37. See, e.g., NS to GCS, 20 Dec. [1812]; in EAS, op. cit., 71–72. He had two students prepare an index "to everything relating to medicine or medical men . . . in the several works."

38. NS to Benjamin Silliman, 31 Mar. 1813; in EAS, op. cit., 85.

39. Yale University Corporation Minutes, 22 Apr. 1817, p. 195.

40. Dartmouth College v. Woodward, 17 U.S. (4 Wheat.) 518 (1819).

41. Francis Brown to NS, 12 Aug. 1817; Mss. 817462, DCA.

42. NS to Francis Brown, 21 Aug. 1817; Mss. 817471, DCA.

43. NS to MO, 14 Aug. 1817; Mss. 817464, DCA.

44. NS to MO, 5 Nov. 1818; Mss. 818605, DCA.

45. NS to MO, 28 Feb. 1822; Mss. 822278, DCA. The Rev. Bennet Tyler was appointed president on 13 Feb. 1822, following the Rev. Dr. Daniel Dana, who had been president after Francis Brown (from 3 Oct. 1820).

46. NS to MO, 31 Mar. 1818; Mss. 818231, DCA.

47. NS to MO, 25 May 1819; Mss. 819325.4, DCA. The struggle would continue for several years. In 1824, in reaction against the law passed by the Connecticut legislature, Dr. Elisha North jumped into the fray—publishing three essays under the pen name "Vesalius." See Sebastian R. Italia, "Elisha North: Experimentalist, Epidemiologist, Physician (1771–1843)," in *Bull. Hist. Med.* 31, no. 6 (Nov.–Dec. 1957): 505–36.

48. NS to EDC, 28 June 1819; EDC Papers (Folder 7), M&A, YUL.

49. NS to GCS, 16 Aug. 1824; BRBML.

50. NS to GCS, 8 Dec. 1827; BRBML. In EAS, op. cit., 137.

51. NS to MO, 19 Nov. 1823; Mss. 823619, DCA.

52. Datus Williams to Mason Cogswell, 1 Mar. 1823; BRBML.

53. NS to LS, 6 Mar. 1818; Mss. 818206.3, DCA. In JAS, op. cit., 293.

54. Henry Ingersoll, "Lectures on the Theory and Practice of Physic & Surgery . . . ," p. 6; Mss. 811602.3, DCA.

55. NS to MO, 7 Mar. 1825; MS 436, Box 4 (Folder 65), DCA.

56. Edward Lind Morse, *Samuel F. B. Morse: His Letters and Journals*, 2 vols. (Boston: Houghton Mifflin, 1914) 1:261. The portrait has been much copied (see, e.g., the jacket and the frontispiece of this book), since it is the only known image of NS done from life. The original hangs in the rotunda outside the C/WML at Yale, along with portraits of several other Yale Medical School worthies (e.g., Ives, Knight, Silliman, and Munroe are all there).

57. "Charter of the General Hospital Society of Connecticut, An Act To Establish A State Hospital, Passed, May 26, 1826," Appendix I in *General Hospital Society of Connecticut, Centenary* (New Haven: [no publ.], 1926), 155.

58. Jonathan Knight, *An Eulogium on Nathan Smith, M.D.* (New Haven: Hezekiah Howe, 1829), reprinted in NRS, ed., *Medical and Surgical Memoirs, by Nathan Smith, M.D.* (Baltimore: Wm. A. Francis, 1831), 21.

59. Gordon A. Donaldson, "The First All-New England Surgeon," *Amer. Jrnl. Surg.* 135, no. 4 (Apr. 1978): 475.

60. Knight, in NRS, ed., op. cit., 20–21.

Chapter 12. A Growing Reputation

1. *Hippocrates* (W.H.S. Jones, trans.), "Law" §I and §II (Cambridge, Mass.: Harvard Univ. Press, 1981), Loeb Classical Library, 2:263, 265 (English); 262, 264 (Greek).

2. See NS to MO, 14 Apr. 1821; Mss. 821264, DCA.

3. Nehemiah Cleaveland, *History of Bowdoin College* (Boston: James Ripley Osgood, 1882), 12.

4. Louis C. Hatch, *The History of Bowdoin College* (Portland, Me.: Loring, Short & Harmon, 1927), 461.

5. Herbert Thoms, "Nathan Smith," *Jrnl. Med. Ed.* 33, no. 12 (Dec. 1958): 824.

6. NS to GCS, 14 Feb. 1818. Oliver S. Hayward cited this letter in manuscript notes, but its current location has not been discovered.

7. NS to Mason F. Cogswell, undated letter [early 1813?]; in EAS, *The Life and Letters of Nathan Smith, M.B., M.D.* (New Haven: Yale Univ. Press, 1914), 84.

8. NS to MO, 28 Dec. 1819; Mss. 819678, DCA.

9. NS to MO, 31 Jan. 1820; Mss. 820131, DCA.

10. NS to GCS, 18 Apr. 1823; BRBML. In EAS, op. cit., 122.

11. JAS, *Life of Dr. Lyman Spalding* (Boston, Mass.: W. M. Leonard, 1916), 2.

12. N. Cleaveland, op. cit., 10.

13. Hatch, op. cit., 461.

14. NS to GCS, 7 Jan. 1821; BRBML. In EAS, op. cit., 109–10, 110.

15. Vote of Bowdoin Trustees, 24 Feb. 1821; Board of Trustees: votes and records, BCL.

16. NS to GCS, 7 Jan. 1821; BRBML. In EAS, op. cit., 110–11.

17. NS to MO, 14 Apr. 1821; Mss. 821264, DCA.

18. NS to Harvey Bissell, 17 Apr. 1821; Mss. 821267, DCA.

19. NS to MO, 23 May 1822; Mss. 822323, DCA.

20. *Harvard University: Quinquennial Catalog of the Officers and Graduates, 1636–1930* (Cambridge, Mass.: Pub. by the Univ., 1930), 853.

21. "Memoir of Dr. Wells," *Boston Med. & Surg. Jrnl.* 2 (3 Aug. 1830): 400. See also Stephen W. Williams, "Dr. John Doane Wells," in his *American Medical Biography, or Memoirs of Eminent Physicians* (Greenfield, Mass.: L. Merriam, 1845), 616–17.

22. "Memoir of Dr. Wells," 400. For more on Wells's career at Brunswick and later at the Berkshire Medical Institute, see the complete article in Williams, op. cit., 615–24, which consists almost entirely of what Williams acknowledges is a long quotation from the eulogium of Wells given at Berkshire by Professor H. H. Childs.

23. NS to GCS, 18 Apr. 1823; BRBML. In EAS, op. cit., 122.

24. NS to MO, 16 Nov. 1821; Mss. 821616, DCA.

25. Vote of Bowdoin Trustees, votes of 21 May 1821 and 13 Feb. 1822; Board of Trustees: votes and records, BCL.

26. N. Cleaveland, op. cit., 13.

27. NS to Parker Cleaveland, 2 June 1822; Parker Cleaveland Papers, Manuscripts and Archives Div., NYPL.

28. N. Cleaveland, op. cit., 138.

29. NS to MO, 14 Mar. 1823; Mss. 823214, DCA.

30. NS to William Leffingwell, 1 May 1823; Misc. Papers (Smith, Nathan), Manuscripts and Archives Div., NYPL.

31. *General Catalogue of Bowdoin College and the Medical School of Maine: A Biographical Record of Alumni and Officers 1794–1950* (Brunswick, Me.: Pub. by the College, 1950), 437–39.

32. NS to Parker Cleaveland, 15 Aug. 1822; Chamberlin Collection, Rare Book Dept., BPL.

33. NS to William Allen, 14 July 1824; Misc. Papers (Smith, Nathan), Manuscripts and Archives Div., NYPL. Though the letter in question carries the date "1824," it seems more probable that it was written in 1825.

34. NS to Parker Cleaveland, 9 Apr. 1826; Parker Cleaveland Papers, Special Collections, BCL.

35. Part of the class that entered Dartmouth Medical School in 1810, Woodward is listed as a nongraduate. *Dartmouth College and Associated Schools General Catalogue, 1769–1940* (Hanover, N.H.: Dartmouth College Publ., 1940), 893.

36. NS to Parker Cleaveland, 9 Apr. 1826; Parker Cleaveland Papers, Special Collections, BCL. On Bond, see *Dartmouth College*, 840.

37. Hatch, op. cit., 462.

38. NS to Benjamin Silliman, 6 Aug. 1814; Mss. 814456, DCA.

39. NS to GCS, 22 Apr. 1826; BRBML (copy in Shattuck Papers, MHS). In EAS, op. cit., 133.

40. Faculty vote at Bowdoin College, 9 Sept. 1825; Faculty: records, minutes, and reports, BCL.

41. Reuben D. Mussey to Parker Cleaveland, 12 Oct. 1830; Parker Cleaveland Papers, Special Collections, BCL.

42. NS to Parker Cleaveland, 22 Aug. 1826; Parker Cleaveland Papers, Manuscripts and Archives Div., NYPL.

43. NS to GCS, 6 Jan. 1826; BRBML (copy in Shattuck Papers, MHS). In EAS, op. cit., 131.

44. Faculty resolution at Bowdoin College, drawn by John D. Wells and Parker Cleaveland, 6 Mar. 1829; Faculty: records, minutes, and reports, BCL.

Chapter 13. Surgeon to New England

1. A. T. Lowe to Oliver P. Hubbard, 7 April 1879; Mss. 879257, DCA.

2. *General Catalogue of Bowdoin College and the Medical School of Maine: A Biographical Record of Alumni and Officers 1794–1950* (Brunswick, Me.: Pub. by the College, 1950), pp. 439–40. See also E. H. Leffingwell, P[rinted] D[ocument]; CLM.

3. NS to William Leffingwell, 1 May 1823; Misc. Papers (Smith, Nathan), Manuscripts and Archives Div., NYPL.

4. *General Catalogue of Bowdoin College*, 439–40.

5. A photograph of this ticket appeared in Oliver S. Hayward, "Dr. Nathan Smith (1762–1829)—American Pioneer," *NEJM* 261, no. 10 (3 Sept. 1959): 492. Note 24, indicating the ticket was to be found in the DCA, is in error; it is in fact in the C/WML, Steiner Room. On the same page, Hayward also said Leffingwell was a graduate of Bowdoin—which he was not. See *supra*, n2.

6. LS, *An Address Delivered at Fairfield, VII December MDCCCXIII, at the Inauguration of the Officers of Physicians and Surgeons of the State of New York* (New York: Wm. Treadwell, 1814), 11.

7. See, e.g., Lester J. Wallman, "The UVM Medical Department: 1804–1836," in Robert V. Daniels, ed., *The University of Vermont: The First Two Hundred Years* (Hanover, N.H.: UPNE [for UVM], 1991), 162.

8. Lyman Allen, "A Sketch of Vermont's Early Medical History," *NEJM* 209, no. 16 (19 Oct. 1933): 796. We know that NS and John Pomeroy had corresponded with each other at least as early as 1811. See NS to John Pomeroy, 30 Jan. 1811 "on the disease called white swelling"; NYAML. Pomeroy may have known of NS considerably earlier. JAS quotes from LS's diary in 1797 when the latter visited Pomeroy in Burlington and then comments that Pomeroy "must have been glad enough now, to get an opinion from a scholar of Nathan Smith"; JAS, *Life of Dr. Lyman Spalding* (Boston, Mass.: W. M. Leonard, 1916), 9, n1. JAS did not reveal on what he based this speculative observation.

9. The idea had durability. A century and a half later, in 1964, the then-dean of UVM's College of Medicine, Robert J. Slater, reportedly said, "Here in Burlington . . . located in the mid-Northern and New England region, it is easier for us to understand the problems of the somewhat remote rural practice. We share many of the concerns of the rural physician." NS would have loved it. Editorial, "Small Medical College Helps Mold Future of Rural Practice," *JAMA* 189, no. 12 (21 Sept. 1964): 40.

10. John King, "Dr. John Pomeroy and the College of Medicine of the University of Vermont," *Jrnl. Hist. Med. and Allied Sciences* 4 (Autumn 1949): 398, 401, 400, 393 (in that order). See also Martin Kaufman, *The University of Vermont College of Medicine* (Hanover, N.H.: UPNE, 1979): 11, 12.

11. UVM Trustees Minutes, Vol. 2, pp. 162, 167; B/HL.

12. NRS to GCS, 28 Sept. 1820; BRBML.

13. See, e.g., Oliver P. Hubbard, *Dartmouth Medical College and Nathan Smith: An Historical Discourse* (Concord, N.H.: Evans, Sleeper, & Evans, 1879): 7, for a reference to the four terms NS taught in Burlington. King, op. cit., 401, n40, makes a point of saying Smith was never "a regular faculty member."

14. NS to MO, 29 Sept. 1822; Mss. 822529, DCA. Also NS to MO, 19 July 1824; Mss. 824419.1, DCA.

15. See King, op cit., 393–406, for more on Pomeroy's role. King's only reference to NS is, surprisingly, the note already quoted in part (see *supra*, n13); NS deserves more than this footnote, even in a discussion of Pomeroy. King continues dismissively, saying NS is "frequently referred to as the founder of the Medical College"—the clear implication being that King does not share the view. It is, of course, true that NS was not the *sole* founder of the Medical College in Burlington.

16. William A. R. Chapin and Lyman Allen, eds., *History: University of Vermont College of Medicine* (Hanover, N.H.: Dartmouth Printing, 1951), 31.

17. NS to MO, 29 Sept. 1822; Mss. 822529, DCA. Porter was also a Dartmouth product. Given that he earned his M.D. in 1818 (see *Dartmouth College*

and Associated Schools General Catalogue, 1769–1940 [Hanover, N.H.: Dartmouth College Publ., 1940], 840), he probably was present for NS's fall 1816 course of lectures.

18. NS to MO, 28 Apr. 1822; Mss. 822278, DCA.

19. NS to Parker Cleaveland, 23 Aug. 1822; Mss. 822473, DCA.

20. NS to MO, 19 July 1824; Mss. 8244191.1, DCA.

21. NS to MO, 5 Jan. 1823; Mss. 823105, DCA.

22. NS to MO, 14 Mar. 1823; Mss. 823214, DCA.

23. NS to MO, 19 Oct. 1822; Mss. 822569, DCA.

24. NS to GCS, 18 Apr. 1823; BRBML. In EAS, *The Life and Letters of Nathan Smith, M.B., M.D.* (New Haven: Yale Univ. Press, 1914), 122. This sentiment could help explain his not having responded affirmatively to overtures apparently made by Middlebury College—also in Vermont—to establish such a department there. See, e.g., Chapin and Allen, op. cit., 31. See also Frederick C. Waite, "Three Episodes in Medical Education at Middlebury College [1810–1837]," *NEJM* 206, no. 14 (7 Apr. 1932): 729–30.

25. NS to GCS, 16 Aug. 1824; BRBML. In EAS, op. cit., 132.

26. Chapin and Allen, loc. cit.

27. JAS, *Life* (Boston: W. M. Leonard, 1916), 131–32, n3, gives a brief account of this "hitherto overlooked episode in the life of Dr. Smith."

28. The newspaper account says "step-mother"; JAS, loc. cit., says "mother-in-law." The discrepancy is insignificant. John R. Gillis, *A World of Their Own Making* (Cambridge, Mass.: Harvard Univ. Press, 1997), 15, point outs that the two terms "were often used interchangeably" during this period.

29. The unanimous opinion of the "jury of doctors"—that Fay had been poisoned—was reported in the Walpole, N.H., *Political Observatory* 3, no. 153 (17 Oct. 1806): 3. (Fay's death notice had appeared in the same paper two weeks earlier: 3, no. 151 [3 Oct. 1806]: 3.)

30. NS, "State of New-Hampshire *vs.* Margery Fay: Examination," Walpole, N.H., *Farmer's Museum* 14, no. 5 (6 Mar. 1807): 4. The lengthy disquisition was preceded by an editorial note indicating the piece had been submitted "by the friends of the person conceived injured" and expressing a disinclination to publish any more on the case, while promising space for self-defense if "either of the faculty conceives his professional skill doubted." Much of the first part of the article as it appeared seems to have been written by those who submitted it, not by NS. JAS, op cit., 132, in the continuation of n3, purports to be quoting from the newspaper account—but it certainly was not *The Farmer's Museum* version. Though substantively not at variance, JAS's text tells the story in very different language.

31. NS to LS, 12 Mar. 1807; LS Papers, NHHS. In JAS, op. cit., 131–32.

32. Already in January, the other Walpole paper—the *Political Observatory*—had published a notice reporting that after "several witnesses" (NS was not named) had been examined, Mrs. Fay's "innocence [was] completely established (4, no. 165 [9 Jan. 1807]: 3). Why Mrs. Fay's supporters thought it was still important to publish NS's remarks three months later is unclear.

33. NS to GCS, 20 May 1823; in EAS, op. cit., 123 (dated 5 May 1823). JAS, op. cit., 314, also makes a passing reference to NS having been involved in "a case of murder."

34. "Trial of Patrick Cole," Portland, Maine, *Eastern Argus* (13 May 1823): 2. The preceding two brief quotations are from this same news item.

35. Lowell v. Faxon and Hawkes, Washington County Court of Common Pleas, March Term 1823, Docket #118, Vol. 3, p. 482. A detailed review of the case can be found in JAS, "Lowell vs. Faxon and Hawkes. Celebrated Malpractice Suit in Maine," *Bull. Amer. Acad. Med.* 11, no. 1 (Feb. 1910): 4–31; that account has been heavily relied on here. Even more complete is the 120-page account in *Report of the Trial of an Action, Charles Lowell against John Faxon and Micajah Hawks, Doctors of Medicine, Defendants for Malpractice in the Capacity of Physicians and Surgeons at the Supreme Judicial Court of Maine, Holden at Machias for the County of Washington, June Term, 1824: Before the Hon. Nathan Weston, Jun., Justice of the Court* (Portland, Me.: Printed for J. Adams, Jr., by David and Seth Paine, 1825).

36. In a lecture on "Reduction of Luxated Humerus," NS explicitly observed that the "practice of giving tobacco &c. is improper where the reduction can be affected [sic] without"—though he went on to say that giving "antimony or tobacco to produce the necessary relaxation" was preferable to bleeding. He also commented that "[n]o pulley or screws should be used," nor "any great force." Worham L. Fitch, "Extracts From Lectures on Surgery Delivered at the Medical Institution at New Haven by Nathan Smith, 1824," pp. 401, 402; YRG 47-J, M&A, YUL.

37. JAS, "Lowell vs. Faxon and Hawkes," 11.

38. Ibid., 19.

39. [NS], "Deposition A," in John C. Warren, *A letter to the Hon. Isaac Parker, containing Remarks on the dislocation of the hip joint, occasioned by the publication of a trial which took place at Machias [Maine,] June, 1824* (Cambridge, Mass.: Hilliard & Metcalf, 1826), 130–31.

40. JAS, "Lowell vs. Faxon and Hawkes," 26.

41. Ibid., 27.

42. Warren, op. cit. See, e.g., 24: "My situation as defendant in this affair, obliges me further to remark upon two other opinions which . . . if correct . . . go directly to diminish the confidence in my testimony"; also p. 128, "Note.—On reviewing my deposition, I find myself not altogether satisfied with the degree of precision in the expression of some parts . . . ."

43. JAS, "Lowell vs. Faxon and Hawkes," 30.

44. Oliver S. Hayward made this presentation at the Boston Medical Library on 13 Apr. 1959. For brief references to the case, see his "Dr. Nathan Smith (1762–1829)—American Pioneer," *NEJM* 261, no. 10 (3 Sept. 1959): 492–93, and "A Search for the Real Nathan Smith," *Jrnl. Hist. Med. And Allied Sciences* 15, no. 3 (July 1960): 275–76. The debate about Charles Lowell's hip had a modest revival in 1990 when three physicians in California, independent of each other, examined photographs of the X-rays and concluded that a dislocation had surely taken place. David Spring to Mary Hayward, 17 May 1990; personal communication. In the files of C. E. Putnam, Concord, Mass.

45. JAS, "Lowell vs. Faxon and Hawkes," 30—citing the remarks appended to the postmortem report by Henry K. Oliver of Boston—acknowledges the possibility that the jury was swayed by the fact that "a distinguished surgeon [NS] asserted that there was no dislocation."

46. Ibid., 24. The reference to a "recent trial" helps give credence to the supposition that NS had been involved in Patrick Cole's case the previous year. There could, of course, have been still another case.

47. Editorial note (unsigned, but certainly by NRS), in *Phila. Monthly Jrnl. of Med. and Surg.* 1, no. 1 (June 1827): 43.

48. Warren, op. cit., 24.

49. NS to GCS, 6 Jan. 1826; BRBML (copy in the Shattuck Papers, MHS). In EAS, op. cit., 131.

50. Samuel Cowls to Mason F. Cogswell, 28 Aug. 1827. Oliver S. Hayward's notes indicated he saw this letter at Yale; recent efforts to locate it were unsuccessful. (Cowls in this letter quotes NS's entire affidavit.)

51. A. Scott Earle, "Nathan Smith and his contributions to surgery," *Surgery* 54, no. 2 (Aug. 1963): 414.

52. Willard Arms to NS, 24 June 1812; DA-3, Box 15 (A–B Folder), DCA.

53. NS to Mason F. Cogswell, 18 Dec. 1815; Mason Fitch Cogswell Papers, M&A, YUL.

54. Thomas Chadbourne to NS, 26 June 1815; DA-3, Box 15 (Accounts Relating to DMS Folder), DCA.

55. See, e.g., John P. Kimball, "Lectures on Surgery, Delivered at New-haven . . . ," p. 30; CLM.

56. [?] Hall to NS, 24 July 1814; DA-3, Box 15 (H Folder), DCA. Several documents having to do with individuals named "Hall" (Benjamin, Nathaniel, etc.) are to be found here; this is the only one where the first name is illegible.

57. Daniel Webster to E[zekiel Webster], 8 Jan. 1828; Mss. 828108, DCA.

58. NS to LS, 4 Apr. 1819; in JAS, *Life*, 313–14.

59. NS to Dr. [?] Fuller, 4 Oct. 1826; Rare Book and Manuscript Library, Columbia University.

60. William A. Benedict and Hiram A. Tracy, *History of the Town of Sutton, Massachusetts, from 1704 to 1876* (Worcester, Mass.: Sanford, 1878), 413.

61. Levi W. Leonard, *The History of Dublin, N.H.* (Cambridge, Mass.: University Press, for the town of Dublin, 1919), 560.

Chapter 14. *A Man of Many Parts*

1. Joseph Perry to GCS, 4 Aug. 1852; Shattuck Papers, MHS.

2. "Obituary," *Amer. Jrnl. Sci. and Arts* 16, no. 1 (July 1829): 213; quoted in Oliver P. Hubbard, *Dartmouth Medical College and Nathan Smith: An Historical Discourse* (Concord, N.H.: Evans, Sleeper, & Evans, 1879), 22–23 (where he—probably correctly—attributes the unsigned obituary notice to Benjamin Silliman, founding editor of the journal).

3. Roswell Shurtleff to GCS, 3 Jan. 1810; Shattuck Papers, MHS.

4. Nehemiah Cleaveland, *History of Bowdoin College* (Boston: James Ripley Osgood, 1882), 138–39.

5. NS to Jonathan Hall, 19 May 1804; Mss. 804319, DCA.

6. NS to GCS, 18 Apr. 1823; BRBML (copy in Shattuck Papers, MHS). In EAS, *The Life and Letters of Nathan Smith, M.B., M.D.* (New Haven: Yale Univ. Press, 1914), 122. A few weeks earlier, on 4 Apr. 1823, NS had written much the same to his wife: "I shall write another [book,] on Surgery, which I hope to have nearly completed before I leave this place"; quoted in Hubbard, op. cit., 26, note.

7. NS to GCS, 8 Dec. 1827; BRBML. In EAS, op. cit., 137.

8. We know a prospectus for a work to be entitled "Practical Observations on Surgery by Nathan Smith, M.D." appeared in one journal. The description of the

content makes clear it was to consist, at least in part, of papers NS did write and publish (elsewhere): "The work will contain an account of the author's mode of operating in Amputation; his mode of treating Dislocations and Fractures, and his practice in Necrosis Wounds of the Joints and Abscesses. Also his peculiar doctrine of the spontaneous stopping of Haemorrhage from wounded Arteries." Perhaps some new papers would also have been included; the book was to be three hundred pages in length. The prospectus is undated, but—judging from the letters quoted above—it was probably some time in 1823. A search of 1823 and 1824 journals has not turned up the ad; it may have appeared on the back page, typically removed when journals were bound. Photostat copy in NS (h1798) Alumni File, DCA.

9. [John] E[berle], "Smith on Typhous Fever," *Med. Rev. and Analectic Jrnl.* 1, no. 1 (June 1824): 63.

10. Ibid., 73, 74. Much later it would be understood that this "able" paper of NS's had foreshadowed by more than a decade Jacob Bigelow's deservedly famous 1835 paper on self-limited diseases (see *supra*, ch. 5, n72); Richard Harrison Shryock, *Medicine and Society in America, 1660–1860* (New York: New York Univ. Press, 1960), 127, 131.

11. E[berle], op. cit., 70, 72.

12. According to a note written by Oliver S. Hayward in the 1960s, Thomas Miner's annotated copy of NS's *Practical Essay on Typhous Fever* was at that time in the "rare book room" at Yale. A recent search has not turned it up in the BRBML, C/WML, or M&A, YUL, however. That Miner had strong views on the subject is not surprising; he was co-author with William Tully of *Essays on Fevers, and other Medical Subjects* (Middletown, Conn.: E. & H. Clark, 1823).

13. Anonymous review of NS, *Practical Essay on Typhous Fever,* in *N.Y. Med. & Physical Jrnl.* 3, no. 3 (1824): 347–63. For a discussion that places this work by NS in historical context, see John R. Paul, "Nathan Smith and Typhoid Fever," *Yale Jrnl. Biol. & Med.* 2, no. 3 (1929–30): 169–81.

14. *Amer. Med. Rev., and Jrnl.* 2, no. 1 (Sept. 1825): 140–50 and 168–69.

15. [John] E[berle], editorial note, *Amer. Med. Rev., and Jrnl.* 2, no. 1 (Sept. 1825): 150.

16. *Amer. Med. Rev., and Jrnl.* 2, no. 2 (Dec. 1825): 355–58 and 370–71; 3, no. 2 (Aug. 1826): 396–97.

17. NS, "Observations on the pathology and treatment of necrosis," *Phila. Monthly Jrnl. of Med. and Surg.* 1 (1827): 11–19, 66–75; in NRS, ed., *Medical and Surgical Memoirs by Nathan Smith, M.D.* (Baltimore: Wm. A. Francis, 1831), 39–96.

18. *Memoirs of the Med. Soc. of London* 6 (1805): 227–31; *Trans. of the Med. Soc. of London* 1, Part 1 (1810): 179–85.

19. The author was A. Philips Wilson until he added "Philip" as a surname, in compliance with certain Scottish laws, to allow him to become chief of his clan; William H. McMenemey, "Alexander Philips Wilson Philip (1770–1847), Physiologist and Physician," *Jrnl. Hist. Med. and Allied Sciences* 13, [no. 3] (July 1958): 289, 297. Citing *Berrow's Worcester Jrnl.* 5648, McMenemey gives the date of the name change as 7 Mar. 1811.

20. A. T. Lowe to Oliver P. Hubbard, 7 Apr. 1879 and 16 Apr. 1879; Mss. 879257 and Mss. 879266 respectively, DCA.

21. NRS, ed., op. cit., 42.

22. A. P. Wilson Philip, *A Treatise on Febrile Diseases, Including the Various*

Species of Fever and All Diseases Attended with Fever, 2d Amer. ed., from the 3d London ed. 1813, edited and with notes by NS, 2 vols. (Hartford, Conn.: Cooke & Hale, 1816), 2:450 and 389–408. See also Benjamin Moseley, *Observations on the Dysentery of the West-Indies, with A New and Successful Manner of Treating It* (London: T. Becket [from the 2d ed.], 1781).

23. NS to LS, 11 Sept. 1817; in JAS, *Life of Dr. Lyman Spalding* (Boston: W. M. Leonard, 1916), 285.

24. Wilson Philip, op. cit., 1:75.

25. Ibid., 333.

26. Ibid., xiii (oddly, the roman-numeraled pages come at the end of the book). Lachlan MacLean, *An Inquiry Into The Nature, Causes, and Cure of Hydrothorax*, 1st Amer. ed. (Hartford, Conn.: Hale & Hosmer, 1814), was another of the books NS gave to Yale (see *supra*, ch. 1, n47).

27. Wilson Philip, op. cit., 2:309.

28. Ibid., 361.

29. Wilson Philip, op. cit., 1:219–20.

30. NS to GCS, 28 Nov. 1808; BRBML (copy in Shattuck Papers, MHS). In EAS, op. cit., 43–44.

31. The statement of the Boylston topic and the announcement of the deadline of 20 Nov. 1808 appear in a newspaper clipping (cut and mounted in a way that makes it impossible to tell which newspaper it was) in LS's scrapbook "Medical Portfolio," p. 185; CLM.

32. The manuscript of NS's unpublished "Dissertation of scirrhous & Cancerous Affections" is at the BRBML (a typescript copy of it is in the CLM). The paper is notable for the two dozen case reports in it, which give valuable insights into NS's understanding of cancer. For a discussion of some features of work NS did in this area, see A. W. Oughterson, "Nathan Smith and Cancer Therapy," *Yale Jrnl. Biol. & Med.* 12, no. 2 (1939): 123–36 (esp. 130–34), discussed *supra*, ch. 10, n57.

33. NS to GCS, 28 Nov. 1808; BRBML (copy in Shattuck Papers, MHS). In EAS, op. cit., 44.

34. JAS, op. cit., 248, n1. Closer to the time in question—and possibly the source for JAS's claim—is Lyman Bartlett How's comment that "In 1811, Dr. Smith went to Exeter, and read several papers [on the topics JAS names]." See Lyman Bartlett How, *The Story of the New Hampshire Medical Society Taken to 1854 . . .* (1891; rev. ed., Nashua, N.H.: Phaneuf Press, 1941), 28. But How also provides no evidence and does not claim to have seen the papers.

35. NS to LS, 21 Mar. 1808; CLM. (Not in JAS, op. cit.)

36. NS to LS, 10 Apr. 1811; Mss. 811260, DCA. In JAS, op. cit., 248.

37. See, e.g., Asa Porter to MO (on the discounting of some notes belonging to NS), 8 Feb. and 18 Feb. 1805; MS-436, Box 1 (Folder 14), DCA. See also George Woodward to MO (on the same subject), 18 Apr. and 20 Apr. 1807; MS-436, Box 2 (Folder 21), DCA.

38. See NS to MO ("I suppose I owe him nearly a hundred dollars"), 4 Sept. 1807; Mss. 807504.1, DCA. Also NS to MO (saying he had enclosed "fifty dollars . . . . The sum due is not far [from that]"), 23 Apr. 1821; Mss. 821273, DCA. Further, NS to MO ("I had a note . . . of 20 dollars I think . . ."), 4 Oct. 1821; DA-3, Box 15 (W–Z Folder), DCA.

39. NS to GCS, 18 Mar. 1811; BRBML. In EAS, op. cit., 55.

40. Memorandum for 9 Aug. 1801; DA-3, Box 15 (S Folder), DCA.

41. Among these were the following: NS vs. Benjamin West Trustee for Benjamin Waterhouse, Charlestown, N.H., Court of Common Pleas: Dec. 1795, No. 70 (case continued); Mar. 1796, No. 59 (ditto); June 1796, No. 18 (ditto); Sept. 1796, No. 11 (found for NS); appealed (by Benjamin West) to Superior Court, Cheshire Cty., Oct. Term 1796, *Cheshire Records*, Vol. 4, p. 127 (case continued); and finally dismissed May Term 1797, *Cheshire Records*, Vol. 4, p. 194. Also NS v. Bela Fitch (for nonpayment), Superior Court, Cheshire Cty., Oct. Term 1797, *Cheshire Records*, Vol. 4, pp. 414–15. Court Records, Keene, N.H. Although many cases (including these) went in NS's favor—more often than not because the defendant defaulted by failing to appear—there are also instances of NS being hauled into court himself for failure to pay bills; see, e.g., Mss. 796103, DCA (at issue was a debt of $32.50).

42. NS to MO, 29 Aug. 1815; Mss. 815479, DCA. For earlier examples, see entries for 26 Feb. 1803, Sept. and June 1804, Aug. 1805, Feb. 1806, and on and on; Account Books, Hanover, 41: MO Accounts of his law practice, 1800–1840, Vol. 2, 1807–1825, p. 9 (Vol. 1, 1800–1807, p. 42, also has several), DCA.

43. Receipt for Hezekiah Ensworth payment of $8.25 due for services 11 June — 13 July 1816; DA-3, Box 15 (D–F Folder), DCA.

44. NS to Benjamin Silliman, 6 Aug. 1814; Mss. 814456, DCA.

45. NS to MO, [?] Oct. 1815; Mss. 815590.1, DCA.

46. One hopes this was not money still owed from the trip abroad! See *supra*, ch. 3, n31.

47. NS to MO, 22 Dec. 1817; Mss. 817672, DCA. The "500. Dollar premium" appears to be money voted by the Yale Board over and above the $400 increase in annual salary also voted for NS. See *supra*, ch. 11, n39.

48. NS to MO, 21 Nov. 1828; Mss. 828602, DCA.

49. NS to MO, [?] May 1818; Mss. 818340.1, DCA.

50. Land Records: Chester, Windsor County, Vt., Vol. B, pp. 181, 186, 187, 279, 300.

51. See, e.g., receipts from 5 Apr. 1798 and 22 Dec. 1800; DA-3, Box 15 (C Folder), DCA. See also the note dated 3 Sept. 1803; DA-3, Box 15 (Miscellaneous Items Folder), DCA. On the prior point, see also, e.g., receipts signed by Jonathan Chase (14 Feb. 1801 and 4 Jan. 1812) and a running account between NS and Dudley Chase (22 Oct. 1797 to 20 Feb. 1798); DA-3, Box 15 (C Folder), DCA.

52. See, e.g., James Morven Smith to MO, 27 Mar. and 18 May 1830, and Catherine C. Smith to MO, 5 Feb. and 21 Sept. 1830; MS-436, Box 4 (Folder 77), DCA. See also Probate Records of the City of New Haven, Vol. 39, pp. 155, 170, 404–405, 462; Vol. 40, pp. 204, 215–16.

53. Will of Jonathan Chase, 15 Jan. 1801; Mss. 801115, DCA. See *supra*, Ch. 8, n5.

54. Documents concerning NS's land purchases in Hanover include the following: 7 Dec. 1806; Mss. 806657. 15 Dec. 1806; Mss. 806665. 18 Dec. 1806 (acknowledged before a Justice of the Peace, 1 Apr. 1807); Mss. 806668. 28 July 1807; Mss. 807428.1. 1 Sept. 1807; Mss. 807501. All DCA.

55. NS to MO, 3 Sept. 1815; Mss. 815503, DCA.

56. NS to MO, 14 Mar. 1822; Mss. 822214, DCA.

57. NS to MO, 10 Mar. 1821; Mss. 821210, DCA.

58. Baxter Perry Smith, *The History of Dartmouth College* (Boston: Houghton, Osgood, 1878), 393.

59. NS to Sally Smith, 14 Mar. 1814; in EAS, op. cit., 95–96..

60. EAS, op. cit., 11.

61. NS to Sally Smith, 17 Dec. 1796; in EAS, op. cit., 17–18.

62. NS to Sally Smith, 23 Feb. 1797; in EAS, op. cit., 19–20.

63. NS to Parker Cleaveland, 23 Aug. 1822; Mss. 822473, DCA.

64. In a careful study of NS's near contemporary Elisha North—the doctor who had written on Connecticut's anatomy law under the pen name "Vesalius"—we learn that he was married. But all we are told about his wife is that she "smoothed [his life] for him" and that they "raised a family of eight children, four boys and four girls." Sebastian R. Italia, "Elisha North: Experimentalist, Epidemiologist, Physician, 1771–1843," *Bull. Hist. Med.* 31, no. 6 (Nov.–Dec. 1951): 533.

65. Copy (dated 23 Nov. 1838) of the deed of "1st day of June ano [sic] Domini 1811"; Mss. 811351, DCA.

66. Deed to Pew No. 1, $100, 11 May 1811; Mss. 811311, DCA. NS must have been in a mood to do business with Baldwin at the time, for on the same day he also bought a piece of land from Baldwin; see receipt, DA-3, Box 15 (Receipts and Oaths Folder), DCA.

67. William A. Benedict and Hiram A. Tracy, *History of the Town of Sutton, Massachusetts, from 1704 to 1876* (Worcester, Mass.: Sanford & Co., 1878), 318.

68. George H. Lyman, *A discourse commemorative of the life & religious experience of the late David Solon Chase Hall Smith of Providence, R.I., formerly of Sutton, Mass., delivered in the Congregational Church, Sutton, April 24, 1859* (Worcester, Mass.: Edward R. Fiske, 1859), 5.

69. Malleville Allen to William Allen, 23 July 1814 (emphasis in original); Mss. 814423, DCA.

70. A. T. Lowe to Oliver P. Hubbard; 16 Apr. 1879, Mss. 879266, DCA.

71. NS to MO, 12 Jan. 1816; Mss. 816112, DCA.

72. NS to MO, 22 Dec. 1817; Mss. 817672, DCA. See also *supra*, n47.

73. NS to MO, 22 Dec. 1817; Mss. 817672, DCA.

74. NS to MO, 19 July 1824; Mss. 824419.1, DCA.

75. See NS to MO, 12 Aug. 1826; Mss. 826462.1, DCA. Also NS to MO, 15 Oct. 1826; Mss. 826265, DCA.

76. EAS, op. cit., 100. She gives no evidence beyond saying there "seems to have been nothing that the devoted father and skilled physician could do to save the precious life of his child" (99), and no relevant letters appear to be extant. But of course it is plausible. Smith did carefully record the date of young Sally's death—"June 13th 1815"—in the family Bible, according to EAS (ibid., 102); she was not yet sixteen. As for expressions of grief by Smith, see NS to GCS, 3 July 1828; Shattuck Papers, MHS (see earlier reference *supra*, ch. 2, n49).

77. NS to GCS, 20 [sic: postmarked 15] Apr. 1811; Mss. 811265, DCA. In EAS, op. cit., 62.

78. NS to GCS, 6 Jan. 1826; BRBML (copy in Shattuck Papers, MHS). In EAS, op. cit., 131.

79. NS to MO, 19 July 1824; Mss. 824419.1, DCA.

80. EAS, op. cit., 13, says "Solon" came from the poetry of Ossian, like some of the other names Sally and Nathan chose for their children. It appears she is mistaken, however; a careful search did not turn up the name in Ossian. "Solon" is, of course, a classical name.

81. EAS, op. cit., 106.

82. NS to GCS, 8 Dec. 1827; BRBML. In EAS, op. cit., 137.

83. "To determine the nature of disease and its cause is the most difficult part

of medical practice," we are told in a passage about Solon. "To understand the complicated and intricate mechanism of the human system requires . . . intuition, genius, judgment and skill. All these Dr. [Solon] Smith possessed in a remarkable degree. So when other physicians had a human machine on their hands that they could not keep going, they used to send for him to find out what cog was broken, pin loose or what pulley disbanded." Benedict and Tracy, op. cit., 316.

84. Ibid, 317.

85. See Ronald H. Fishbein, "Nathan Smith and the Johns Hopkins Connection," in *Md. Med. Jrnl.* 38, no. 6 (June 1989): 471. The archives of Jefferson Medical School are strangely silent on NRS, and no photograph of him appears in James F. Gayley, *A History of the Jefferson Medical College of Philadelphia . . . , with Biographical Sketches of the early Professors illustrated with portraits & engravings* (Philadelphia: Joseph M. Wilson, 1858). It should be noted that the claims by various writers that NS assisted his son, NRS, in the founding of Jefferson Medical School (see, e.g., John Pollard Bowler, "Master Surgeons of America: Nathan Smith," in *Surg., Gyn., and Ob.* 48, no. 6 [June 1919]: 833), are based more on flights of fancy or wishful thinking than on reality. No evidence has been found that NS ever went to Philadelphia or had anything to do with the establishment of Jefferson Medical School.

86. The journal was variously called (or referred to as) *Medical Review and Analectic Journal, American Medical Review and Journal, American Medical Review*, and *Medical Review Analectic.*

87. In his "Remarks on Dislocations of the Hip-Joint," NRS at least opened with a note acknowledging that the principles he was presenting were "derived from my father's lectures." See NRS, ed., op. cit., 163. In his "Hints on the Operation of Lithotomy," before launching into his own experience, he spent four pages discussing his father's work—apparently as a kind of excuse for including his own paper. Ibid., 241–44.

88. NRS to one of his sisters [not here named], 19 Jan. 1829; Shattuck Papers, MHS. In EAS, op. cit., 138–39.

89. Warfield T. Longcope, "Smith, Nathan Ryno," in *Dictionary of American Biography*, Dumas Malone, ed. (New York: Charles Scribner's Sons, 1935), 17:328. See also Eugene F. Cordell, "Smith, Nathan Ryno (1797–1877)," in Howard A. Kelly and Walter L. Burrage, eds., *American Medical Biographies* (Baltimore: Norman, Remington, Co., 1920), 1076–78; and C. Donegan, "Smith, Nathan Ryno," in Martin Kaufman, Stuart Galishoff, and Todd L. Savitt, eds., *Dictionary of American Medical Biography*, 2 vols. (Westport, Ct.: Greenwood Press, 1984), 2:697.

90. *An Essay on the Diseases of the Middle Ear* (Baltimore: Hatch & Dunning, 1829). See Longcope, op. cit., 328.

91. Donegan, op. cit., 697.

92. Alexius McGlannan, "The Surgical and Anatomical Works of Nathan Ryno Smith," *Univ. of Md. Bull. School of Med.* 9, no. 4 (Apr. 1924–25): 138.

93. *Treatment of Fractures of the Lower Extremity by the Use of an Anterior Suspensory Apparatus* (Baltimore: Kelly and Piet, 1867).

94. Longcope, op. cit., 328; Cordell, op. cit., 1078; and EAS, op. cit., 163.

95. S. D. Gross, *An Address Delivered Before the Alumni Association of the Jefferson College of Philadelphia* (Philadelphia: Collins, Printer, 1871), 14.

96. T.[sic] Morven Smith, "Cases of Necrosis illustrating the Practice of Ex-

posing and Perforating the Diseased Bone at an early period in the progress of the malady," in *Amer. Jrnl. Med. Sciences* 23, no. 45 (Nov. 1838): 93–96.

97. *New-York Daily Times* 2, no. 511 (9 May 1853): 1 *et seq.* For the initial account of the accident, see the same paper, vol. 2, no. 510 (7 May 1853): 1. EAS, op. cit., 160, tells of Morven's death but (inexplicably) has the date wrong by ten days.

98. EAS, loc. cit.

99. Mary M. Smith to GCS, 25 Oct. 1852; Shattuck Papers, MHS.

100. "Genealogy"; Shattuck Papers, MHS. A handwritten note about John Derby (who died on 5 Dec. 1812) is inserted in the Shattuck genealogy booklet. It reads in part as follows: "Childless, the fatherless found in him a father. Blind in his old age, he was led by an orphan child of his adoption. The 'visual ray' was let into his sightless orbs by a surgeon [NS], a son of whom baptized with his name, has been educated from means saved by his prudence."

101. GCS to Benjamin Silliman, 6 Feb. 1829; Shattuck Papers, MHS.

102. GCS to John D. Smith, 6 Feb. 1829; Shattuck Papers, MHS.

103. NRS to GCS, 12 May 1829; Shattuck Papers, MHS.

Chapter 15. Epilogue

1. Jonathan Knight, "A Lecture Introductory to the Course of Instruction in the Medical Institution of Yale College . . . ," bound in *Kingsley Misc. Papers* (New Haven: B. L. Hamlen, Printer, 1839) 27:20; BRBML. That Knight should be moved to speak this way a full decade after his predecessor's death shows that the words of high praise spoken in the immediate aftermath of NS's death (see *infra*, n2, e.g., for Knight's own words at that earlier point) need not be discounted as nothing more than kind words uttered only to avoid speaking ill of the dead.

2. Jonathan Knight, *An Eulogium on Nathan Smith, M.D.* (New Haven: Hezekiah Howe, 1829), reprinted in NRS, ed., *Medical and Surgical Memoirs by Nathan Smith, M.D.* (Baltimore: Wm. A. Francis, 1831), 21. The two quoted passages that follow are from the same source, pp. 21 and 21–22, respectively.

3. Alan Gregg, personal communication to John Sloan Dickey (then-president of Dartmouth College), April 1948, as noted by Oliver S. Hayward; in the files of C. E. Putnam, Concord, Mass. Quoted by John F. Fulton (who surely got it from Hayward) in his "Foreword" to Oliver S. Hayward and Elizabeth H. Thomson, eds., *The Journal of William Tully, Medical Student at Dartmouth 1808–1809* (New York: Science History, 1977), xii.

4. Henry I. Bowditch, *Memoir of Amos Twitchell, M.D.* (Boston: John Wilson and Son, 1851), 16, 30.

5. Oliver Wendell Holmes, "The Medical Profession in Massachusetts," in his *Medical Essays* (Boston: Houghton Mifflin, 1883), 350.

6. Oliver P. Hubbard, *Dartmouth Medical College and Nathan Smith: An Historical Discourse* (Concord, N.H.: Evans, Sleeper, & Evans, 1879), 7, 18.

7. John P. Bowler, "Master Surgeons of America: Nathan Smith," in *Surg., Gyn. and Ob.* 48, no. 6 (June 1929): 829.

8. William Allen, *An Address Occasioned by the Death of Nathan Smith, M.D. . . .* (Brunswick, Me.: G. Griffin, Printer, 1829), 8.

9. Harvey Cushing, *The Medical Career: An Address in The Ideals, Opportu-*

nities, and Difficulties of the Medical Profession . . . (Hanover, N.H.: Dartmouth College, 1929), 37–38.

10. Knight, in NRS, ed., op. cit., 24, 25, 35.

11. Samuel D. Gross, "Surgery," in Edward H. Clarke, Henry J. Bigelow, Samuel D. Gross, et al., *A Century of American Medicine* (Philadelphia: Henry C. Lea, 1876), 121.

12. William H. Welch, "Introduction" to EAS, *The Life and Letters of Nathan Smith, M.B., M.D.* (New Haven: Yale Univ. Press, 1914), [v].

13. William H. Welch, "The Relation of Yale to Medicine," *Yale Med. Jrnl.* 8, no. 5 (Nov. 1901): 141–42. Here Welch shows familiarity with Knight's *Eulogium*.

14. Frederic S. Dennis, "Smith, Nathan (1762–1829)," in Howard A. Kelly and Walter L. Burrage, eds., *American Medical Biographies* (Baltimore: Norman, Remington, 1920), 1076.

15. George Washington Corner, *Two Centuries of Medicine: A History of the School of Medicine, University of Pennsylvania* (Philadelphia: J. B. Lippincott, 1965), 57.

16. Samuel L. Knapp, *Lectures on American Literature with Remarks on Some Passages of American History* (New York: Elam Bliss, 1829), 123–24.

17. Bowler, op. cit., 833.

18. Knight, in NRS, ed., op. cit., 19.

19. Carleton B. Chapman, *Dartmouth Medical School: The First 175 Years* (Hanover, N.H.: UPNE, 1973), 19.

20. Warfield T. Longcope, "Smith, Nathan," in Dumas Malone, ed., *Dictionary of American Biography* (New York: Scribner's, 1935), 17:325.

21. Knight, in NRS, ed., op. cit., 23.

Bibliography

Chronological List of Works by Nathan Smith

"A dissertation, on the causes and effects of spasm in fevers; pronounced . . . before the President, Medical Professors, and Governors of Harvard University, at Cambridge, July 5th, 1790." *Massachusetts Magazine* 3, no. 1 (Jan. 1791): 33–35; 3, no. 2 (Feb. 1791): 81–83.

"Dr. Smith's Reply." *Massachusetts Magazine* 4, no. 5 (May 1792): 314–15.

"Dr. Smith's Replication to Philozetemia." *Massachusetts Magazine* 5, no. 4 (Apr. 1793): 218–21.

"Observations on the Position of Patients in the Operation for Lithotomy, with a Case." *Memoirs of the Medical Society of London* 6 (1805): 227–31.

"Valedictory Charge," in Ellsworth, "Extracts from the Lectures," pp. [29–31].

"State of New-Hampshire *vs.* Margery Fay: Examination." *The [Walpole, N.H.] Farmer's Museum* 14, no. 51 (6 Mar. 1807): 4.

"Dissertation on scirrhous & Cancerous affections." Unpublished Mss., ca. 1808 (48 pp.); BRBML (typescript copy in CLM).

[Miscellaneous Notes on Medical Subjects, 2 vols.]: "Book [Lecture Notes on Chemistry]," 1809 (56 pp.); lecture notebook [n.d.] (204 pp.). Mss.; BRBML.

"On the medicinal properties of sanguinaria Canadensis, or Blood Root." *Transactions of the Medical Society of London* 1, part 1 (1810): 179–85. Reprinted in *Edinburgh Medical and Surgical Journal* 8, no. 30 (Apr. 1812): 216–17; also, in French, in *Annales cliniques ou Journal des sciences médicales* (Montpellier) 26 (1811): 394–95.

A Treatise on Febrile Diseases, Including the Various Species of Fever, and All Diseases Attended with Fever, by A. P. Wilson Philip. 2d American edition, with notes and additions by Nathan Smith, M.D., from the 3d London edition of 1813. Hartford, Conn.: Cooke & Hale, 1816.

"A Nosological Arrangement of Diseases." In Nathan Smith, ed., *A Treatise on Febrile Diseases,* vol. 1, pp. 29–42.

"[Of the Typhus Fever.]" In Nathan Smith, ed., *A Treatise on Febrile Diseases,* vol. 1, pp. 213–18.

"Dr. Smith's Treatise on Dropsy." In Nathan Smith, ed., *A Treatise on Febrile Diseases,* vol. 1, Appendix 2, pp. xiii–xxvii.

"[Pneumonia Typhoidea.]" In Nathan Smith, ed., *A Treatise on Febrile Diseases,* vol. 2, pp. 206–10, note.

"[Acute Rheumatism.]" In Nathan Smith, ed., *A Treatise on Febrile Diseases,* vol. 2, p. 251, note.

"[The causes of hemorrhage.]" In Nathan Smith, ed., *A Treatise on Febrile Diseases,* vol. 2, pp. 309–12, note.

"[Respecting Epidemic Catarrh.]" In Nathan Smith, ed., *A Treatise on Febrile Diseases,* vol. 2, p. 361, note; vol. 2, pp. 162–63, note.

"Dr. Smith's Note on Dysentery." In Nathan Smith, ed., *A Treatise on Febrile Diseases,* vol. 2, pp. 389–408.

"Dr. N. Smith's Appendix: Of the Modus Operandi of morbid poisons, and other exciting causes of disease." In Nathan Smith, ed., *A Treatise on Febrile Diseases*, vol. 2, pp. 449–53.

"Case of Ovarian Dropsy, Successfully Removed by Surgical Operation." *American Medical Recorder* 5, no. 17 (1822): 124–26. Reprinted in Nathan R. Smith, ed., *Medical and Surgical Memoirs*, pp. 227–30; in *Edinburgh Surgical and Medical Journal* 18, no. 70 (Oct. 1822): 532–34; in French, in *Archives générales de médecine* 1 (1823): 126–27; and in A. Scott Earle, ed., *Surgery in America: From the Colonial Era to the Twentieth Century*, 2d ed. (New York: Praeger, 1983), pp. 108–10.

"Directions to the Accoucher [sic]," as taken down by Abraham Lines Smyth (1823). Reprinted in Annan, pp. 528–34.

A Practical Essay on Typhous Fever. New York: E. Bliss and E. White, 1824. Reprinted in Nathan R. Smith, ed., *Medical and Surgical Memoirs*, pp. 39–96; and in *Medical Classics* 1, no. 8 (Apr. 1937): 781–819.

"Deposition A." In John C. Warren, *A letter to the Hon. Isaac Parker, . . . June, 1824*, pp. 130–31. Cambridge, Mass.: Hilliard & Metcalf, 1826.

"Account of a New Instrument for the Extraction of Coins & Other Foreign Substances from the Oesophagus." *American Medical Review, and Journal* 2, no. 1 (Sept. 1825): 168–69. Reprinted in Nathan R. Smith, ed., *Medical and Surgical Memoirs*, pp. 239–40 (with the title "Description of a New [etc.]"); and in A. Scott Earle, ed., *Surgery in America: From the Colonial Era to the Twentieth Century*, 2d ed. (New York: Praeger, 1983), pp. 106–108.

"Observations on Fractures of the Femur, with an account of a New Splint." *American Medical Review, and Journal* 2, no. 1 (Sept. 1825): 140–50. Reprinted "with a cut" (and an acknowledgement that it had been previously published) in *Philadelphia Monthly Journal of Medicine and Surgery* 2, no. 2 (Jan. 1828): 51–59; and in Nathan R. Smith, ed., *Medical and Surgical Memoirs*, pp. 129–41.

"Observations on Fractures of the Leg, with an account of a new support." *American Medical Review, and Journal* 2, no. 2 (Dec. 1825): 355–58.

"On Amputation at the Knee-joint." *American Medical Review, and Journal* 2, no. 2 (Dec. 1825): 370–71.

"Suture of the Palate." *American Medical Review, and Journal* 3, no. 2 (Aug. 1826): 396–97.

"Remarks on the Spontaneous Suppression of Hemorrhage, in Cases of Divided and Wounded Arteries, With Comments on the Physiology and Pathology of the Circulating System." *Philadelphia Monthly Journal of Medicine and Surgery* 1, no. 5 (Oct. 1827): 201–206; 1, no. 6 (Nov. 1827): 249–53; 2, no. 2 (Jan. 1828): 59–61. Reprinted in Nathan R. Smith, ed., *Medical and Surgical Memoirs*, pp. 187–201. Translated and published as "Remarques sur la suppression spontanée de l'hémorrhagie dans les cas de section et de plaies des artères," in *Journal des progrès des sciences et institutions médicales* (Paris) 9 (1828): 118–30.

"Case of Dislocated Humerus reduced ten and a half months after the Displacement." *Philadelphia Monthly Journal of Medicine and Surgery* 1, no. 5 (Oct. 1827): 214–17. Translated and published as "Luxation des Humerus zehn und einen halben Monat nach der Luxation eingerichtet," in Ludwig Friedrich v. Froriep, ed., *Notizen aus dem Gebiete der Natur- und Heilkunde* 21, no. 456 (Juli 1828): 255.

"Observations on the Pathology and Treatment of Necrosis." *Philadelphia Monthly Journal of Medicine and Surgery* 1, no. 1 (June 1827): 11–19; vol. 1, no. 2 (July 1827): 66–75. Reprinted in Nathan R. Smith, ed., *Medical and Surgical Memoirs*, pp. 97–121; in *Medical Classics* 1, no. 8 (Apr. 1937): 820–38; and in *Reviews of Infectious Diseases* 8, no. 3 (May–June 1986): 505–10.

"Remarks on Amputation." In Nathan R. Smith, ed., *Medical and Surgical Memoirs* (1831), pp. 215–25.

"Ligature of the External Iliac Artery, for the Cure of Aneurism." In Nathan R. Smith, ed., *Medical and Surgical Memoirs* (1831), pp. 235–37.

"Heads of Lectures on Anatomy. Lectures on Anatomy." Unpublished Mss. Notebook, [n.d.], (158 pp.); BRBML.

"Introductory Lecture on the Progress of Medical Science." Mss., [n.d.], 25 pp.; BRBML. In Emily A. Smith, *The Life and Letters of Nathan Smith*, pp. 169–79.

Student Notebooks on Nathan Smith's Lectures

Allen, Ezekiel. "A Memorandum of the Lectures given at the Medical Institution of Hanover," 1816 (165 pp., including notes on two lectures by Cyrus Perkins). Vault Mss., DCA.

Anon. "Extracts from a course of Chimical [sic] Lectures delivered at Dartmouth College by Nathan Smith Oct. 1st 1806" (ca. 30 pp.). Vault Mss., DCA (typescript copy in C/WML).

———. "Lectures by Eli Ives MD and Nathan Smith MD" [ca. 1820] (50 pp.). YRG 47-J, M&A, YUL.

———. "Lectures in Surgery by Nathan Smith M.D. Jan. 14th 1825" (78 pp.). YRG 47-J, M&A, YUL (typescript copy in C/WML).

———. "Lectures in Surgery By Professor Smith . . . in 1825 & 6 December 14" (44 pp.). BRBML.

———. "Lectures in Surgery by N. Smith M.D. (115 pp., including notes on lectures "given in Burlington Vt Autumn of 1822" [pp. 1–96] and notes on lectures "in Yale College, the winter of 1822–3" [pp. 97–115]. Mss., BRBML.

———. "Nosological Arrangement of Diseases by Nathan Smith M.D. Delivered in the term of 1819–20" (342 pp.). YRG 47-J, M&A, YUL.

———. "Notes on the Theory and Practice of Physic by Nathan Smith, M.D." [n.d.] (50 pp., including notes on lectures by Eli Ives). Clendenning History of Medicine Library, University of Kansas Medical Center.

———. "Notes on the Theory and practice of Physic from the lectures of Doct. Smith Nov 8th 1825" (65 pp., 9 pp. of drug recipes). YRG 47-J, M&A, YUL.

——- [presumed to be by a student of Nathan Smith]. "Phthisis pulmonalis, Auscultation, . . ." [n.d.] (16 pp., in five sections, unbound). Mss. 001322, DCA.

———. "Theory and practice of physic: Nathan Smith M.D. . . . Professor of the Theory and Practice of Physic, Surgery, and Obstetrics. Yale College, 1815" (69 pp.). Edward G. Miner Library, University of Rochester Medical Center.

Barrett, Benjamin. "Notes from the Lectures of Nathan Smith M.D. C.S.M.S. Lond., Professor of the Theory & Practice of Physic, Surgery, & Obstetrics In the Medical Institution of Yale College," 1821 (2 vols. bound together, titled "Notes"; 140 pp., including 3 pp. Table of Contents). BRBML.

Bedford, Andrew. "A Course of Lectures on Theory & Practice of Physic By Nathan Smith M.D., Medical Institution of Yale College AD 1823 & 4" (ca. 83 pp.). YRG 47-J, M&A, YUL.

Bird, Isaac. "Lectures of Dr. Smith [signed: Nathan Smith, M.D.]" [1816] (66 pp.). M&A, YUL.

Carpenter, Elijah W. "Lectures at New Haven on Surgery, Midwifery, Theory and Practice of Physic, By Nathan Smith, M.D.," Nov. 10th 1813 (175 pp.). YRG 47-J, M&A, YUL (typescript copy—with those of the next four entries—in C/WML).

———. "Notes From *Lectures* on the Theory & Practice of Physic, Surgery, and Obstetrics, Delivered at NewHaven, Conn. A.D. 1813 & 14, By Nathan Smith, M.D. (26 pp.). YRG 47-J, M&A, YUL.

———. "Notes on Doct. Smith's Lectures -1814- Newhaven Jan. 12" (79 pp.). YRG 47-J, M&A, YUL.

———. "Notes on Doct. Smiths Lectures on Surgery & Theory & practice of Physic—N.Haven, 14th March 1814" (57 pp., plus Index). YRG 47-J, M&A, YUL.

———. "New Haven Jan'y 1814 Operations performed by Dr. Smith" (12 pp.). YRG 47-J, M&A, YUL.

[Carrington, Edwin W. (?)]. "Lectures on the Theory and Practice of Medicine By Nathan Smith, M.D." [1827–28] (pp. 247–379 of 665 pp.), in William Tully, "Outlines of a course of lectures on the theory and practice of medicine . . . ," bound with other lecture notes in a volume entitled *Medical Lectures*. MS 19th, C/WML.

[Chadbourne, Thomas]. "Notes taken from Dr Smiths lectures—1815." Smith, Nathan, "Notes taken . . ." (92 pp. plus 9 pp. at back, reverse direction); Vault Mss., DCA.

Champion, B. "Notebook Containing Excerpts of Lectures given at Dartmouth Medical College by Drs. S. Sumner, Eli Todd, and Nathan Smith, together with Prescriptions and Receipts, Hanover, N.H. 1809" (143 pp.). NYAML.

Clark, Job. ["Lecture Notebook of Medical Instruction . . . 1816–1817"] (224 pp., including notes [interspersed] on lectures by Eli Ives and Benjamin Silliman). Job Clark Papers: Group No. 18, Series I, Box 1 (Folder 7); M&A, YUL.

Cushing, Rufus King. "Notes on the Theory & Practice of Physic February-May 1823, from the Lectures Delivered by Nathan Smith . . . ." (110 pp.). Special Collections, BCL.

Edwards, David Shelton. "Theory & Practice of Physic by Nathan Smith MD . . . [1815?]" (50 pp.). In Nathan Smith, "Lectures in the Theory and Practice of Physic." MS C 300, NLM.

Elder, Samuel. "Medical Notebook, containing notes of lectures by Nathan Smith and Cyrus Perkins at Dartmouth Medical College" [NS lectures from 27 Nov. 1811 through 9 Dec. 1811] (ca. 100 pp.). Vault Mss., DCA.

Ellsworth, William C. "Chemical Lectures As delivered in a Course of Lectures at Dartmouth College Oct. 1st AD 1806 by Nathan Smith MD" (ca. 65 pp.). Smith, Nathan, "Wm. C. Ellsworth, Chemical Lectures . . ." Vault Mss., DCA.

———. "Extracts from the Lectures on the Theory & Practice of Physic, As Delivered in a Course of Lectures at Dartmouth College, Oct. 1, 1806, by Nathan Smith, M.D." (ca. 57 pp.). Smith, Nathan, "William C. Ellsworth, Extracts . . ." Vault Mss., DCA.

Farnsworth, Samuel. "Lectures by Dr Smith Dartmouth University [sic], Oct. 20th AD 1812" (54 pp.). Vault Mss., DCA.

Fitch, Worham L. "Extracts From Lectures on Surgery Delivered at the Medical Institution At New Haven by Nathan Smith 1824" [sic: inside front cover says "Nov. 12th 1825 No. 2," and the lectures in this notebook end "May 9th 1826"; thus it appears the cover is wrong, the date having been inadvertently confused with that for the other book of notes—see next entry], (468 pp., plus

Index). YRG 47-J, M&A, YUL (typescript copy—also of the next entry—in C/WML; a second typescript copy in CLM).

———. "Lectures on the Practice of Physic and Surgery by Nathan Smith M.D. C.S.M.S. Prof. . . . in the Medical Institute of Yale College, 1825" [sic: see note on previous entry; this should have read "1824"—the lecture notes end "Feb. 16th 1825"] (450 pp., plus Index). YRG 47-J, M&A, YUL (typescript—with those of previous entry—in C/WML; a second typescript copy in CLM).

Gillette, Horace C. "Lectures on Surgery By Nathan Smith MD Yale College New-haven Connecticut 1828" (291 pp.). YRG 47-J, M&A, YUL.

Goodwin, J. S. "Extracts from Lectures delivered at Dartmouth Medical Theatre by Nathan Smith, M.D. CSMS Lond . . . AD 1812, 1813" (156 pp.). Vault Mss., DCA.

Gorham, Calvin. "Extracts from Nathan Smith's Lectures Delivered at Dartmouth University [sic], AD 1811–12 (ca. 140 pp). Vault Mss., DCA.

Grosvenor, William. "Lectures from Nathan Smith MD" [1827–28], includes *inter alia* "Lectures delivered by Doct Smith on Theory & practice of Medicine—New Haven" and "Nathan Smith on Surgery" (42 pp. and 65 pp. respectively of 362 pp.). YRG 47-J, M&A, YUL.

Hall, David E. "Notes from Lectures of Dr. N. Smith Prof. of Theor. & Pract. of medicine etc. at Yale College 1818–9" (166 pp. of 268 pp., including notes from lectures by Eli Ives). YRG 47-J, M&A, YUL.

Heffron, John jun. "Extracts from a course in Chemical lectures delivered at Dartmouth College by Doct Nathan Smith Hanover, N.H. Oct. 4th 1809" (40 pp. of ca. 134 pp. [pp. 41–102 headed "Lectures on Surgery" but including "Theory and Practice" as well]; followed by pp. 1–31 [new numbering] with records of visits to patients, etc.). Medical Mss. Collection, Group No. 346, Box 3 (Folder 7); M&A, YUL.

———. "Receipts & Materia medica etc. [1809] (ca. 40 pp. of drug recipes, including 7 from "Doct. Smith" on pp. 3–8). Medical Mss. Collection, Group No. 346, Box 3 (Folder 7); M&A, YUL.

Humphrey, Phelps. "Notes Taken from the Lectures of Nathan Smith M.D. C.S.M.S. Lond Prof. Of the Theory & Practice of Physic Surgery & Obstetrics For the Medical Institution of Yale College . . . November 1821" (81 pp.). YRG 47-J, M&A, YUL.

Hunt, Orrin. "Lectures on the Theory & Practice of Physic by Nathan Smith MD C.S.M.S. Lond, Professor of Surgery Obstetrics & Theory & Practice of Physic Yale College" [1818–19] (122 pp.). YRG 47-J, M&A, YUL (typescript copy in C/WML).

Ingersoll, Henry. "Lectures on the Theory and Practice of Physic & Surgery. Delivered at Dartmouth Medical Theatre AD 1811 By Nathan Smith MD" (127 pp.). Mss. 811602.3, DCA.

Kellogg, Alfred. "Notes from the Surgical Lectures of Nathan Smith, M.D., During the course of 1821–22" (209 pp.). YRG 47-J, M&A, YUL.

Kimball, John P. "Lectures on Surgery, Delivered at Newhaven, Connecticut, By Nathan Smith, Professor of the Theory and Practice of Physic & Surgery. Taken as Delivered by John P. Kimball 1819. Copied from Dr. J. P. Kimball's Manuscript, November 1821" (302 pp. plus Table of Contents [6 pp.]). CLM (typescript copy in C/WML).

King, Dan. "Notes From Lectures on the Theory & Practice of Physic given at the Medical College, New Haven in 1814.15. By Nathan Smith. M.D. C.S.M.S." (ca. 155 pp.). M&A, YUL.

Lay, Willoughby Lynde. "Lectures on the Theory and Practice of Physic by Nathan Smith MD, Professor of Surgery, Midwifery, Theory & Practice of Physic, Yale College, New Haven," January 12th AD 1814 (ca. 150 pp.). YRG 47-J, M&A, YUL.

Lufkin, A[aron]. "Lectures by Dr. Smith Book No. 2, March 14, 1822 Brunswick Maine" (ca. 240 pp. in five separate booklets; half sheets). Special Collections, Galter Health Sciences Library, Northwestern University.

Mack, Andrew. "Journal kept during a course of chemical . . . lectures given by Dr. Nathan Smith . . . ," 1810 (17 pp.). Vault Mss., DCA.

Murdoch, Ellice. "Notes on Surgery Taken from Lectures delivered at the Medical Institution of Yale College By Nathan Smith MD. CS.MS.Lond. [1815, 1816, & 1817]" (ca. 207 pp. [pp. 165–72 have been carefully excised], including transcription by Murdoch of notes John Titsworth took in lectures by [Valentine] Mott). Edward G. Miner Library, University of Rochester Medical Center.

Skilton, Avery J. "Lectures on the Theory and Practice of Physic, by Nathan Smith, M.D., CSMS Lond Professor of the Theory and Practice of Physic in the Medical Institution of Yale College"; "Medical Jurisprudence by Nathan Smith MD CSMSL; Nosological Arrangement of Diseases"; and "Directions to the Accoucheur by Nathan Smith MD [1826–27]" (102 pp. of 169 including notes on lectures by Eli Ives and Jonathan Knight). In Eli Ives, "Lectures on the Diseases of Children." MS F 12, NLM.

Skinner, Roger S. "Notes on the lectures of Nathan Smith, M.D., professor of surgery, theory and practice of physic, and midwifery, at Yale college, New Haven" [after 1813], (265 pp. [some blank]). M&A, YUL.

Smyth, Abraham Lines. "Notes from Lectures [on the Theory and Practice of Physic by Nathan Smith] delivered in Yale College, New Haven, 1823" (108 pp.). NYAML.

Talcott, William Olmstead. "Lectures on Theory and Practice by Nathan Smith MD Professor of Theory and Practice, Surgery and Obstetricks in the Medical Institution of Yale College" [n.d.] (176 pp.). YRG 47-J, M&A, YUL.

Thomson, Asahel. "Sketches of the Lectures of Nathan Smith M.D. . . . [And Eli Ives . . .] Delivered in the course Of 1816 and 1817 [at Yale]" (331 pp. [headed "Lectures of Prof. Smith on the Theory & Practice of Medicine And Surgery"] of 777 pp.). BRBML.

Turner, Rufus. "Directions to the Accoucheur by Dr. Smith," "On Midwifery," and "On Obstetrics" [n.d.] (32 pp. of ca. 125 pp., including notes on lectures by others). YRG 47-J, M&A, YUL (typescript copy in C/WML).

Woodbury, Peter L. "Medical Institution of Yale College, Lectures on Theory and Practice of Medicine, and on Surgery and Midwifery, by Nathan Smith, M.D. November 26, 1813–14 . . ." (Vol. I, 366 pp.; Vol. II, 321 pp. [some blank pages in each]. YRG 47-J, M&A, YUL (microfilm copy of both volumes at the C/WML).

Works on Nathan Smith

Adcock, Louis C. "Early American Chemistry Teachers." *Chemistry* 48, no. 10 (Nov. 1975): 15–16.

Aievoli. "Storia della Medicina: Nathan Smith e l'ovariotomia." *La Riforma Medica* 45, no. 31 (3 agosto 1929): 1065.

Allen, Lyman. "A Sketch of Vermont's Early Medical History." *NEJM* 209, no. 16 (19 Oct. 1933): 792–98.

Allen, William. *An Address Occasioned by the Death of Nathan Smith, M.D., First Lecturer in the Medical School of Maine at Bowdoin College, Delivered by Appointment of the Faculty of Medicine.* Brunswick, Me.: G. Griffin, 1829.

Allibore, S. Austin. *A Critical Dictionary of English Literature and British and American Authors* (3 vols.), vol. 2, p. 2152. Philadelphia: J. B. Lippincott, 1877.

Anglem, T. J. "Nathan Smith" (typescript, ca. 1927), 5 pp. Nathan Smith (h1798) Alumni File, DCA.

Annan, Gertrude L. "Advice of Nathan Smith, 1762–1829, on the Conduct of the Accoucheur." *Bulletin of the New York Academy of Medicine*, 2d series, 12, no. 9 (Sept. 1936): 528–34.

Anon. "American Physicians: Nathan Smith." *American Journal of Surgery* 16, no. 3 (June 1932): 539.

———. "Broadcast to Honor U.V.M. Medical Founder." *[Brattleboro, Vt.] Phoenix* (7 Feb. 1947). Photocopy in Nathan Smith (h1798) Alumni File, DCA.

———. "Dr. Nathan Smith." *Boston Medical and Surgical Journal* 2, no. 20 (30 June 1829): 312–16.

———. "Dr. Nathan Smith Established Medical School 131 Years Ago." Photocopy of unidentified newspaper clipping (7 Dec. 1928) in Nathan Smith (h1798) Alumni File, DCA.

———. "The Exile permitted to return!" *New Hampshire Patriot* 8, no. 23 (10 Sept. 1816): [3]. Photocopy in Nathan Smith (h1798) Alumni File, DCA.

———. "Heroes of American Medicine XII. Nathan Smith." *Hygeia* 6, no. 5 (May 1928): 244.

———. ["It is seldom the lot of any man . . . ."] Photocopy of unidentified newspaper clipping in Nathan Smith (h1798) Alumni File, DCA.

———. "Nathan Smith." *Transactions of the [New Hampshire Medical] Society* (June 1891): 131–35. Concord, N.H.: Republican Press Association, 1891.

———. "NH Country Doctor Will Be Dramatized On Radio Saturday." *Concord [N.H.] Monitor & Patriot* (6 Feb. 1947): 1, 6. Photocopy in Nathan Smith (h1798) Alumni File, DCA.

———. [Obituary notice.] *Connecticut Journal* 52, no. 3196 (27 Jan. 1829).

———. [Obituary notice.] *[New Haven] Columbian Register* (31 Jan. 1829).

———. "Our Boston Literary Letter, As to Medicine and Medicos" (review of Emily A. Smith, *The Life and Letters of Nathan Smith*). *Springfield [Mass.] Republican* (22 July 1914). Photocopy in Nathan Smith (h1798) Alumni File, DCA.

———. "Pay Tribute to Circuit Riding N. E. Doctor." *Hillsborough [N.H.] Messenger* (6 Feb. 1947). Photocopy in Nathan Smith (h1798) Alumni File, DCA.

———. Review of Emily A. Smith, *The Life and Letters of Nathan Smith*. *[Brattleboro, Vt.] Phoenix* (24 Feb. 1915). Photocopy in Nathan Smith (h1798) Alumni File, DCA.

———. "Review of [Jonathan] Knight's Eulogium." *Quarterly Christian Spectator* 1, no. 1 (Mar. 1829): 204–208.

———. Review of Nathan Smith, *Practical Essay on Typhous Fever*. *New York Medical & Physical Journal* 3, no. 11 (1824): 347–63.

———. "Smith, Nathan." R. French Stone, ed., *Biography of Eminent American Physicians and Surgeons*, 2d rev. ed., p. 475. Indianapolis, Ind.: C. F. Hollenbeck, 1898.

———. ["We are happy to be informed . . . ."] *Dartmouth Gazette* 16, no. 885 (4 Sept. 1816): [3].

Bell, Whitfield J., Jr. "The Medical Institution of Yale College, 1810–1885." *Yale Journal of Biology and Medicine* 33, no. 3 (Dec. 1960): 169–83.

Bowler, John Pollard. "Master Surgeons of America: Nathan Smith." *Surgery, Gynecology, and Obstetrics* 48, no. 6 (June 1929): 829–33.

Burr, Harold Saxton. "The Founding of the Medical Institution of Yale College." *Yale Journal of Biology and Medicine* 6, no. 3 (Jan. 1934): 333–40.

Chapin, William A. R., and Lyman Allen, eds. *History: University of Vermont College of Medicine,* pp. 30–32. Hanover, N.H.: Dartmouth Printing, 1951.

Chapman, Carleton B. *Dartmouth Medical School: The First 175 Years,* pp. iv–24 *(passim).* Hanover, N.H.: University Press of New England, 1973.

———. "1797–1812 Phase One: The Smith Era," Part II.B. of "Development 1797–1968: The Next Logical Step." *Dartmouth Medical School Quarterly* (Special Issue) 5, no. 1 (Summer 1968): 8–15.

Child, William H. "Nathan Smith," in *History of the Town of Cornish, New Hampshire, with Genealogical Record, 1763–1910.* Vol. I, *Narrative,* pp. 274–75; Vol. 2, *Genealogy,* pp. 334–35. [Concord, N.H.:] General Rumford Press, [1911?]; Spartanburg, S.C.: The Reprint Company, 1975.

Cleveland, Mather, and Oliver S. Hayward. "Nathan Smith (1762–1829) on Amputations." *Journal of Bone and Joint Surgery* 43-A, no. 8 (Dec. 1961): 1246–54.

Colby, Virginia Reed, and James B. Atkinson. "Dr. Nathan Smith, 1762–1829, Founder of Four Medical Colleges," in *Footprints of the Past: Images of Cornish, New Hampshire, and the Cornish Art Colony,* pp. 40–44. Concord, N.H.: New Hampshire Historical Society, 1996.

Conner, Phineas Sanborn. "Historical Address," in Dartmouth Medical College, *Centennial Exercises.* Hanover, N.H.: Dartmouth Press, 1907.

Crockett, Walter H. "Founders of and Teachers in the Medical College [University of Vermont]: Sketches of Dr. Nathan Smith, Dr. Nathan Ryno Smith and Dr. Benjamin Lincoln." *Vermont Alumni Weekly* 15, no. 24 (14 Apr. 1926): 378–79.

Crosby, A. B. *A Contribution to the Medical History of New Hampshire.* Nashua, N.H.: Moore and Langley, 1870.

Cushing, Harvey. *The Medical Career: An Address on The Ideals, Opportunities, and Difficulties of the Medical Profession, Containing a Tribute to Dr. Nathan Smith, Founder of Dartmouth Medical School.* Delivered at Dartmouth, Nov. 20, 1928. Hanover. N.H.: Dartmouth College, 1929 (2d ed., Brattleboro, Vt.: Ichabod Crane, 1930).

———. "Remarks . . . at the Unveiling of the Nathan Smith Tablet" (typescript, 6 pp.). Nathan Smith (h1798) Alumni File, DCA.

Dennis, Frederic S. "Smith, Nathan (1762–1829)," in Howard A. Kelly and Walter L. Burrage, eds., *American Medical Biographies,* pp. 1073–76. Baltimore: Norman, Remington Co., 1920.

———. "Nathan Smith (1762–1829)," in Howard A. Kelly and Walter L. Burrage, eds., *Dictionary of American Medical Biography,* pp. 1132–35. New York: D. Appleton and Co., 1928.

Donaldson, Gordon A. "The First All-New England Surgeon." *American Journal of Surgery* 135, no. 4 (Apr. 1978): 471–79.

———. "The Legacy of Nathan Smith." *Harvard Medical Alumni Bulletin* 55, no. 1 (Feb. 1981): 20–28.

Earle, A. Scott. "Nathan Smith and his contributions to surgery." *Surgery* 54, no. 2 (Aug. 1963): 410–16.

E[berle, John]. "Smith on Typhous Fever." *Medical Review and Analectic Journal* 1, no. 1 (June 1824): 63–80.

———. [Editorial accompanying Nathan Smith's "Observations on Fractures of the Femur . . ."]. *Medical Review and Analectic Journal* 2, no. 1 (Sept. 1825): 150.

Edwards, Bela Bates. "Nathan Smith," in *Biography of Self-Taught Men* (2 vols.), 2:109–17. Boston: Benjamin Perkins & Co., 1846, 7.

Field, William W. *The Good Doctor Smith: Life and Times of Dr. Nathan Smith 1762–1829.* New Haven: Advocate Press, 1992.

Fishbein, Ronald H. "Nathan Smith and the Johns Hopkins Connection." *Maryland Medical Journal* 38, no. 6 (June 1989): 469–75.

French, Edward. "Four Medical Men of New Hampshire." *Transactions of the [New Hampshire Medical] Society* (June 1891): 167–72. Concord, N.H.: Republican Press Association, 1891.

Frost, C. P. "Medical Education in New Hampshire." *Transactions of the [New Hampshire Medical] Society* (June 1891): 157–66. Concord, N.H.: Republican Press Association, 1891.

Gordon, Maurice Bear. *Aesculapius Comes to the Colonies,* pp. 128–41. Ventnor, N.J.: Ventnor Publishers, Inc., 1949.

Graham, Robert. "A Firm Foundation." *Dartmouth Medicine* 16, no. 1 (Fall 1991): 14–21.

Hahn, L. "Smith (Nathan)," in A. Deschambre, ed., *Dictionnaire Encyclopédique des Sciences Médicales,* vol. 10, p. 82. Paris: G. Masson and P. Asselin, for the Libraire de l'Académie de Médecine and the Libraire de la Faculté de Médecine (respectively), 1881.

Halpert, Brenda. "Historical Profile: Dr. Nathan Smith 1762–1829." *Massachusetts Physician* 36, no. 9 (Sept. 1977): 11–12.

Harrington, Thomas Francis. "Nathan Smith," in J. G. Mumford, ed., *The Harvard Medical School: A History, Narrative and Documentary: 1782–1905* (3 vols.), 1:335–54. New York: Lewis Publishing Co., 1905.

Harvey, Samuel C. "The Education of Nathan Smith." *Yale Journal of Biology and Medicine* 1, no. 5 (Mar. 1929): 259–68.

Hayward, Mary L., and Oliver S. Hayward. "Nathan Smith's Family" (typescript, ca. 1960, 22 pp.). Nathan Smith (h1798) Alumni File, DCA.

Hayward, Oliver S. "The Basis in Syndenham, Rush, and Armstrong for Nathan Smith's Teaching." *Annals of Internal Medicine* 56, no. 2 (Feb. 1962): 343–48.

———. "Dr. Nathan Smith (1762–1829)—American Pioneer." *NEJM* 261, no. 10 (3 Sept. 1959): 489–94.

———. "Essay on William Tully," in Oliver S. Hayward and Elizabeth H. Thomson, eds., *The Journal of William Tully: Medical Student at Dartmouth 1808–1809,* pp. xiii–xxiv. New York: Science History Publications, 1977.

———. "The History of Oncology: III: America, and the Cancer Lectures of Nathan Smith." *Surgery* 58, no. 4 (Oct. 1965): 745–57.

———. "Jo Gallup, Epidemiologist—1769–1849." *JAMA* 189, no. 6 (10 Aug. 1964): 81–82.

———. "Jo Gallup, New England Epidemiologist (1769–1849)." *NEJM* 269, no. 10 (7 Nov. 1963): 1015–18. Reprinted in *Dartmouth Medical School Alumni Magazine* [6, no. 1] (Fall 1981): 30–32, 44–45.

———. "Nathan Smith's Medical Practice or Dogmatism versus Patient Inquiry." *Bulletin of the History of Medicine* 36, no. 3 (May-June 1962): 260–67.

———. "Nathan Smith (1762–1829), Politician." *NEJM* 263, no. 24 (15 Dec. 1960): 1235–43; 263, no. 25 (22 Dec. 1960): 1288–91.

———. "A Search for the Real Nathan Smith." *Journal of the History of Medicine and Allied Sciences* 15, no. 3 (July 1960): 270–81.

———. "A Student of Dr. Nathan Smith [William Tully]." *Connecticut Medicine* 24, no. 9 (Sept. 1960): 553–59.

———. "Three American Anatomy Letters (1817–1830)." *Bulletin of the History of Medicine* 38, no. 4 (July–Aug. 1964): 377–78.

———. "Two Nineteenth Century Medical Professors: Nathan Smith and his Son, Ryno." *Bulletin School of Medicine University of Maryland* 48, no. 4 (Oct. 1963): 39–58.

———. "What Nathan Smith Means To Me." *JAMA* 176, no. 1 (July 1961): 202, 204, 206.

———, and Mather Cleveland. *See* Cleveland, Mather, and Oliver S. Hayward.

———, and Elizabeth H. Thomson, eds. *The Journal of William Tully, Medical Student at Dartmouth 1808–1809*. New York: Science History Publications, 1977.

How, Lyman Bartlett. *The Story of the New Hampshire Medical Society Told to 1854 . . . at the Centennial of the Society in 1891*. Rev. and cont. by Henry O. Smith. Nashua, N.H.: Phaneuf Press, 1941.

Hubbard, Oliver P. *Dartmouth Medical College and Nathan Smith: An Historical Discourse. A Lecture Introductory to the Eighty-Third Course of the New Hampshire Medical Institution at Dartmouth College*, July 31, 1879. Concord, N.H.: Evans, Sleeper & Evans, 1879. Reprinted as *The Early History of the New Hampshire Medical Institution*. Washington, D.C.: Globe Publishing, 1880.

Hurd, Henry M. "Nathan Smith, Nathan R. Smith, and Alan P. Smith. A Medical Family." *Maryland Medical Journal* 59, no. 3 (1916): 56–59.

Ifkovic, J. W. "Smith, Nathan," in Martin Kaufman, Stuart Galishoff, and Todd L. Savitt, eds., *Dictionary of American Medical Biography*, p. 696. Westport, Conn.: Greenwood Press, 1984.

Joyce, Terrence J. "Nathan Smith, Joseph Smith, and the Seeds of Mormonism." Unpublished Mss., 13 pp.

[Kelly, Emerson Crosby, comp.]. "Nathan Smith: Biography; Bibliography of Writings; Bibliography of Biographies" (plus editorial note). *Medical Classics* 1, no. 8 (Apr. 1937): 773–81.

Kimball, Gilman. "The President's Annual Address: A Biographical Sketch of Dr. Nathan Smith, Founder of the Dartmouth Medical College." *Gynecological Transactions* 8 (1883): 27–42. An abstract of this "Address" appeared in *Medical News of Philadelphia* 43, no. 12 (22 Sept. 1883): 324–25.

Knight, Jonathan. *An Eulogium on Nathan Smith, M.D.* New Haven: Hezekiah Howe, 1829. Reprinted in Nathan R. Smith, ed., *Medical and Surgical Memoirs*, pp. 12–36.

Kohorn, Ernest I. "The Department of Obstetrics and Gynecology at Yale: the First One Hundred Fifty Years, from Nathan Smith to Lee Buxton." *Yale Journal of Biology and Medicine* 66, no. 2 (Mar.–Apr. 1993): 85–105.

Lindskog, Gustaf E. "Yale's first professor of Surgery: Nathan Smith, M.D. (1762–1829)." *Surgery* 64, no. 2 (Aug. 1968): 524–28.

Longcope, Warfield T. "Smith, Nathan," in Dumas Malone, ed., *Dictionary of American Biography*, vol. 16, pp. 324–29. New York: Scribners, 1935.

Longo, Lawrence D. "Classic Pages in Obstetrics and Gynecology: Nathan Smith, 'Case of ovarian dropsy, successfully removed by a surgical operation.'" *American Journal of Obstetrics and Gynecology* 126, no. 4 (15 Oct. 1976): 506.

Mandrey, William H. "Dr. Nathan Smith Medical Pioneer." Photocopy of unidentified newspaper clipping (22 Aug. 1954). Nathan Smith (h1798) Alumni File, DCA.

Mercer, Sir Walter. "The Contributions of Edinburgh to early American Medicine." *Journal of the Royal College of Surgeons Edinburgh* 7, no. 3 (Apr. 1962): 183–84.

Morain, William D. *The Sword of Laban: Joseph Smith, Jr., and the Dissociated Mind*. Washington, D.C.: American Psychiatric Press, 1998.

Mumford, James Gregory. *A Narrative of Medicine in America*, pp. 298–307. Philadelphia: J. B. Lippincott Co., 1903.

Nye, Robert E., Jr. "Nathan Smith's Time in London: A Better Investment?" *Dartmouth Medical School Alumni Magazine* [10, no. 1] (Fall 1985): 12–15.

———. "Nathan Smith's Trip to Edinburgh: A Waste of Time?" *Dartmouth Medical School Alumni Magazine* [8, no. 1] (Fall 1983): 24–27.

Osler, William. "Men and Books: Nathan Smith." *Canadian Medical Association Journal* 4, no. 12 (1914): 1109–11.

Oughterson, A. W. "Nathan Smith and Cancer Therapy." *Yale Journal of Biology and Medicine* 12, no. 2 (Dec. 1939): 122–36.

[Painter, Charles F.]. "Dr. Nathan Smith, 1762–1829." *NEJM* 199, no. 2 (12 July 1928): 103–104.

Parsons, John W. "Nathan Smith." *Transactions of the [New Hampshire Medical] Society* (June 1891): 131–35. Concord, N.H.: Republican Press Association, 1891. Reprinted as "Dr. Nathan Smith." *The Granite Monthly* 14, no. 10 (Oct. 1892): 313–16.

Paul, John R. "Nathan Smith and Typhoid Fever." *Yale Journal of Biology and Medicine* 2, no. 3 (Jan. 1930): 169–81.

Philozetemia. "Critique of Dr. Smith's Theory of Spasm." *Massachusetts Magazine* 3, no. 8 (Aug. 1791): 478–79.

———. "Philozetemia's Reply to Dr. Smith." *Massachusetts Magazine* 4, no. 8 (Aug. 1792): 487–88.

Powers, Samuel [Leland]. "Character Sketches of Dartmouth Men" (Speech at Symphony Hall, Boston, 26 Jan. 1922). Typescript copy in Samuel Powers (1874) Alumni File, DCA.

Putnam, Constance E. "The Apples of His Eye." *Dartmouth Medicine* 21, no. 1 (Fall 1996): 34–39.

———. "A Feverish Enterprise." *Wellcome History*, no. 7 (Dec. 1997): 5.

———. "To Promote Useful Science." *Dartmouth Medicine* 22, no. 1 (Summer–Fall 1997): 22–29.

———. "The Rockingham Roots of Dartmouth Medical School: Samuel Whiting and Nathan Smith" (Address at Annual Pilgrimage, Rockingham [Vt.] Old Meeting House, 3 Aug. 1997). Unpublished mss., 20 pp.

———. "Smith, Nathan," in John A. Garraty, ed., *American National Biography* (24 vols.). New York: Oxford University Press, 1999.

———. "What Happened to Nathan Smith's 'New Splint'?" Paper given at the 1994 MEPHISTOS Conference, Harvard University. Unpublished mss., 35 pp.

———. "What a Riot! Raising Corpses for Students at Dartmouth Medical School in the Early 19th Century—and How Ezekiel Dodge Cushing Took the Heat for his Mentor, Nathan Smith." Paper given at the 1996 MEPHISTOS Conference, University of Toronto. Unpublished mss., 25 pp.

———. "The Doctor's Wife: Now, Then, and In Between." Paper given at the 1996 Women's Voices Conference, Simmons College. Unpublished mss., 32 pp.

[Silliman, Benjamin.] "Obituary," in *The American Journal of Science and Arts* 16, no. 1 (July 1829): 211–14. The same text had appeared earlier in the *New Hampshire Statesman & Concord Register* 5, no. 49 (25 Apr. 1829), and in the *Woodstock [Vt.] Observer* (28 Apr. 1829).

Smith, Bryce A. "Notes on the Materia Medica of Nathan Smith." *Yale Journal of Biology and Medicine* 11, no. 3 (1939): 189–205.

Smith, Emily A. *The Life and Letters of Nathan Smith, M.B., M.D.* New Haven: Yale University Press, 1914.

Smith, Nathan R. "Biographic Memoir of the Author [i.e., Nathan Smith]." In Nathan R. Smith, ed., *Medical and Surgical Memoirs*, pp. 9–12, 36–37.

———, ed. *Medical and Surgical Memoirs, by Nathan Smith, M.D.* Baltimore: William A. Francis, 1831.

Spalding, James A. "The Friendship of Dr. Nathan Smith and Dr. Lyman Spalding." *Bulletin of the American Academy of Medicine* 7, no. 10 (Dec. 1906): 714–34.

———. *Life of Dr. Lyman Spalding.* Boston: W. M. Leonard, 1916.

Stearns, Carl M. "Dr. Nathan Smith," in Carl M. Stearns, *The Early History of Medicine in Sullivan County, N.H.*, pp. 121–25. Springfield, Vt.: Hurd's Offset Printing, 1974.

Steiner, Walter Ralph. "Historical Address: The Evolution of Medicine in Connecticut, with the Foundation of Yale Medical School as its Notable Achievement," from the *Memorial of the Centennial of the Yale Medical School, 1814–1914.* New Haven: Yale University Press, 1915.

Stone, R. French, ed. "Smith, Nathan," in *Biography of Eminent American Physicians and Surgeons*, p. 475. Indianapolis: Carlon & Hollenbeck, 1894.

[Talbott, John], Editorial. "Nathan Smith of Dartmouth (1762–1829)." *JAMA* 199, no. 2 (9 Jan. 1967): 158–59.

Thoms, Herbert. *The Doctors of Yale College 1702–1815 and The Founding of the Medical Institution.* Hamden, Conn.: Shoe String Press, 1960.

———. "Nathan Smith." *Journal of Medical Education* 33, no. 12 (Dec. 1958): 817–26.

———. "Nathan Smith and Ovariotomy." *International Abstracts of Surgery* 48 (Apr. 1929): 305–307.

Tully, William. *The Journal of William Tully, Medical Student at Dartmouth 1808–1809*, Oliver S. Hayward and Elizabeth H. Thomson, eds. New York: Science History Publications, 1977.

Van Antwerp, Lee D. "Nathan Smith and Early American Medical Education." *Annals of Medical History* n.s. 9 (Sept. 1937): 449–63.

Wade, Hugh Mason. *A Brief History of Cornish 1763–1974* (with a "Genealogical Section" by Stephen P. Tracey and Dwight C. Wood), pp. 19–22. Hanover, N.H.: University Press of New England, 1976.

Waterson, Davina. "Smith, Nathan (1762–1829)," in Howard A. Kelly, ed., *Cyclopedia of American Medical Biography* (2 vols.), vol. 2, pp. 388–90. Philadelphia: W. B. Saunders, 1912.

Welch, William H. "Introduction," in Emily A. Smith, *The Life and Letters of Nathan Smith, M.B., M.D.*, pp. [i–vi]. New Haven: Yale University Press, 1914.

———. "The Relation of Yale to Medicine." *Yale Medical Journal* 8, no. 1 (Nov. 1901): 127–58. Reprinted in William H. Welch. *Papers and Addresses* (3 vols.), vol. 3, pp. 243–72. Baltimore: Johns Hopkins University Press, 1920.

Wheelock, Seymour E. "A First-Rate Tale." *Dartmouth Medicine* 15, no. 1 (Fall 1990): 48–51.

———. "The Prophet, the Physicians and the Medical School." *Dartmouth Medical School Magazine* 8, no. 3 (Spring 1984): 25–27.

Wikoff, Jerrold. "The Medical Genius of Nathan Smith," with sidebar, "Nathan Smith's Cure Saved Joseph Smith." *[Lebanon, N.H.] Valley News* (22 Sept. 1981): 13.

Williams, Stephen West. "Dr. Nathan Smith," in Stephen W. Williams, *American Medical Biography, or Memoirs of Eminent Physicians*, pp. 524–45. Greenfield, Mass.: L. Merriam, 1845.

Wirthlin, LeRoy S. "Joseph Smith's Boyhood Operation: An 1813 Surgical Success." *Brigham Young University Studies* 21, no. 2 (Spring 1981): 131–54.

———. "Nathan Smith (1762–1828[sic]) Surgical Consultant to Joseph Smith." *Brigham Young University Studies* 17, no. 3 (Spring 1977): 319–338.

Index

Some of the same abbreviations used for institutions and persons in the Notes (see p. 275) are also used internally within the Index.

178, 179–80, 181–82, 186–87, 187,
293n41, 294n70, 312nn48/51,
319n91, 377n36; Kimball, J., 83,
233; King, D., 160–61; Mack, 76–77;
Skilton, 69–70, 157; Turner, 66; style
of, 62–64, 66–67, 67–74, 75, 77–80,
167, 207; tickets for, 213, 221,
296n14 (photo of, 84, 222)
Leffingwell, Edward Henry, 221, 222,
305n74, 325n5
Leffingwell, William, 221
Leonard, Levi W.: quoted, 234
Lettsom, John Coakley (1744–1815),
20, 45–56, 82, 240; NS friendship
with, 45
Lincoln, Levi, 175, 211
Lincoln, Nathan Smith (1828–1898),
273
Lister, B. C.: quoted, 91
Lithotomy, 103, 166, 168, 170, 173,
184, 187, 215, 240, 314n3; NRS
and, 256, 333n87
Long & Clement, 134
Longcope, Christopher, 274
Longcope, David, 274
Longcope, Warfield T., 274; quoted, 266
Loudon, Irvine: quoted, 150
Louis, Pierre-Charles-Alexandre, 312n45
Lowe, A. T.: quoted, 64, 171, 221, 240
Lowell, Charles, 229, 230, 231, 327n44
Lubec, Me., 229, 230
Lyman, George H.: quoted, 252

McClellan, George, 239
McDowell, Ephraim (1771–1830), 185–
86, 318nn80–81/87, 319nn88–89
Mack, Andrew, 95
McKinstry, Nathan, 118, 105n68
MacLean, Lachlan, 242, 330n26
Magner, Lois N.: quoted, 296n21
Maimonides, Moses: quoted, 143
Maine State Legislature, 131, 209–10,
211, 212
Map of New England, 2
Massachusetts General Hospital, 230,
231, 314n2
Massachusetts Medical Society, 20, 70,
87–88, 96, 116, 144

Materia medica, 22, 24, 52, 54, 55, 67,
69, 74, 105, 111, 115, 152, 161, 194,
198, 224; defined, 13, 68
Medical College (Memphis, Tenn.), 119
Medical education, 61–66, 85, 104,
121–22, 191–93, 212, 221–22, 225,
226, 267; content of, 37–38, 49; cost
of, 24–25, 84, 213, 283n41; courses
taught by NS as part of, 52, 136,
195, 198, 199, 213, 216, 221, 265;
in Edinburgh, 39, 42–45, 149, 192,
287n43; in Glasgow, 42, 49; at Harvard, 21, 23–24, 35, 66, 163; in
London, 45–46, 49; in New York,
308n55; payment for, 12, 55–56,
195, 213, 218; in Philadelphia, 23,
37, 64, 75, 89, 95, 106, 116, 138,
192, 256, 333n85; "reading with the
doctor," 12, 13 (*see also* Medical libraries); "riding with the doctor," 12,
14, 34–35, 56, 104, 107–8, 169, 174,
187, 240; in rural America, 37, 50–
51, 56, 102–3, 119, 223, 264, 265,
305n74, 325n9. *See also* Anatomy,
teaching of; Apprenticeship, medical;
Chemistry; Dartmouth Medical
School; Lectures by NS; Medical Institute of Yale College; Medical
School of Maine; Smith, Nathan,
teaching skill of; "Theory and practice"; University of Vermont
Medical Institute of Yale College, 100,
119, 131, 188, 221–22, 273, 322n56;
curriculum at, 198, 205; first faculty
at, 194–96; founding of, 191–98;
library at, 13, 280n47; NS begins
teaching at, 201; NS considered for
faculty at, 192, 195–98; photo of
medical building at, 202; quality of
students at, 206, 213. *See also* Yale
College, Board of Trustees at
Medical libraries, 7, 12–13, 35, 36, 45–
46, 126–27, 196, 203, 216, 278n23,
280n47, 286n19, 322n37
Medical practice (NS's), 143–64; boarding patients and students as part of,
31, 33, 108, 121; in Cornish, N.H.,
16–18, 23, 32–36, 120; geographical

Continued from page iv

"The History of Oncology: I, Early Oncology and the Literature of Discovery; II, The Society for Investigating Cancer, London; III, America and the Cancer Lectures of Nathan Smith," in *Surgery* 58, nos. 2, 3, and 4 (Aug., Sept., and Oct. 1965): 460–68, 586–99, and 745–57, respectively.

In addition, it should be noted that an earlier version of chapter 4, "The Founding of Dartmouth Medical School," was published by Constance E. Putnam in *Dartmouth Medicine* 22, no. 1 (Summer–Fall 1997): 22–29, under the title "To Promote Useful Science"; similarly, an earlier version of chapter 7, "Students, Colleagues, and Friends," was published by Constance E. Putnam in *Dartmouth Medicine* 21, no. 1 (Fall 1996): 34–39, under the title "The Apples of His Eye."

Permission to quote from letters and other documents owned by various libraries and archives was also graciously granted by courtesy of the following: Trustees of the Boston Public Library; Bowdoin College Library; Rare Book and Manuscript Library, Columbia University; Francis A. Countway Library of Medicine, Harvard University; Dartmouth College Archives at Baker Library; Massachusetts Historical Society; National Library of Medicine; New Hampshire Historical Society; New York Academy of Medicine Library; New York Public Library; the University of Vermont Bailey/Howe Library; and at Yale University by the Harvey Cushing/John Hay Whitney Medical Library, the Beinecke Rare Book and Manuscript Library, and the Yale University Library.

UNIVERSITY PRESS OF NEW ENGLAND publishes books under its own imprint and is the publisher for Brandeis University Press, Dartmouth College, Middlebury College Press, University of New Hampshire, Tufts University, and Wesleyan University Press.

Library of Congress Cataloging-in-Publication Data
Hayward, Oliver S., M.D.
    Improve, perfect, & perpetuate : Dr. Nathan Smith and early
American medical education / Oliver S. Hayward and Constance E.
Putnam ; foreword by C. Everett Koop ; introduction by Philip Cash.
        p.   cm.
    Includes bibliographical references and index.
    ISBN 0-87451-860-1 (alk. paper)
    1. Smith, Nathan, 1762-1829.   2. Physicians—New England—
Biography.   3. Surgeons—New England—Biography.   4. Medical
teaching personnel—New England—Biography.   5. Medical education—
New England—History—19th century.   I. Putnam, Constance E.,
1943-   .   II. Title.
R154.S6H39   1998
610'.92—dc21   97-47155
[B]